Social Issues
in Diagnosis

Social Issues in Diagnosis

AN INTRODUCTION FOR STUDENTS AND CLINICIANS

EDITED BY

Annemarie Goldstein Jutel
Associate Professor
Victoria University of Wellington
New Zealand

Kevin Dew
Professor
Victoria University of Wellington
New Zealand

Johns Hopkins University Press
Baltimore

© 2014 Johns Hopkins University Press
All rights reserved. Published 2014
Printed in the United States of America on acid-free paper
9 8 7 6 5 4 3 2 1

Johns Hopkins University Press
2715 North Charles Street
Baltimore, Maryland 21218-4363
www.press.jhu.edu

Library of Congress Cataloging-in-Publication Data

Social issues in diagnosis : an introduction for students and clinicians / edited by
Annemarie Goldstein Jutel, Kevin Dew.
    p. ; cm.
  Includes bibliographical references and index.
   ISBN 978-1-4214-1300-6 (pbk. : alk. paper) — ISBN 1-4214-1300-0 (pbk. : alk. paper) —
ISBN 978-1-4214-1301-3 (electronic) — ISBN 1-4214-1301-9 (electronic)
   I. Jutel, Annemarie, editor of compilation.   II. Dew, Kevin, editor of compilation.
   [DNLM: 1. Diagnosis.   2. Culture.   3. Physician-Patient Relations.
4. Power (Psychology) WB 141]
  RC71.5
  616.07'5—dc23
                                  2013028967

A catalog record for this book is available from the British Library.

*Special discounts are available for bulk purchases of this book. For more information, please
contact Special Sales at 410-516-6936 or specialsales@press.jhu.edu.*

Johns Hopkins University Press uses environmentally friendly book materials, including
recycled text paper that is composed of at least 30 percent post-consumer waste, whenever
possible.

Contents

Medical Advisors

Joel Lexchin received his MD from the University of Toronto in 1977 and for the past twenty-six years has been an emergency physician at the University Health Network. He is currently a professor in the School of Health Policy and Management at York University in Canada and an associate professor in the Department of Family and Community Medicine at the University of Toronto. From 1992 to 1994 he was a member of the Ontario Drug Quality and Therapeutics Committee, and he was the chair of the Drugs and Pharmacotherapy Committee of the Ontario Medical Association from 1997 to 1999. He has been a consultant for the province of Ontario, various arms of the Canadian federal government, the World Health Organization, the government of New Zealand, and the Australian National Prescribing Service. He is the author or coauthor of over 125 peer-reviewed articles on topics such as physician prescribing behavior, pharmaceutical patent issues, the drug approval process, and prescription drug promotion. He is a coauthor of *Drugs of Choice: A Formulary for General Practice* and author of *Drug Therapy for Emergency Physicians*.

Kathryn L. Weise trained in pediatrics at Rainbow Babies and Children's Hospital in Cleveland, Ohio, followed by further training in pediatric intensive care at Children's Hospital National Medical Center in Washington, DC. Between 1987 and 2009, she was an attending physician in pediatric critical care at Rainbow Babies and Children's Hospital, the University of Virginia, and the Cleveland Clinic. In 2000, she completed a master's degree in bioethics at Case Western Reserve University. She currently attends as a hospitalist at the Cleveland Clinic Children's Hospital for Rehabilitation, directs the Cleveland Fellowship in Advanced Bioethics, participates in ethics consultation for adults and children, and chairs the Pediatric Ethics Committee at the Cleveland Clinic Foundation. She is a member of the American Academy of Pediatrics Committee on Bioethics and serves as an ethicist on research data safety monitoring boards. She has published in the areas of pediatric critical care, pediatric palliative care, and bioethics.

Contributors

Sudeepa Abeysinghe is a research fellow at the London School of Hygiene and Tropical Medicine. Her research interests include the sociology of pandemics, risk and scientific uncertainty, and the politics of evidence use in policy making.

Christian Bröer is an associate professor of sociology at the University of Amsterdam. He researches the relation between people's experience of health and other problems and how that experience shapes or is shaped by collective problem solving. He has published on noise annoyance, attention deficit hyperactivity disorder, environmental health risks, electrohypersensitivity, mobilization, professionalism, and care policy. His current projects involve the investigation of the interplay between health risk perception and policy interventions concerning mobile phone mast siting and rethinking medicalization theory through international comparative research on attention deficit hyperactivity disorder. Bröer is chair of the research group Dynamics of Citizenship and Culture and a member of the Centre for Social Science and Global Health.

Kevin Dew is a professor of sociology at Victoria University of Wellington and before that was a lecturer in the Department of Public Health at the Wellington School of Medicine and Health Sciences. Current research activities include studies of interactions between health professionals and patients, health inequalities, the social meanings of medications, and the role of public health in contemporary society.

Mary Ebeling is an associate professor of sociology in the Department of Culture and Communication at Drexel University. Her research is focused on pharmaceutical and medical marketing, emerging translational medicine and technologies, and the social shaping of diagnosis.

John Gardner is a PhD candidate at the Centre for Biomedicine and Society, Department of Sociology and Communications, Brunel University, London. His research interests are the social implications of innovative health technologies, pharmaceuticalization, and empirical bioethics. He is currently undertaking qualitative research into the use of deep brain stimulation to treat children with neurological disorders.

Dawn Goodwin is a senior lecturer in social science and medicine and an ethnographer of health care whose previous research has explored the relationship between knowledge, action, and professional accountability, resulting in the book *Acting in*

Anaesthesia: Ethnographic Encounters with Patients, Practitioners and Medical Technologies. She publishes in the fields of science and technology studies and medical sociology, and has edited a collection of studies focusing on diagnosis across different contexts of work titled *Ethnographies of Diagnostic Work: Dimensions of Transformative Practice.*

Andrew Greenberg is a doctoral student at the City University of New York Graduate Center. He is also an organizer with the Doctors Council SEIU, a labor union for doctors based in New York City. His current research examines how evidence-based medicine is transforming the power relations in the New York City public hospital system.

Jennifer Hemler is a PhD candidate in the Department of Sociology at Rutgers, the State University of New Jersey, specializing in culture and cognition and medical sociology. Jennifer has written about the medicalization of compulsive buying and its use as a coping mechanism for different types of social strain. She has also coauthored articles on disparities in cancer treatment, physician preferences, and other issues in cancer survivorship. Her current research explores how women "move on" or proceed to a "new normal" after a diagnosis of breast cancer.

Tania M. Jenkins is a doctoral candidate at Brown University, supervised by Phil Brown. She teaches a course on the sociology of diagnosis aimed at precollege students contemplating careers in medicine through the Summer@Brown program. She is currently working on a National Science Foundation–supported ethnography that examines the construction of prestige and hierarchy within the medical profession.

Annemarie Goldstein Jutel is an associate professor at Victoria University of Wellington. Author of *Putting a Name to It: Diagnosis in Contemporary Society*, she has published widely on the sociology of diagnosis. Her publications have appeared in journals such as the *Journal of the American Medical Association*, *Social Science and Medicine*, and *PLoS Medicine*. Jutel is also a registered nurse.

Thomas McConnell initially studied psychology before studying medicine at Lancaster University. He is currently working as an academic junior doctor in trauma and orthopedics at the University of Oxford. His interest in the sociology of diagnosis developed out of a research module on the subject, undertaken as part of his medical degree.

Rebecca Olson has a PhD in sociology from the Australian National University and is currently a lecturer in public health at the University of Western Sydney, Campbelltown. Her research interests lie in the sociologies of cancer, diagnosis, and emotions; public health; and interprofessional health education. She is currently involved in research on improving health protection information for caregivers of cancer patients and understanding socialization in university-based interprofessional health education.

Lindsay Prior is a professor of sociology in the School of Sociology, Social Policy and Social Work and a principal investigator and member of the management committee of the Centre of Excellence for Public Health at Queen's University Belfast. During the last few decades, he has undertaken observational and interview studies in primary care practices, psychiatric hospitals, medical and cancer-genetic clinics, and various community-based health-care facilities. Among other things, he is currently studying the concept of "well-being" and its implications for health policy.

Barbara Katz Rothman is a professor of sociology at the City University of New York, where she also serves on the faculties of public health, women's studies, and disability studies. She holds visiting professorships at Plymouth University in the United Kingdom, where she held a Leverhulme professorship; at Ryerson University in Toronto in the International Midwifery Preparation Program; and at the Charite in Berlin in the Health and Society Master's Program. She has served as the Maria Gompart Mayer Professor at Osnabrueck University in Germany and as a Fulbright professor at the University of Groningen in the Netherlands. Her books, with Germany, Finnish, and Japanese translations, include *In Labor: Women and Power in the Birthplace*; *Laboring On* with Wendy Simonds; *The Tentative Pregnancy*; *Recreating Motherhood*; *The Book of Life*; and *Weaving a Family: Untangling Race and Adoption*.

Lisa Sanders is a board-certified internist. She was educated and trained at the Yale School of Medicine and remains on the faculty there, teaching medical students and residents. She is the author of the popular *New York Times Magazine* "Diagnosis" column, the inspiration for the hit television series *House, M.D.* and the best-selling book *Every Patient Tells a Story: Medical Mysteries and the Art of Diagnosis*. In book, column, and blog, Sanders explores the messy process of diagnosis, filled with red herrings, false leads, and dead ends, from which—despite the difficulty—the answer is often reached and lives are saved. She practices medicine and teaches internal medicine residents in Waterbury, Connecticut.

Gordon Schiff is a general internist and the associate director of Brigham and Women's Center for Patient Safety Research and Practice and an associate professor of medicine at Harvard Medical School. He worked for three decades at Chicago's Cook County Hospital, where he directed their general medicine clinic. He is author of numerous articles on patient safety, diagnosis error, test management, laboratory-pharmacy linkages, health information technology, and medication quality improvement. He is a member of the editorial boards of *Medical Care, Journal of Public Health Policy*, and *BMJ Quality and Safety*. He is past co-chair of the International Diagnosis Errors in Medicine conferences.

Ilina Singh is a professor of science, ethics, and society in the Department for Social Science, Health and Medicine at King's College London, with a cross-appointment to the Institute of Psychiatry. Her work examines the psychosocial and ethical implications of advances in biomedicine and neuroscience for young people and families. Her research has several goals: to investigate the benefits and risks of biomedical and neuroscience technologies for children; to enable evidence-based policy making in child health and education; and to bring social theory and ethical insights into better alignment with children's social, emotional, and behavioral capacities.

Recent projects include: Voices on Identity, Childhood, Ethics and Stimulants (www.adhdvoices.com); Survey of Neuroenhancement Attitudes and Practices among British Young People; and an edited volume on biomarkers and bioprediction, *Bioprediction, Biomarkers, and Bad Behavior: Scientific, Legal, and Ethical Challenges*, published in 2013 by Oxford University Press.

Dena T. Smith is an assistant professor of sociology at Goucher College. She has written about sociological contributions to medical understandings of suffering, specifically the way in which psychiatry (and the medical field more generally) classifies particular illnesses and how these diagnostic categories lead to particular perceptions of illness and particular treatments. Smith's work involves interviews with psychiatrists about their practice and the lack of resistance to medicalization in contemporary psychiatry. She also examines the waning use of talk therapy and the reliance on medication-based treatments. Smith is currently researching gender differences in mental health.

Sandra H. Sulzer is a postdoctoral fellow at the Cecil G. Sheps Center for Health Services Research, University of North Carolina at Chapel Hill. She has a PhD in sociology from the University of Wisconsin–Madison. Her current research projects include studies of the diagnostic process in borderline personality disorder and doctor-patient communication in the context of patient self-advocacy. Additionally, she is researching clinical communication around pediatric attention deficit hyperactivity disorder. Her past research has included the study of online support groups and the development of better methodological tools for analyzing online discourse.

Catherine Trundle lectures in anthropology at Victoria University of Wellington. She obtained her doctorate in social anthropology from Cambridge University. Her research interests include the intersection of medical and legal anthropology, human rights, and the military. She currently researches claims for health compensation made by nuclear test veterans in New Zealand and the United Kingdom.

Acknowledgments

We would like to thank the colleagues, friends, and family who have challenged our thinking and forced us to clarify our ideas. Particular thanks to Ellen Goldstein for putting a name to it and to Kelley Squazzo, from Johns Hopkins University Press, for her unabated enthusiasm.

Social Issues
in Diagnosis

Introduction

Annemarie Goldstein Jutel and Kevin Dew

This book is written for those who work, or are studying to work, in a clinical setting. It does not teach how to diagnose, or what groups of diseases emerge from particular social settings. It demonstrates how society influences the clinician's diagnosis, how sick people think about disease and illness, why some treatment plans fail despite their technical suitability to a particular disease, and why the relationship between layperson and professional is so pivotal to care. This book also explains the social impact of diagnosis on the individual—patient, doctor, or both—well beyond the reach of the physical symptoms.

Diagnosis serves an important social role. It confers social status to those who diagnose, and can have a remarkable impact on the social status of those diagnosed. Medical professionals can, through diagnosis, apportion resources and reimbursements, legitimize patient complaints, and determine whether someone who commits a crime goes to prison or receives therapy. The medical diagnosis and its associated prognostications determine what treatment is chosen and whether someone receives curative or palliative intervention. For the patient, however, the diagnosis gives permission to act in normally unacceptable ways (not going to work, staying in bed). It can also transform someone's identity, flagging impending decline, permanent incapacity or lifelong risk. In this light, the capacity to diagnose can be seen as having power over life and death, freedom and incarceration, assistance and penury.

Diagnosis is a clinical act *par excellence*. It is an event that places the doctor in front of the patient, drawing on a deep and specialized knowledge base in order to identify the cause of a specific case of human discomfort or dysfunction, and to identify a remedy. Being able to label illness is an important responsibility of medicine (and, increasingly, of other allied health fields).

But diagnosis is also a social activity. The labels that doctors or other diagnosticians are allowed to use are decided by consensus before they enter classification systems or become approved medical taxonomies. Social boundaries are established by diagnosis: lay and professional, sick and not sick, endocrinologist and rheumatologist.

Diagnosis has social consequences. While a diagnosis can explain, it can also stigmatize and terrify. The sufferers of both mental and physical illnesses may be marginalized and ostracized because of their diagnosis. Schizophrenia, borderline personality disorder, and Alzheimer disease have negative connotations, but so do lung cancer, gout, and obesity—they are physical disorders that may limit one's horizons or carry the stigma of presumed lack of control. A diagnosis can shake the very foundations of one's being.

Studying diagnosis from a sociological perspective offers clinicians and students a rich and sometimes provocative view of medicine and the cultures in which it is practiced. A sociological perspective is one that considers how individuals function within a wider social context. Rather than seeing each case as one isolated problem, it attempts to see social patterns of behavior, reaction, cause, and effect. While the doctor's appointment appears, on the surface, to be between one doctor and one layperson, even this intimate interaction has much wider social foundations. The attitude of the layperson (and of the clinician) as well as the reaction to, and compliance with, treatment plans may hinge on educational, gendered, cultural, and demographic factors. What treatment is available depends on diagnostic code, insurance coverage, and state of residence. The distribution of disease and the chance that this patient, as compared to another, may suffer from a particular condition depends on similar social factors.

If you are a medical student reading this book, it may be because the Medical College Admissions Test will evaluate social science knowledge, for the first time, starting in 2015. This change in MCAT content is an acknowledgment that understanding different populations, social settings, and cultural context has an important impact on the quality of care that a doctor is able to provide. If you are already a clinician, you are well aware that the medical task is not always so clear-cut as simply performing the task. Diagnosing and providing a treatment plan is only the start of what can be a messy process. Figuring out how to achieve the best possible outcomes requires more than just knowing your patient. Why clinicians have poor outcomes with particular diseases, specific population groups, or certain diagnoses can often be understood with an eye to social influences. And, for a nonmedical clinician reading this book, understanding the social power of the diagnosis will help to explain the status of medicine, its reluctance to relinquish diagnostic authority, and the reasons for medicalization of conditions that might not at first glance seem to be medical at all.

Mary Ebeling, in chapter 9, refers to the "crowded room" in which diagnosis takes place. The examination room, which appears to harbor only the clinician and the patient, is influenced by other forces, structures, and players that, while not physically present, shape how the diagnosis takes place. While Ebeling makes specific reference to commercial players, we extend this metaphor to describe the general social nature of the diagnosis and the purpose of this book. We aim to describe how both diagnostic labels and the process of diagnosis are phenomena that are anchored in groups and structures as much as they are in the interactions of the patient and doctor.

To speak of diagnosis today is to make reference to diagnosis as either classification or process. A diagnostic classification is an agreed-upon label for a condition officially recognized by medicine as being disease. A diagnostic process is the means by which the physician ascertains the presence of such a condition. Both the classification and the process are framed by social and political forces and have social and political consequences.

Many social forces and agents interact to frame diagnoses and their conse-quences. The development and economics of new technologies, the "discovery" or recognition of symptom clusters as discrete diseases, the negotiation of diagnostic recognition by sanctioning bodies, and the historical structure of disease taxono-mies all contribute to creating the diagnostic classifications that are available for use by contemporary medicine.

But these factors are not independent, in their own genesis, from their social consequence: it is a kind of chicken-and-egg situation. While diagnoses cannot import a social consequence until they become standardized as a label, the impact of the label continues to feed into the framing of diagnostic categories as they are or as they will become. With each revision of the *Diagnostic and Statistical Manual of Mental Disorders* or of the *International Statistical Classification of Diseases*, there are drawn-out debates about how changing a diagnostic category will affect the treat-ment of disease or the experience of those diagnosed with it, or about how current categories either achieve or fail to fulfill their promise.

These social consequences are diverse, and both positive and negative. To have a recognized disease may activate (or not) a range of services, treatments, and re-sources. But it may also, as mentioned above, mark the individual with stigmata, or prime her for exploitation. Diagnoses are the stuff of the disease mongers who sell anything from, historically, Dr. Williams's *Pink Pills for Pale People* and *Pennyroyal and Steel Pills for Females* to Zyprexa and Paxil today.

But this is not a one-way model. Just as the social consequences of diagnosis mold the disease classifications, so do the classifications frame the experiences of diagnosis, a point that hardly needs amplification. As one example, state employ-ees of Alabama have been compelled since 2009 to subject themselves to an annual medical examination, including measuring body mass index (BMI). Patients with high BMI values who are subsequently diagnosed as obese face an increased insur-ance premium (Fernandez 2008), which results in the immediate consequence of financial penalty. Diagnosis may also be at the heart of reimbursement or disability contests. Incapacitating, medically unexplained symptoms that are not recognized as clear diagnoses rarely result in disability determination despite the incapacity they might engender. An individual seeking disability payments would see the diag-nosis as key in their pursuit.

In both of these cases, the consequences of the diagnosis (stigmatization for the obese and resources for those with medically unexplained symptoms) feed into the circular relationship described above. Patient advocacy groups, researchers, and insurers will all have their ideas about how better to frame problems such as fibro-myalgia or obesity.

The dynamic social nature of diagnosis and the diagnostic process is an important point of academic reflection precisely because diagnoses are not prior, ontological entities but social categories that organize, direct, explain, and sometimes control our experience of health and illness. Bowker and Star (1999, 50) describe classifi-cations as a kind of "work practice," but an invisible one, valorizing some points of view and silencing others. The inevitable privileging of certain voices over others in medical classification is opaque and must be made visible. Sociological analysis of diagnosis provides a tool for revealing the points of view that are contained in a disease label.

The power of sociological analysis is its potential to reveal the deep layers of negotiation, compromise, and interests that cover and surround the scientific evidence of a disease. What tools does sociology have at its disposal to help us reveal these deeper layers of understanding? We can consider two broad responses to this. Sociology is a richly theoretical discipline that over the last 150 years has developed and refined a range of concepts and models that can be informative, insightful, and revealing. And it has many perspectives. There are a variety of sociologies, and the dialogue and debate that are their consequences further enrich the field of sociological inquiry. But the core task of all sociologies is the systematic and theoretically informed analysis of patterns of social interaction.

Sociology is a discipline that was born during a time of upheaval and massive social change in Western society. There was the cultural revolution of the Enlightenment, the French political revolution, and the economic revolution of industrialization. In the attempt to understand these transformations, to diagnose the causes, and to prognosticate the results of these developments, the discipline of sociology emerged. The newly created discipline engaged many issues, from trying to understand the causes of conflict and cohesion to exploring the roles and functions of institutions like religion, family, and medicine to understanding what determines an individual's life chances, constraints, and opportunities. It is clear that all these questions have a direct bearing on the profession of medicine and its tasks.

Under the broad umbrella of sociology there are many subdisciplines, of which medical sociology is a lively and productive example. Medical sociologists ask a wide range of questions, but all have in common the principle of not taking phenomena at face value. There is no assumption in sociology that medical decisions are grounded only in the world of biology. There is no assumption that commonsense explanations that are based on individual beliefs and actions provide sufficient explanations of decision making. For sociologists, the context in which decisions are made and actions are undertaken is all-important. To understand the context, we need to take into consideration the history of ideas and institutions, the cultural understandings that are at play, the particular social circumstances of participants, and the way in which social order is shaped by the taken-for-granted elements of everyday interaction (how we present ourselves to each other, how we achieve communication, how moral forces shape interactions between people).

Sociologists may ask whether the medical profession in particular, and the health-care system in general, help to overcome social inequalities or reinforce them (Navarro 1978; Wilkinson 1996). They may ask how the profession came to gain its status, at whose expense, and with what consequences (Dew 2003; Willis 1983). They may ask questions about communication between medical practitioners and their clientele and how that limits or fosters interaction (Silverman 1997). This interest has been intensified by the realization that most healing takes place in contexts removed from formal contact with the established health professions (Nettleton 1995; Stacey 1988). As such, a great deal of diagnosis takes place in nonmedical settings, too.

So what might we achieve by undertaking a sociological analysis of diagnosis? A sociological perspective will assist clinicians and student clinicians in examining their own assumptions and in relating their own experiences to broader social and cultural concerns. This capacity to see our own world in the context of wider social forces enhances our capacity to be self-critical, to examine the assumptions of others, and to consider the consequences of social action, both intended and unintended. And it does more than this. By having a greater range of tools and concepts that help us to understand why we act in the way we do and the outcomes of our actions, we can also consider in greater depth that question central to the sociological imagination: "How could it be otherwise?" (Willis 1994, 4).

Historically the state has conferred great authority on the medical profession, establishing it as an autonomous profession with powers to regulate itself and to order the conditions of clinical practice. One might initially think that this assessment of the profession was a consequence of superior science and diagnostic capabilities. But this is far from the case. Medical treatment during the eighteenth and nineteenth centuries was not diagnostically driven but included bloodletting and the administration of large doses of calomel (mercurous chloride) and other dangerous mineral drugs, purgatives, emetics, and venesection (Coulter 1975; Duffy 1979; Kaufman 1971). This form of treatment was based on the theory of humors, where, for example, miasmas or noxious substances arising from filth and putrefying matter that corrupted the natural humors of the body caused fever. Treatment was aimed at driving out the vitiated humors (Duffy 1979), and this driving-out could be quite drastic.

An extreme and influential exponent of this style of medicine was Benjamin Rush, who in the early 1800s was considered the greatest physician of his day (Duffy 1979). He ascribed all disease to "capillary tension," and its only cure was bloodletting and purging. "He had such confidence in the lancet that he was willing to remove up to four-fifths of the blood in the body if necessary to alleviate the symptoms" (Kaufman 1971, 2). For Rush, desperate diseases required desperate remedies. Patients were bled until they fainted, and then on recovery were bled again.

Blistering was also a treatment of choice, where a second-degree burn would be created, and would then become infected and suppurate. The pus was seen as a sign of the infection being drawn out of the system (Kaufman 1971). Purging was carried out by the use of emetics to induce vomiting and cathartics to evacuate the bowels. Calomel was also given in large doses for a variety of conditions. These massive doses produced salivation, loosening of the teeth, falling-out of the hair, and other symptoms of acute mercury poisoning. Because calomel would also irritate the bowel, it was sometimes given with opium.

Within the worldview of the time the *materia medica* worked because it produced visible and predictable physiological effects: purges purged, emetics induced vomiting, opium soothed pain and moderated diarrhea. Bleeding, too, seemed obviously to alter the body's internal balance, as evidenced both by a changed pulse and the very quantity of blood drawn (Rosenberg 1992, 15).

Drugs used by medical practitioners in the nineteenth century were not standardized. Therefore practitioners could only estimate the potency of the drugs they were giving. In was not until 1910 that the idea of the "biological assay" was first mooted to measure the biological activity of a remedy. At this time it was suggested that the biological potency of digitalis (from the leaves of the foxglove) could be assessed by a "cat unit." That is, pharmacists making up the potion could test the potency of the leaves by determining how many leaves it took to kill a cat (Porter 1995). But it was only a partial solution to finding the strength of medicinal preparations, as different cats varied in their tolerance for drugs. From then on, however, more effort was put into standardizing medicines, and it was not until they were that one could put any faith in tests of therapeutic effectiveness. Without standardizing the drug, one could not tell whether the effect of giving the drug (negative or positive) was a result of the regime of treatment or of the potency of the particular dose given.

In the nineteenth century, as medicine was increasingly given state patronage, physicians resisted the idea that statistical methods should be employed to "decide if the differences in rates of cure between two populations of patients should in fact be attributed to the treatment regimes" (Porter 1995). To accept the notion of a controlled trial would be to subordinate clinical judgments and medical ideas to the dominance of numbers. Although attempts were made in the first half of the twentieth century to assess the outcomes of some treatments by subjecting them to statistical tests, the practice was rejected, as medicine was "always concerned with the individual" and not "facts without authenticity" (Hacking 1990, 85). The use of statistical methods in medicine only began after 1900, and it was not until the 1940s that statistical tests gained a firm foothold in medical research.

The idea of comparing groups to look for statistically significant differences was a style of reasoning that was foreign and alien to nineteenth-century medical men. Many more concepts needed to be accepted before clinical trials could become the norm. One important concept was the notion of "normal" that could be compared with the deviant (Hacking 1990). Without a notion of a normal distribution of the population, it was not possible to establish whether the responses one got from a therapeutic intervention were due to chance (therefore not outside the normal distribution) or to some real effect (therefore "deviating" in a positive way from a normal distribution). The notion of "normal" that we use today, which is both a comparison with the pathological and an ideal for which we strive (as in norms of behavior), did not take a hold on medical and social thought until the late nineteenth century. Once a notion of normal had been established, the deviant could be identified and the constraints around normality would become narrower and narrower. The shift in the style of reasoning that occurred in the twentieth century can be seen today in the powerful standardizing forces of applied genetic knowledge, where for example "deviant" fetuses can be identified early and aborted, leading to an increasingly "standardized" population.

So historically the relationship between authoritative medical diagnosis and science has been tenuous; even today knowledge that is trusted changes, and so do diagnoses. But with the nineteenth-century medical armamentarium and worldview the medical profession successfully embarked on the process of professionalization, achieving state patronage and a level of clinical autonomy.

Since the 1980s this medical autonomy has been increasingly under challenge. For example, allied health professions have found opportunities to develop new strategies designed to contest the dominance of doctors. Nurses and other medical professionals have acquired both diagnostic and prescribing rights. Another important development since the 1980s has been the rise of consumerism, with the users of health services demanding greater accountability, better quality of service (Williamson 1992), and a more egalitarian relationship with their doctors (Pringle 1998).

Some theorists suggest that consumers are increasingly gaining information and knowledge about health and medicine that rival the knowledge of the medical profession. But the advances in general education, and the increasing access that consumers have to information through such media as the Internet, do not necessarily mean that the doctor and patient are on a more equal footing. Although the average consumer is capable of evaluating much more specialized technical information today, the quantity and quality of specialized knowledge has also increased (Freidson 1994).

The rise of consumerism and the feminist critique of what has historically been a male-dominated medicine have played their part in bringing about changes in the work practices of physicians. Doctors believe that their status has diminished in recent years, with patients more demanding and more likely to challenge a diagnosis by asking for a second opinion (Lupton 1997). Another important element in this change since the 1970s has been managerialism's impact on medical practice, whereby attempts have been made to give increasing authority to management and to introduce market competition to the health system (Traynor 1996). Historically the medical profession has been able to retain a marked level of autonomy that has freed it from control by the state or other professional groups. This autonomy has prompted concerns about variations among general practitioners; for example, in patterns of clinical practice, which have in turn raised questions about the scientific basis of medical practice (Daniels 1992; Eddy 1984; Rosenthal 1995).

Inroads on the clinical autonomy of medical practitioners are now increasingly apparent. The drive toward evidence-based medicine and the development of treatment protocols represent dimensions of this trend (Berg 1997). The establishment of quality-assurance programs for medical practitioners is another aspect. These programs can involve the review of a doctor's practice by peers and the auditing of a doctor's medical procedures. The way this affects autonomy is that clinicians' decisions are more accountable and made more transparent, and potentially they are more standardized.

Technology is another important feature that influences health-care practice and diagnostic processes. The twentieth century has seen unprecedented development in technological intervention in health practices (Uttley 1991). Scientific and technological developments have provided the basis for safer practices; they have also been a source of controversy. Debates have been sparked by any of a range of technological advances—from the impact of the polluting consequences of industrial development on the health status of the population (Doyal and Pennell 1979) to the possible adverse effects of new drugs (Abraham 1995). Diagnosis is a central issue here, because to diagnose is often to identify the cause. Is the patient's diagnostic label a result of chemical exposure, an adverse event to a changed medication, and so on? The new developments of genetic technology pose another set of questions. For what sort of conditions should we screen? If we find people with a genetic susceptibility to certain conditions, what impact will that have on their lives? Will it affect their prospects of gaining medical insurance? How will it affect their prospects in the labor market? Questions of this sort will become increasingly important in the future as new medical technologies enter standard practice (Willis 1998).

As noted above, there are many different sociological perspectives. We won't set out to identify the full range here, but it is worth noting that some sociologists focus on the issue of how social order is maintained and what functions different institutions have in maintaining that order. Some sociologists focus on issues of power and conflict and how these play out in relation to certain social structures, such as class, gender, and ethnicity. Some sociologists focus on how we experience and negotiate our social world and the meanings that we have available to us to understand it.

A term associated with sociology and other social sciences is social construction. This is a term that is often incorrectly ascribed an antibiophysical bent. Social constructionism is an important principle in our aim to understand diagnosis and its role in medicine and society, as well as in our understanding of health and illness. It interrogates how social factors influence what we accept as truth. Some social constructionists would argue that basic categories we assume are natural (such as time and space) are the product of social interaction and organization. Using time as an example, we don't need this concept until we have to participate in some socially organized event such as communal rituals, hunting, harvesting. Less dauntingly, we can think of social constructionism as an approach that focuses on how social factors shape our ideas, beliefs, actions, and institutions. Focusing on the social does not mean that it is only social forces that shape our world. We are obviously shaped by the physical, the biological, the material world.

You will encounter many useful concepts as you read this book. One orienting concept that is implicitly or explicitly drawn on is socialization. Socialization is a concept used to describe how we come to learn certain roles in our society. For example, how do we come to behave like girls and boys, men and women, students and health professionals? There are many elements involved in the process of socialization, such as education, social attitudes, cultural rituals, and so on. The concept of socialization goes to the heart of our sense of identity and self. A number of studies have shown how medical students are socialized into the culture of medical practice in the hospital setting (Atkinson 1997; Bosk 1979; Fox 1957). This process involves learning the codes of conduct of medical practice, dealing with the uncertainty of clinical practice, and coping with the events of life, death, and dying in the clinical setting. But patients are socialized into the patient role, too. They learn, usually from a young age, how to conduct themselves in the consultation, what to say and what not to say, and when to say it. Being socialized into a particular role does not mean we have no choice about how we behave in that role. Most sociologists do not deny individual choice and freedom of will, but they seek to explain how factors outside of the individual influence those choices and one's life course.

The contributors to this book are often called upon by clinicians to determine why a particular group of patients seem loath to follow treatments, present communication problems, or don't achieve the expected health outcomes. "What's going on here?," a clinician might ask us. "How can I manage this differently, or what should be done?" The sociological perspective can explore the forces that convene in the particular setting to result in the situation before the individual clinician and her patient. There are methodological tools to research the social world. Sociologists can be interested in the prevalence of a phenomena (using something like a survey, longitudinal research, or cohort studies), identifying specific causes (perhaps implementing some form of experimental design), how something is done (so might use some form of observation), or how people respond to or experience a situation (so might conduct interviews, examine diaries, and so on). To understand change over time in ideas and institutions, archival sources and documents might be the sources of analysis. Researchers can also be creative, getting people to take photos, do drawings, create montages, and any number of other possibilities to get at people's stories, understandings, and experiences.

It should now be clear that a sociological perspective can question and unsettle our assumptions and get us to consider processes, like diagnosis, in a different light. While this book focuses on the sociological, it has its foundations firmly in the clinical. By looking at social process, structures, and questions, we intend to provide more options for clinicians to understand their practice and obstacles to its success. We hope that these sociological descriptions resonate in your own understanding of your work. Glaser and Strauss (1968), in their seminal work on diagnostic disclosure of terminal illness, described the contribution of the sociologist as being one wherein the sociologist "reports what he observes in a way which rings true to an insider . . . but in a fashion they [the insider] would not have written it" (9). The sociological perspective is informative, detailed, and different from what the student of medicine, or of other diagnostic professions, learns in a pathophysiology or clinical assessment course. It is precisely this difference that should help enrich your professional experience.

MAKING THE ROUNDS: INSIDE THIS BOOK

As you will discover in chapter 1, much of diagnosis hinges on the vagaries of classification and how medicine determines similarity and difference. Classification is, as Eviatar Zerubavel has written, a way of carving up the continuum of nature in to chunks. These divisions help us to organize our lives and our tasks. Just as medicine cuts up disease into diagnostic categories, assembling symptoms, causative agents, and therapeutics into logical parcels that serve as the basis for treatment and care, so too have the contributors to this book classified the social aspects of diagnosis into discrete areas of reflection. In the paragraphs that follow, we describe these concepts as a way to provide you with a road map for the use of this book.

Chapter 1 goes to the heart of what diagnosis aims to achieve: the classification of illness. It introduces the notion that diagnosis is a thoroughly social activity that changes not only with different scientific understandings, but also with cultural shifts and social influences. We show how systems of classification are the product of historical, cultural, and social circumstances, and that what classification systems, or schemas, we use influences how we intervene in the world. But it is not just major cultural shifts in medicine that lead to different classification schemes; more mundane matters like what conditions are funded and the particular specialty of the person doing the classifying have a great bearing. Once a particular classification has taken hold, we tend to see any other signs or symptoms in relation to that classification.

Chapter 2 moves from our understandings of diagnostic classifications to the process of diagnosis—emphasizing its dynamic, contingent, and interactional nature. Diagnosis is an outcome of collaborations near and at a distance; it is an ongoing process and it is mixed up with interventions and treatment plans. The process of diagnosis shifts through stages of greater uncertainty and certainty—for both the patient and the clinician. Understanding the time dimension of diagnosis can be clinically important; the clinician must attune to its importance to allow patients to adjust to a shift in their reality. Seeing diagnosis in this way has important implications, as it reveals the social systems and players that make up the outcome of a diagnosis as well as the nonlinear and dynamic nature of the diagnostic process.

Chapter 3 grapples with the pervasive phenomenon of uncertainty that patients and practitioners alike would prefer to eliminate. Even with increasingly powerful medical diagnostic technologies, the uncertainty of diagnosis and prognosis is still part of the everyday experience of medical practitioners. As we demonstrate, however, efforts to eliminate uncertainty may have detrimental effects, including misdiagnosis, increased morbidity, and even mortality. Chapter 3 demonstrates how acknowledging and even accepting uncertainty can often add to, rather than detract from, the outcomes medical consultation seeks to achieve.

The immediate diagnostic relationship is the topic of chapter 4, which begins with a discussion of why we refer to the people who seek diagnosis as "patients" proposing other ways of considering the relationship between lay and professional, but we review how the relationship has changed over time, and how some of these changes have challenged the professional identity of doctors. Part of a profession's status is gained through its capacity to hold and distribute information and knowledge—actions that have been challenged by the explosion in health information now available in myriad outlets. Chapter 4 also notes the importance of prediagnostic work undertaken by the layperson even before turning up at doctor's office, and how the diagnostician might understand this as an important diagnostic preliminary.

Chapter 5 covers the incredible power a diagnostic label can convey. We explore how giving a name to a condition can have an effect upon a person's identity: how they see themselves, the goals they set for themselves, and the roles they assume. Even though their physical condition has not changed, the receiving of a life-altering diagnosis may cleave their lives into "before" and "after," altering their direction. While clinicians cannot necessarily predict how a patient will respond to a diagnosis, knowing about the life world of the patient—what they do, what they value, how they see themselves—improves the communication and impact of an unwelcome diagnosis.

Chapter 6 digs into the murky world of discrimination, the outcome of another form of classification. Given the huge diversity in the population of patients, clinicians can't help but categorize and stereotype. This is one way in which humans deal with a complex social world. As chapter 6 reveals, however, research shows us that we are likely to make different diagnoses depending on the social group of the patient, that men and women are treated differently, as are people of different ethnic and cultural backgrounds. Chapter 6 makes an argument not to treat everyone in the same way, but to treat everyone with dignity. To do so, clinicians need to be cognizant of the differences in how they see various groups, and increase their understanding of others.

The monopoly that physicians have enjoyed in the diagnostic arena gives medical practitioners an authority like no one else, and puts patients and others who rely on a diagnosis in a position where they are dependent upon medical practitioners. Chapter 7 considers medical authority and some of its important contemporary challenges. In order for medical specialisms to gain credibility, diagnostic capacities have been developed and honed. Today this is still a powerful basis of the high social status of medical practitioners, but like everything else in society there are changes and shifts that affect this authority. Other health professionals, such as nurses, have taken on some diagnostic capability; patients have better access to diagnostic information; people with particular conditions have greater opportunities to organize and lobby; legal systems have changed to empower patients; quality assurance goals can constrain clinical autonomy; and clinicians have become increasingly reliant on diagnostic technologies.

Chapter 8 introduces us to the pervasive social process of medicalization, or the expansion of medical categories and broadening of diagnostic and treatment activities. While medical professionals are clearly involved, they are not necessarily (perhaps rarely!) the instigators. To study the process of medicalization is to study the processes by which a medical label gets attached to a particular condition. Depending on what is at stake, for a condition to become medicalized it could mean anything from a victory for those struggling for a recognition of their ailments, to a triumph for pharmaceutical companies as their market expands. But one possible consequence of these powerful medicalizing forces is that what we consider normal is increasingly limited and constrained as more of daily life is experienced or identified as pathological.

Chapter 9 builds on medicalization by focusing on the pervasive influence of marketing on diagnosis. Marketing by purveyors of medical interventions and devices not only pressures clinicians to diagnose in particular ways but also influences the classifications of diseases and conditions. Marketing drives up health costs and fosters overdiagnosis. Diagnosis can be seen as a marketing opportunity, one with a rich history and one that needs to be critically examined.

Technological developments have had a huge impact upon the diagnostic process, an issue that is the focus of chapter 10. How medical practitioners use helpful diagnostic technologies is shaped by a range of institutional, commercial, and political social forces. Technologies do not just evolve in an autonomous fashion driven by some internal logic but are embedded within social practices and relationships, and they of course alter and transform those practices and relationships. Technological diagnostic interventions can also be crucial for patients if the technological outputs give credibility to their experience of symptoms and open up new forms of self-identity. But what we get from diagnostic technologies still needs to be interpreted and can be disputed, as chapter 10 reveals.

So much is vested in diagnosis that it can give rise to contestation, as chapter 11 delineates. Some social groups may identify diseases that others (notably medicine) may dismiss. This takes us to the heart of the scientific enterprise and its limitations: the goal of proving causation. We may take the view that where there is doubt about the relationship between a cause and a symptom, science will eventually find the answer. But there are circumstances where science is not able to be the arbiter, and is unlikely ever to be, as there are inherent limitations in the capacity of science to determine what is going on, and where this occurs, political, economic, cultural, and social factors will determine the outcomes. Contested diagnoses and illnesses can be bewildering for patients suffering from something that is debilitating them but not "recognized" and to clinicians who do not see an intervention path that works for the patient.

Chapter 12 focuses on the patient side of the consultation dyad. In all sorts of ways, patients are forced to diagnose. They are the ones who decide when to see a doctor. Patients make candidate diagnoses, and the clinician may confirm them or come up with a different determination. But more than this, the patients make sense of their illness through the stories they tell about that experience based on everyday understandings of diagnosis, and chapter 12 shows how clinicians can learn by attending to the narratives of their patients. Clinicians should perhaps tread lightly when dismissing patients' diagnoses, as they are potentially unraveling powerful explanatory stories. To push the argument a little, one thing a clinician can take from chapter 12 is that the clinical diagnostic work and lay diagnostic work may not always serve the same purpose, and that a greater awareness of the sense-making activities of lay diagnosis may facilitate relationships in the consultation.

It is clear that diagnosis is a thoroughly social process. But how can we learn more about this process, and how should we study the complex world of social forces? To understand the social world, we are forced to go beyond research approaches designed to test pharmaceuticals. Chapter 13 provides us with some direction here. There are many systematic and rigorous approaches to the study of the social world, some of which require a great commitment in time and resources to learn and apply. Chapter 13 offers an overview of some important ways of gaining insight into the social processes in diagnosis.

Finally, we conclude with stories from the frontline of diagnosis. The words of two prominent general practitioners describe the central role of diagnosis in day-to-day doctoring and reveal concerns about misdiagnosis, the emotional investment in diagnosis by patients and clinicians, the unnoticed centrality of diagnosis in everyday clinical practice, and the vigilance required to keep attuned to the social shaping and social consequences of diagnosis.

Our final section provides readers with the CLASSIFY mnemonic, which is designed to help keep the social overlay to clinical diagnosis in the foreground of clinical thinking. It's not enough to know how bodies work to do the best possible diagnostic work; one must also know how society understands disease and how disease affects those who have it, who label it, and who work with those thus labeled.

Finally, throughout the book, words in **boldface** indicate terms defined in the glossary.

REFERENCES

Abraham, John. 1995. *Science, Politics and the Pharmaceutical Industry: Controversy and Bias in Drug Regulation*. New York: St. Martin's Press.

Atkinson, Paul. 1997. *The Clinical Experience: The Construction and Reconstruction of Medical Reality*. 2nd ed. Aldershot: Ashgate.

Berg, Marc. 1997. *Rationalizing Medical Work: Decision-Support Techniques and Medical Practices*. Cambridge, MA: MIT Press.

Bosk, Charles. 1979. *Forgive and Remember: Managing Medical Failure*. Chicago: University of Chicago Press.

Bowker, Geoffrey, and Susan Leigh Star. 1999. *Sorting Things Out: Classification and Its Consequences*. Cambridge, MA: MIT Press.

Coulter, Harris. 1975. *Divided Legacy: A History of the Schism in Medical Thought*. Vol. 1, *The Patterns Emerge: Hippocrates to Paracelsus*. Washington: Weehawken.

Daniels, Stephen. 1992. "The Pragmatic Management of Error and the Antecedents of Disputes over the Quality of Medical Care." In *Quality and Regulation in Health Care: International Experiences*, edited by Robert Dingwall and Paul Fenn, 112–40. London: Routledge.

Dew, Kevin. 2003. *Borderland Practices: Regulating Alternative Therapies in New Zealand*. Dunedin: University of Otago Press.

Doyal, Lesley, and Imogen Pennell. 1979. *The Political Economy of Health*. London: Pluto.

Duffy, John. 1979. *The Healers: A History of American Medicine*. Champaign: University of Illinois Press.

Eddy, David. 1984. "Variations in Physician Practice: The Role of Uncertainty." *Health Affairs* 3(2): 74–89.

Fernandez, Don. 2008. "Alabama 'Obesity Penalty' Stirs Debate." *WebMD*, August 25, http://www.webmd.com/diet/news/20080825/alabama-obesity-penalty-stirs-debate.

Fox, Renée. 1957. "Training for Uncertainty." In *The Student Physician: Introductory Studies in the Sociology of Medicine*, edited by Robert Merton, 207–41. Cambridge, MA: Harvard University Press.

Freidson, Eliot. 1994. *Professionalism Reborn: Theory, Prophecy and Policy*. Chicago: University of Chicago Press.

Glaser, B. G., and A. L. Strauss. 1968. *Awareness of Dying*. New Brunswick, NJ: Aldine.

Hacking, Ian. 1990. *The Taming of Chance*. Cambridge: Cambridge University Press.

Kaufman, Martin. 1971. *Homeopathy in America: The Rise and Fall of a Medical Heresy*. Baltimore: Johns Hopkins University Press.

Lupton, Deborah. 1997. "Doctors on the Medical Profession." *Sociology of Health and Illness* 19(4): 480–97.

Navarro, Vincente. 1978. *Class Struggle: The State and Medicine*. London: Robertson.

Nettleton, Sarah. 1995. *The Sociology of Health and Illness*. Cambridge: Polity.

Porter, Theodore. 1995. *Trust in Numbers: The Pursuit of Objectivity in Science and Public Life*. Princeton, NJ: Princeton University Press.

Pringle, Rosemary. 1998. *Sex and Medicine: Gender, Power and Authority in the Medical Profession*. Cambridge: Cambridge University Press.

Rosenberg, Charles. 1992. *Explaining Epidemics and Other Studies in the History of Medicine*. Cambridge: Cambridge University Press.

Rosenthal, Marilynn. 1995. *The Incompetent Doctor: Behind Closed Doors*. Buckingham: Open University Press.

Silverman, David. 1997. *Discourses of Counselling: HIV Counselling as Social Interaction*. London: Sage.

Stacey, Margaret. 1988. *The Sociology of Health and Healing*. London: Unwin Hyman.

Traynor, Michael. 1996. "A Literary Approach to Management Discourse after the NHS Reforms." *Sociology of Health and Illness* 18(3): 315–40.

Uttley, Stephen. 1991. *Technology and the Welfare State: The Development of Health Care in Britain and America*. Cambridge, MA: Unwin Hyman.

Wilkinson, Richard. 1996. *Unhealthy Societies: The Afflictions of Inequality*. London: Routledge.

Williamson, Charlotte. 1992. *Whose Standards? Consumer and Professional Standards in Health Care*. Buckingham: Open University Press.

Willis, Evan. 1983. *Medical Dominance: The Division of Labour in Australian Healthcare*. Sydney: Allen and Unwin.

———. 1994. *Illness and Social Relations: Issues in the Sociology of Health Care*. St. Leonards: Allen and Unwin.

———. 1998. "The 'New' Genetics and the Sociology of Medical Technology." *Journal of Sociology* 34(2): 170–83.

Constructing Order
Classification and Diagnosis

Dena T. Smith and Jennifer Hemler

STARTING POINTS

- Classifying diseases is important for identifying public health priorities.
- Diagnosis is the process of symptom identification, interpretation, and classification.
- Doctors and clinicians need to rely on disease models (guides for how to classify and cluster symptoms) in order to treat patients expediently and effectively.
- Doctors and clinicians are trained how to think about disease according to particular medical models.

A middle-aged **patient** comes into the ER fearing he is having a heart attack. He complains that his "chest hurts," his heart is "pumping too fast," and that he "can't breathe." When you interview him, you notice that his speech seems slightly slurred. He is agitated, talking fast. You also notice that he is sweating. He seems to be having trouble answering your questions, revises his answers, is confused about the sequence of events. It's your job to make a diagnosis so that this patient can be admitted to the proper department and treated appropriately. But how do you perform this task?

Making a diagnosis is a complex process whether you are in an emergency room, clinic, or practice-based setting. What the patient tells you and how he tells you this information are critical parts of this process. Before the patient even reaches you, social factors have shaped his understanding of medicine, disease, and symptom expression. The patient above may fear he is having a heart attack because heart disease "runs" in his family. He may have a fairly well-formed, though not necessarily accurate, idea of what constitutes "heart attack." Consequently, he may only tell you the symptoms he feels are medically relevant to his understanding of heart attack, ignoring others that in tandem with the above presentation could indicate different underlying disease paths: for instance, the addition of vision problems to his symptom set may indicate a transient ischemic attack (TIA), while feelings of anxiety or nausea could indicate a panic attack.

How you make medical sense of what a patient tells you (and any additional information gathered by intake personnel, if you are not the first caregiver to see the patient) is the next step in this process. After the data are filtered through the

PEDIGREE OF MAN.

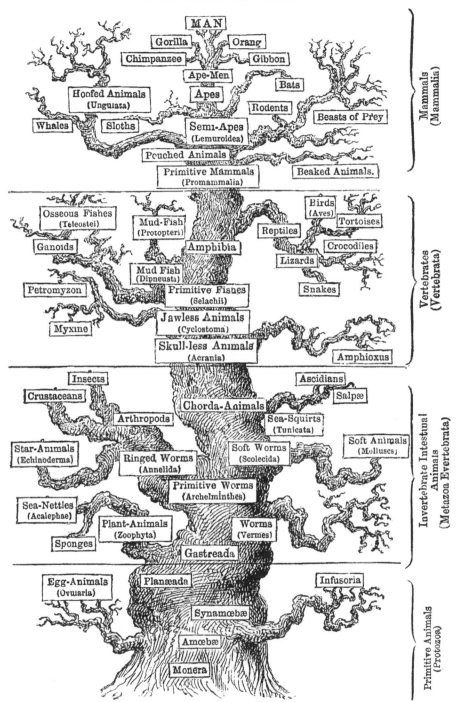

Figure 1-1. Ernst Haeckel's "Pedigree of Man," 1897.

patient's lens, you subject the information to your own processes of mental accounting. When the patient above complains that he "can't breathe," do you attribute this to hyperventilation or to chest pressure? Does his heart "pumping too fast," mean that he has a rapid or an irregular heartbeat? Does the fact that his "chest hurts" mean that he is experiencing pain, tightness, or pounding? How you make these distinctions can lead to different ways of thinking about his condition.

What the patient tells you is also subject to your own interpretive schemas. You noticed the patient's sweating, slurred speech, and confusion. Do you perceive these symptoms to be related or distinct? Do you attribute them to the condition that has landed him in the ER or to yet another medical condition, one independent of his current problem? For example, these particular symptoms could equally indicate a substance abuse problem or a mental illness that has little to do with heart disease or TIA. Or his sweating, agitation, and confusion could be caused by the anxiety of being in the ER, thinking he's having a heart attack. While conducting medical tests can clarify symptoms, doctors need to decide what information is crucial, what information is irrelevant, and what information is missing in order to know which tests to conduct. The patient's demeanor as well as her age, race, class, and gender may also influence how a doctor perceives symptoms and their seriousness, ultimately influencing interpretation of the medical problem at hand (see chap. 6, on diagnosis and diversity).

The truth is that doctors and clinicians have limited and filtered information about their patients (although the longer the length of the relationship between the doctor and her patient, the easier it is to interpret the information received). Diagnosis— the process of symptom identification, interpretation, and classification—is complicated and confounded by many factors. We have shown only a glimpse of how these interactional-level factors lend complexity to making a diagnosis. But other factors, seemingly removed from the direct patient interaction we described above, also add complexity to the diagnostic process.

Organizational-level factors, like the type of medical training you received and the relation of your medical specialty to others in the field, shape how you think about the classification of problems into medical diseases and disorders. Society-level factors—health-care management systems that structure reimbursements, pharmaceutical companies that link drugs to specific disorders, and federal health-care policies that determine access to insurance—clearly affect diagnostic practice. And cultural factors, like the dominant medical model in use at the time, location, and historical moment in which you live, shape medicine and diagnostic practice, too. Many of these factors remain outside the purview of medical personnel at the time of diagnosis: doctors and clinicians need to be able to act expediently and effectively, which means they need to attend to some information and "bracket," or ignore, other types of information. But some factors that influence diagnostic practice remain outside the thought processes of doctors because of the very nature of specialist training. Doctors and clinicians learn particular ways of viewing patients' bodies and interpreting what their patients tell them, which means they learn to *not* view bodies and symptoms through other possible frameworks.

In this chapter we discuss the ways in which systems of medical classification—of categorizing symptoms and diseases—are dependent upon social factors. Classificatory systems do not arise from "natural" or innate properties of disease or medicine alone. Ways of perceiving diseases are subject to **reification** over time. This means that diseases are understood to be distinct, physiological categories without any social or cultural content. The aim of this book (and of this chapter in particular) is to underline how even physically extant conditions always carry a social imprint. Clinicians and laypeople alike should recognize that classification systems, though they reflect the standards of a field, are malleable and socioculturally dependent and have particular, often significant, social and medical consequences.

THE SOCIAL CONSTRUCTION OF ILLNESS

The classification of "symptoms" into organized clusters, which can then be labeled "diseases," is the heart of modern medicine. Diagnostic manuals like the *Diagnostic and Statistical Manual of Mental Disorders* (DSM) and such classification systems as the *International Classification of Diseases* (ICD) or SNOMED Clinical Terms (SNOMED CT) outline the sets of symptoms that are considered to characterize diseases. They also outline how different illnesses relate to each other. But medical classification systems, like other professional and lay practices, adhere to some basic rules of classification. They bear a social imprint: we make decisions about which aspects of a thing are significant (and worth attending to) and which are negligible (and can be ignored); in doing so, we decide which things fit together (are similar) and which do not (are dissimilar; Zerubavel 1997).

If we look again at our scenario above, we have the following symptoms: chest pain, accelerated heart rate or heart palpitations, trouble breathing, slurred speech, sweating, and confusion (and perhaps more we don't know about yet). The above manuals provide guidelines for making diagnoses in terms of specifying symptom clusters, but the clinician must "lump" and "split" (Zerubavel 1997) these symptoms to mirror what the chosen classification schema specifies. Lumping and splitting symptoms in different ways might lead you to make different decisions about your patient's condition. Knowing the severity of each symptom and length of time the patient has been

> All diseases then ought to be reduc'd to certain and determinate kinds, with the same exactness as we see it done by botanic writers in their treatises of plants. For there are diseases that come under the same *genus*, bear the same name, and have some symptoms in common, which, notwithstanding, being of a different nature, require a different treatment. (Sydenham 1769, iii–iv)

suffering from each will help you assign meaning to the symptoms—perhaps helping you decide which symptoms are significant and which are negligible, which are core to a diagnostic category, and which are peripheral—and how to prioritize symptoms vis-à-vis different diagnostic categories.

Heart disease, panic disorder, TIA, and hypertension all share symptoms, so making a diagnosis requires you to mentally differentiate the symptoms into discrete groups and importance levels. Perhaps you decide chest pain and shortness of breath are the most pressing symptoms, so you address those first. Perhaps you decide the heart palpitations, slurred speech, and mental confusion are the "core" symptoms, relegating the others to the background. Or perhaps you differentiate respiratory symptoms from circulatory or nervous system symptoms. These are all ways of lumping and splitting the symptoms into categories to help you make sense and assign meaning to them.

Consider even how we presented the data: we lumped chest pain, shortness of breath, and heart rate into one group; sweating, mental confusion, and slurred speech into another. We did this to distinguish what the patient described versus what might be observed, and we also decided to list the more "concrete" symptoms first and the more ambiguous symptoms second. But perhaps we subconsciously (because of how we've been trained to think about the mind/body split in Western society) presented the data in such a way that might lead you to interpret the first set of symptoms as "physical" and the second as "mental." Mental symptoms are surely not less important than physical symptoms, and they may not be distinct insofar as there is an interaction between biochemistry and mental processes. But mental symptoms may be irrelevant in the context of one diagnosis, like heart disease, and highly relevant to others, like stroke or panic attack. Depending on the kind of doctor you are—psychiatrist or internist—you may prioritize one symptom set over another (after, of course, making sure your patient is not in mortal danger at that moment).

Classifying information in one way often obscures other ways to classify the same data, because classification in and of itself depends on seeing the world in a particular way. Our basic views of the world depend on classification. Think about how—and that—we classify people according to race in America (and that other countries have different ways of classifying race). For instance, during the period of slavery and segregation in the United States, having "one drop" of "black blood" made you black; someone with a black great-grandfather whose other relatives were white would still be considered black despite having more whites in his family tree. We still largely classify race this way today. That we consider President Barack Obama to be the first black president even though half his family is white confirms that the one-drop rule continues to affect how we perceive race. In addition, even though there are several similarities between Obama and other presidents of the past—he graduated from an Ivy League law school, served as a U.S. senator, is married, has children—these similarities were far less relevant to most Americans during his election than his racial classification. The president's African heritage and skin color mark him as black and, because of racial politics in the United States, his blackness is the most salient element of his *identity* to Americans at large.

This process of filtering and classifying information works the same way in medicine: how a practitioner organizes symptoms into a disease is influenced by how she is trained to perceive the data. This way of thinking about symptom classification leads her to make particular kinds of diagnoses and may prevent her from perceiving other possible diagnoses. In our scenario above, lumping symptoms together under the classification of heart disease may make it difficult to perceive those symptoms as independent from each other or as related to another

2. PHILOPROGENITIVENESS.

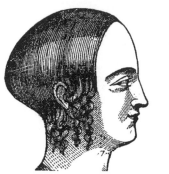 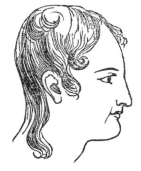

No. 47.   Large.   No 48.   Small.

Figure 1-2. Philoprogenitiveness, or the capacity to love children and small animals, as determined by the shape of the skull (Lavater 1855).

condition. This is both a strength and weakness of any system of classification. The way we view what belongs together and what does not allows us to function according to a certain logic, but it also hinders us from thinking across categories that we perceive to be unrelated. It is usually when faced with our biggest challenges—cases that defy textbook definitions or standard practices—that we need to think across our established categories of knowledge (or "out of the box"). This is one of the reasons why the process of carving out new diagnostic categories is so difficult (and often political), as was the case with HIV and AIDS. This is also why atypical presentations of existing diseases are so hard to identify, as highlighted in the popular television series *House, M.D.*

We need to be reflexive about how we classify symptoms and diseases, because these classificatory systems have consequences for how we see patients, fund research, and proceed with treatment (discussed below). But we first need to take a step back and think about which symptoms and diseases even make it into our classification systems. Symptoms and diseases do not exist in the body or mind alone. Before a symptom, problem, or condition can be classified as (part of) a disease, it needs to be considered undesirable—by individuals experiencing the problem, by the medical community and its powerbrokers (i.e., the people writing textbooks and diagnostic handbooks), and by society at large (Jutel 2011). For example, epilepsy was once thought of as a gift from the gods. Obesity was revered in some cultures and time periods as a sign of wealth or well-being. What we now call bipolar disorder has at times been tied to creativity, romanticized as artistic temperament.

These conditions lost their positive appeal at certain points in different cultures, becoming thought of as problems of the individual, and hence undesirable: epilepsy was confusing and frightening, perceived as a symptom of demon possession, witchcraft, or a sign of internal badness; obesity was **stigmatized** as an outward manifestation of moral depravity or lack of control or will power; and the mercurial habits of individuals suffering from bipolar disorder became less romantic as their behavior became less socially acceptable. These conditions and others, like attention deficit hyperactivity disorder (ADHD) and alcoholism, underwent a shift from "badness" to "sickness" (Conrad and Schneider 1992). Whereas children with excessive energy and focusing problems were once labeled likely future criminals, or more recently "problem children," today these children are thought to be biologically ill, often treated with stimulant medications like Ritalin and Adderall or antipsychotics. While not all conditions are stigmatized as bad, in order to be considered a disease, a phenomenon needs to be recognized and accepted by the established medical community and the surrounding society as something that falls under medical jurisdiction, and this process is often contentious.

Fibromyalgia and homosexuality are both interesting examples to consider in this light. Studies on fibromyalgia can be traced back to the 1970s. It was recognized as a syndrome by the American Medical Association in 1987, and diagnostic criteria for research were outlined by the American College of Rheumatology in 1990. But it was not until 2007 that fibromyalgia was codified as a medical condition, mostly because of sufferers' responses to the targeted drug Lyrica (an anticonvulsant originally approved for use in epilepsy and pain caused by shingles and diabetes; Barker 2011). Fibromyalgia had previously been considered a psychological ailment that affected women, much like hysteria. While accepted as a medical syndrome today, some practitioners continue to question its legitimacy as a disease because its etiology is largely unknown. Sufferers continue to complain that others, family and doctors alike, treat their symptoms as residing "in their head" (see Barker 2005).

Homosexuality also has a complicated history of inclusion and exclusion within medical classification. DSM-I classified homosexuality as a "sociopathic personality disturbance." In 1973, homosexuality was removed from DSM-II, which many date as the declassification of homosexuality as a mental disorder, but "sexual orientation disturbance" was included in its place. This category was then changed to "ego-dystonic homosexuality" in DSM-III, only to be removed in 1986. In the case of both fibromyalgia and homosexuality, their respective medical classification and declassification were largely the results of social pressure from interest groups on the medical profession. Both of these cases called for an investigation into the ways medicine and science are practiced and the types of claims they can make. They also both challenge the rigid divisions that conventional wisdom would have us make between the mind and the body, genetics and the environment. These cases illustrate that what we even consider to be "medical" or "nonmedical" can shift over time in relation to larger cultural shifts, like changes in technological and scientific understandings and social beliefs and attitudes.

Medical classification thus has critical social and medical impact: a diagnosis stamps a set of symptoms as a disease, marking it as real and legitimate, physical or psychological (Jutel 2011). We currently accept epilepsy, fibromyalgia, and obesity as diseases. We no longer accept the notion that homosexuality is a disease. Over time, we reify these classificatory decisions, such that it becomes difficult to think of accepted diseases as nonmedical and vice versa. But physical and mental states come to be thought of as diseases (or not) through a process of *social construction* (Berger and Luckmann 1966).

Social construction refers to the ways in which human beings build meaning: we create categories to classify and make sense of the world around us. These categories are designed in relation to our value systems, our culture and our societies, but they become a part of our taken-for-granted assumptions about the world. Categories like "health" and "illness," as well as what we assign to each category, are social constructions. Can you imagine something like cancer being considered a natural and normal part of human life? Probably not. Yet cancer is a natural biological process. If we did not divide human experience into health and illness, we would not think of cancer as a "disease" to be battled but perhaps just another normal part of the life continuum. To be clear, noting that a phenomenon is socially constructed does not mean that it does not exist or that its meaning is fake, made up, or insignificant. Instead, social construction describes how the meanings attributed to human experiences are social in nature: human beings collectively (usually not purposefully or consciously, but often under the influence of scientists, researchers, and other knowledge brokers) negotiate and accept certain meanings about phenomena over time and rely on these meanings to create order in the world around them.

Social constructions like health and illness (similar to other social constructions like race, gender, and beauty) are higher-order constructions: if we picture a classification tree in our minds, they form the larger, sturdier branches. They provide more of the structure for how we think and as such are more stable constructs, less subject to scrutiny. The "fruit" hanging from these branches, the specific elements we classify as belonging to health and illness, may be more contested and subject to change over time. But the point is that none of these classificatory elements are purely naturally occurring phenomena. They are social categories created and arranged to designate a certain sense of order to the world; they reflect ways of seeing the world that encompass certain power arrangements, moral ideas, and political interests. Social constructions are carried forward in time and transformed through use, new knowledge, and interaction with others, becoming part of our own **socialization** into the world around us. We are socialized into ways of perceiving, interpreting, and understanding (i.e., ways of classifying) the data all around us so that we know how to act in the world. **Professional socialization** involves being trained in a particular field or occupation so that we learn to filter knowledge through this specialist lens, which we discuss below.

PROFESSIONAL SOCIALIZATION

In every profession, newcomers must be inducted into the field. Law students spend grueling years memorizing a vast amount of information about the legal system, its cases, and rulings. Literature students closely study a voluminous canon of work, becoming fluent in theories of language and writing. Students in the social sciences learn methods and tools through which they can analyze groups and world events. In medicine, students must learn how various systems within the body function, which diagnostic codes to use for identifying pathology, and the appropriate treatment regimens for specific conditions. Most importantly, medical students and interns learn how to think like doctors, nurses, and clinicians through explicit training in particular medical classificatory systems. The most major of these systems, learned primarily during the first two years of medical training and internship, are (1) "normal" anatomical and physiological systems of the body (e.g., the immune system) and (2) pharmacological and toxicological properties of medications and their uses.

These classificatory systems provide the basis of medical education, helping the medical student learn not only the data that are the human body, but also how to organize that data in particular ways and apply what one has learned to particular cases. These ways of thinking become ingrained in the student, such that they start to shape how he looks at patients. One aspect of learning how to think like a doctor or clinician involves the formation of schemas, mental frameworks, or tools that help us organize our thinking about people (including ourselves), places, objects, and experiences. Schemas allow us to understand a stimulus (Howard 1995, 93) or "perceive the social scene" (Schuman 1995, 82). In other words, schemas act as shorthand guides or filters for interpreting events and information. We are not able to see, hear, taste, feel, smell, or process cognitively everything in our environments. Thus we learn shortcuts to help us focus on certain stimuli, allowing others to blend into a fuzzy background. In this way, classification is largely about making sense of an otherwise incomprehensibly vast set of experiences and stimuli. Such sense making is particularly important to consider in terms of how doctors and clinicians practice.

The young resident can more easily understand and emotionally tolerate a patient's troubling and perhaps confusing symptoms if she can apply a particular set of schemas to the case. Once a "volatile" patient is labeled schizophrenic, for instance, that patient becomes more understandable and familiar to the resident. The resident can use what she knows about schizophrenia and other patients suffering from it to interpret this patient's future actions. Similarly, a range of severe yet seemingly disjointed symptoms can be frustrating for the doctor (not to mention the patient), as in our opening vignette about the patient with the chest pain or other cases of ambiguous and multiply interpretable symptoms. But if the doctor recognizes a particular symptom—a distinctive rash, perhaps—that she recalls seeing in another patient, the doctor can apply a particular diagnostic schema to the patient. The distinctive rash, with other symptoms like joint pain, fatigue, headache, and neuropathy, enables the doctor to organize her thinking about the patient and the symptoms around the possibility of Lyme disease. Using the rash as the schematic cue, the doctor is able to render the symptoms more manageable and the patient's woes more understandable.

Diagnosis lumps patients together. Doctors use medical classification to identify types of patients so that all patients who exhibit similar characteristics can be compared. Once diagnosed, patients are then thought to be similar to each other in disease course, symptom expression, and behavior. Schemas can be extremely important for organizing thinking, but they can also be a hindrance if doctors perceive everything a patient does as related to an illness. Rosenhan (1973) conducted a study in which several pseudopatients (his graduate students) checked themselves into a psychiatric hospital, claiming to hear sounds and voices. They were diagnosed with schizophrenia, but once they entered the hospital, they acted as they normally would. However, the pseudopatients' "normal" behaviors, like taking notes, were interpreted according to their diagnoses so much so that in some cases Rosenhan needed to rescue his students from the hospitals. Similarly, patients who are obese often complain that doctors perceive that all of their ailments are related to or caused by their obesity (Friedman et al. 2012), and patients who have survived cancer have a difficult time telling if new aches and pains are distinct from or related to their cancer or cancer treatment (Hudson et al. 2012).

In addition to applying different schemas, particularly tools for how to think about data, human beings also employ different "lenses" at different times, depending on the situation, in order to filter perceivable phenomena to a manageable number of stimuli (Zerubavel 1997). We all have different lenses we use to filter information based on what role we are fulfilling at the time. You may have a student or professional lens, a political lens, an artistic lens, or a family-oriented lens, for example. Whereas schemas give us a quick way to interpret information, the perspective or lens we apply determines which schemas we activate. Research shows that our **definition of the situation** (Thomas and Thomas 1928, 571–72) strongly influences the lens we apply, although we may still experience tension between conflicting demands of our different lenses. Doctors often have to negotiate between their personal beliefs and professional oaths, for instance. Consider how your personal religious beliefs (or lack thereof) might clash with a patient's end-of-life decision or how your own beliefs about raising children might interfere with a decision to inform underage patients about their conditions and treatment options with or without consulting their guardians. A doctor might personally choose a different treatment for himself than he would propose to a patient.

The lenses we apply are informed by our memberships in a particular **thought collective**, which is "a community of persons mutually exchanging ideas or maintaining intellectual interaction" (Fleck 1935 [1979], 39). Thought collectives, more often than not, constrain our decision making by directing us to act and think according to the **norms** of a particular community. As Zerubavel (1997) explains, "the cognitive stances we adopt as members of particular social environments . . . constrain our mental 'vision' by exerting upon us tremendous pressure to conform to them" (32). Thought collectives provide **thought styles**, which direct the perception of members of the group. As stated above, doctors are taught to think in particular ways. These ways of thinking, or thought styles, create consistency and continuity within a field over time. Medical students learn to think like doctors, law students to think like lawyers. Medical classification systems are representations of what is considered legitimate illness and thus represent particular ways of seeing. These systems should be considered "historically situated artifacts" that are "learned as part of membership in communities of practice" (Bowker and Starr 1999, 287). Similarly, Goodwin's (1994) notion of professional vision explores the idea that "the ability to see relevant entities is not lodged in the individual mind, but instead within a community of competent practitioners" (626). Though it is true of all residents, Luhrmann (2001) explains of psychiatry residents, "what one learns to do affects the way one sees" (83).

Becoming a professional in any medical field is a matter of learning the knowledge of the group, how that knowledge should be organized, what the appropriate courses of action should be, and how this knowledge should be passed on through particular types of discourse and teaching (Boltanski and Thévenot 1991; Friedland and Alford 1991). In medicine, it is standards that allow for all of this.

MEDICAL STANDARDIZATION

Medicine is a difficult and demanding field because patients rarely suffer from "textbook cases" of disease. Being able to work within uncertainty is part of the art of medical practice (see chap. 3 for more on uncertainty). In fact, how well a practitioner can tolerate uncertainty may be the hallmark of the clinician (Cassell 2004, 214). But the stakes of practicing medicine within uncertainty are high—for both patients and practitioners. Operating under continual uncertainty would not be cognitively sustainable for anyone in any field; it would be paralyzing. Practitioners of medicine need to attach themselves to particular institutional logics and accepted systems of knowledge in order to act. Being able to rely on classification systems is one way of harnessing the uncertainty associated with modern medicine. Light (1980) describes adherence to diagnostic schemes as an "ideological resolution of uncertainty." Cassell (2004) describes how practitioners "turn toward what is seemingly knowable" (217) about the patient's disease rather than focusing on the idiosyncrasies of a patient's case or looking at the patient holistically. In this way, doctors manage to prod and poke the idiosyncratic patient into a less complicated textbook case (Cassell 2004).

Textbooks and diagnostic manuals provide models for understanding illness and treating patients that become detached from their socially constructed roots by their scientific and medical authority. We often fail to consider, for instance, that medical researchers and other experts in a field have set the thresholds for what counts as illness and disease, deciding the ranges of normality for blood work or determining how many symptoms on a checklist or average on a scale qualifies one as having a disorder (see Horwitz and Wakefield 2006; Mullaney 2006). Even determining what is statistically significant is based on a cutoff point agreed upon by convention, be it a confidence interval or a p-value. (We also tend to not think about what medical research gets funded, so that their findings *can* become translated into medical practice.) While perhaps paradoxical, it is not surprising that medical students receive "training for certainty" (Atkinson 1984) rather than being taught medicine as an uncertain science (Cassell 2004; Fox 1997) at such an early stage in their careers. Students "learn to view the science underlying medicine as established 'facts' and soluble 'puzzles,'" perceiving patients' problems as "the result of identifiable diseases," so that "once the 'correct' identification has been made, treatment and related recommendations automatically and predictably follow" (Gerrity et al. 1992, 1027–28). Doctors tend to adhere to similar treatment schemas long after they leave residency and internship programs, partly in attempt to maintain mental control over what can be slippery terrain (Groopman 2008; Klitzman 1995; Smith 2011).

Both Fox (1997) and Cassell (2004) describe medicine's inherent uncertainty as precisely that which makes **evidence-based medicine** so important for doctors. Using reliable practices and categorizations alleviates some of the potential uncertainty or fuzziness involved in the observation of symptoms and classification of disease. Evidence-based practice relies on distinct classification: depression must be distinguished from chronic fatigue syndrome, as must heart disease from anxiety disorders. Classificatory standards allow the clinician to know what he is seeing and to enact a course of action. If a diagnostic system offers valid definitions of an illness that allows a doctor to accurately identify and treat a patient, it is his best hope to avoid the potential uncertainties of human variability. Standards also allow for agreed-upon language that fosters communication between practitioners and for more reliable research in which investigators measure what they perceive to be the same symptoms, course of illness, and utility of treatment.

The primary purpose of classificatory systems in medicine is to create standards for diagnosis and treatment to help practitioners effectively and efficiently understand the symptoms with which their patients present. Standards are important in all branches of medicine as "a measure established by authority, customs, or general consent to be used as a point of reference" (Timmermans and Berg 2003, 24; see chap. 7 for further discussion of the relationship between authority and standards). For instance, after observing psychiatry residents, T. M. Luhrmann (2001) explains that standards or categories used to classify are so crucial because "in medicine . . . diagnosis gives a doctor control because it tells him how he might be able to help a patient" (45). Luhrmann's statement illustrates the necessity of "conventional norms of classification" (Zerubavel 1997, 54) to which doctors can point, particularly important in psychiatry although all types of medicine operate according to similar processes in making diagnoses.

Psychiatry may be a good case study for us to discuss here in regard to the importance of classificatory schemas to the profession. Psychiatry may experience a heightened need for extensive classification schemes, as compared to other fields, because "unlike the case with, for instance, cholera, there is no medical test for a specific disease pathology for any major psychiatric illness" (Luhrmann 2001, 20). In the absence of any other markers of illness and because the field has been subject to criticism about reliability and validity, psychiatrists must rely on diagnostic standards to "ensure stability of meaning over different sites and time and are essential to the aggregation of individual health care data into larger wholes" (25). The DSM is the arbiter of psychiatric medical standards in the United States, and the World Health Organization's ICD is closely synched to it. These standards work to control the possibility that clinicians from different backgrounds with different training might perceive their patients' symptoms in various ways.

Let us take the release of DSM-III in 1980, "one of the most significant events in psychiatry in the last half of the 20th Century" (Kirk and Kutchins 1992, 6), as an example of how standards are used to create homogeneity in diagnosis. The American Psychiatric Association regularly revises the DSM, and its third revision marked a change in approaches in psychiatry from a Freudian, psychodynamic model to a biomedical model. Psychiatrists who supported DSM-III leveled criticisms at earlier versions, and the psychodynamic model of psychiatry in general, because diagnoses could not be verified across psychiatrists and treatments could not be standardized (Horwitz 2002), meaning that the reliability and validity of diagnoses were low. DSM-III presented extensive criteria for diagnosing mental illness that clinicians, social workers, psychologists, and psychiatrists could all

Panic Disorder

A. At some time during the disturbance, one or more panic attacks (discrete periods of intense fear or discomfort) have occurred that were (1) unexpected, i.e. did not occur immediately before or on exposure to a situation that almost always caused anxiety, and (2) not triggered by situations in which the person was the focus of others' attention

B. Either four attacks, as defined in criterion A., have occurred within a four-week period, or one or more attacks have been followed by a period of at least a month of persistent fear of having another attack.

C. At least four of the following symptoms developed during at least one of the attacks:

 1. shortness of breath (dyspnea) or smothering sensations
 2. dizziness, unsteady feelings, or faintness
 3. palpitations or accelerated heart rate (tachycardia)
 4. trembling or shaking
 5. sweating
 6. choking
 7. nausea or abdominal distress
 8. depersonalization or derealization
 9. numbness or tingling sensations (paresthesias)
 10. flushes (hot flashes) or chills
 11. chest pain or discomfort
 12. fear of dying
 13. fear of going crazy or of doing something uncontrolled
    Note: Attacks involving four or more symptoms are panic attacks; attacks involving fewer than four symptoms are limited symptom attacks . . .

D. During at least some of the attacks, at least four of the C symptoms developed suddenly and increased in intensity within ten minutes of the beginning of the first C symptom noticed in the attack.

E. It cannot be established that an organic factor initiated and maintained the disturbance, e.g., amphetamine or caffeine intoxication, hyperthyroidism. **Note**: Mitral valve prolapse may be an associated condition, but does not preclude a diagnosis of panic disorder (American Psychiatric Association, 2000*).

*We use the DSM-III classification in this example to show these extensive criteria. These criteria have been updated in subsequent versions of DSM, including the DSM-IV-TR, though the description is largely identical.

follow. The standard diagnosis of panic disorder, one of many anxiety disorders in DSM-III (as well as DSM-IV, DSM-IV-TR, and the latest DSM-5, which was published in 2013), illustrates how specific classifications provide order and clarity for mental health doctors with different types of training when faced with patients' often troubling symptoms.

Diagnostic criteria for panic disorder allow doctors to easily note and count patients' symptoms. In particular, this diagnostic classification accomplishes three crucial tasks at the heart of the medical model. First, it distinguishes panic disorder from other kinds of anxiety disorders and other mental and physical disorders (points A and E). In other words, phobias are different than panic attacks. Second, it defines the duration of symptoms necessary for a diagnosis (point B). And third, it identifies the specific symptoms, which assesses the severity of the condition (points C and D). Offering specific criteria eases the burden of diagnosis for clinicians and also increases the chances that doctors in different locations understand patients' symptoms in the same way, thus increasing the reliability of diagnostic categories (which are key concerns in an evidence-based paradigm).

Medical professionals seek to avoid the confusion of multiple perspectives for understanding a condition. Historically, debates raged in the nineteenth century about whether illness was the result of miasmas (disease clouds) or some form of physical contagion. Debates today about the etiology of depression, diabetes, obesity, heart disease, and posttraumatic stress disorder (PTSD) highlight the same controversies over which lens we need to use to see these diseases (or nondiseases). Obesity is seen as a medical problem, though it can also be seen as a lifestyle issue or, as many sociologists argue, a social problem, given obesity's high correlation with poverty and lack of availability of healthy foods. These kinds of controversies have always existed within the medical field and between medical professionals and lay perspectives. Within medicine, diagnostic reliability depends upon practitioners perceiving symptoms in similar ways, yet controversies like those above show just how difficult it is to arrive at consensus.

UNINTENDED CONSEQUENCES: THE "SIDE EFFECTS" OF MEDICAL CLASSIFICATION

Classification is not neutral; it has consequences for the doctors who employ the standards and it also deeply affects patients who experience the outcomes of being diagnosed with particular conditions and given particular courses of treatment. And yet most diagnostic systems are not consistently reliable. Variability in diagnosis can never be completely eliminated because of human error, but also because of sub- and cross-cultural variation in populations and practitioners. Further, trying to objectify human experience and disease states that do not present in the same ways presents challenges.

Radiology is a good case in point. Reliability is a central concern in radiology, especially since what one sees on a film (tumors, bone breaks, lack of blood flow to the bowel) can mean the difference between life and death. But what a radiologist observes in one instance is not always what she sees at another moment—and diagnosis across practitioners is far less than 100% reliable (Groopman 2008, 177–82). One study showed that even among specialists, different doctors interpret electrocardiograms (EKGs) in varying ways; what some considered as showing a myocardial infarction, others did not. Likewise, pathologists examining biopsies of the cervix did not come to the same conclusions when they later repeated their readings (Groopman 2008, 182).

Moreover, diseases can have varying presentations in different cultural groups, undermining the reliability of the classification system. One useful example is Vega et al.'s (2004) study in which they show that US-born Mexican Americans have higher rates of depressive disorder than immigrant Mexicans. They conclude that "greater social assimilation increases psychiatric morbidity," meaning that as Mexican immigrants learn American norms, they are more likely to express their unhappiness in typically American, largely psychological ways (Vega et al. 2004, 532). Similarly, Becker (1995) shows that as Fijian society became increasingly westernized, Fijian body image changed to reflect a new, much thinner norm, and anorexia was introduced as a new disorder. The H1N1 influenza pandemic presented with different symptom groups in different countries. While gastrointestinal symptoms were present in Chinese and Japanese patients, they were not noted as significant features in reports from Mexican epidemiologists (Jutel et al. 2011). Similarly, Japanese patients diagnosed with depression have traditionally experienced and expressed more physical symptoms than their Western counterparts, complaining to their doctors of ailments like backaches, neck pains, headaches, and intestinal distress rather than only depressed mood (Waza et al. 1999). Simon et al. (1999) also found that the extent to which people in different countries experience somatic symptoms of depression is at least partly a reflection of cultural differences. Taken together, these studies show that culture is tremendously important in how people experience illness, whether they see their feelings, thoughts, moods, or physical sensations as illness at all, and how these differing symptoms might trouble international classification systems.

CLASSIFYING AS A PERSPECTIVE

In this chapter we explained that the lumping of certain symptoms into diagnostic categories (and the splitting of those categories from others) is a consequential process—a social, cultural, and political endeavor—not a purely medical one. In the vignette that opens this chapter, we discussed several steps doctors and clinicians go through in their process of making a diagnosis. Throughout this chapter we have discussed how students are trained to act and think like doctors or clinicians. In the trajectory from student to doctor or clinician, the steps taken in making a diagnosis may become second nature. Professionals of any sort usually cease questioning the basis of their knowledge at some point in their careers, in order to act expediently or to rein in the uncertainty at the heart of the profession. This act often results in a reification of the terms of the discipline, propping up the sanctity and power of their professional existence.

Though we do not often stop to consider diseases such as cancer, depression, or HIV as medical classifications, these diseases represent the artful construction of certain symptom sets (decisions about how symptoms are lumped together) and diagnostic tools (standards for how measurement scales and technological outputs should be used and deciphered). The medical field determines which symptoms count as illnesses and what severity or number of symptoms constitutes a disease. Medical classifications have dramatic effects on who receives treatment and what kind. Given the central role of medication in the modern world, doctors have a powerful role in applying diagnoses as labels. Medical labels also affect how lay-people and patients see themselves and others. It is important to keep in mind that any classificatory system is but one way in a range of possible perspectives for seeing any phenomenon. It is important to understand the clinician's role in reproducing or altering medical models for how illness is perceived, classified, and treated.

TAKEAWAY POINTS

- Medical classification systems are the outcomes of social processes.
- The interaction between dominant cultural ways of thinking about medicine, disease, and the body and technological advances and scientific discoveries has an important impact on medical practice.
- Specialization enables doctors and clinicians to see symptoms in particular ways, but it also limits their abilities to view symptoms according to different frameworks or models.

DISCUSSION QUESTIONS

1. What does it mean to say that diseases and diagnostic categories are socially constructed?
2. Why is classification so useful and important for medical practice?
3. What are the consequences (both drawbacks and benefits) of medical classification for patients?
4. What kinds of lenses might you need to negotiate when practicing medicine?
5. Do you think your medical training teaches you to view patients and diseases according to particular schema? Can you give examples where schemas helped and hindered your assessment of a patient?

REFERENCES

American Psychiatric Association. 2000. *Diagnostic and Statistical Manual of Mental Disorders*. Rev. 4th ed. Washington, DC: American Psychiatric Association.
Atkinson, Paul. 1984. "Training for Certainty." *Social Science and Medicine* 19(9): 949–56.
Barker, Kristin. 2005. *The Fibromyalgia Story: Medical Authority and Women's Worlds of Pain*. Philadelphia: Temple University Press.
———. 2011. "Listening to Lyrica: Contested Illnesses and Pharmaceutical Determinism." *Social Science and Medicine* 73(6): 833–42.
Becker, Anne-Emmanuelle. 1995. *Body, Self and Society: The View from Fiji*. Philadelphia: University of Pennsylvania Press.
Berger, Peter L., and Thomas Luckmann. 1966. *The Social Construction of Reality: A Treatise in the Sociology of Knowledge*. New York: Anchor.

Boltanski, Luc, and Laurent Thévenot. 1991. *On Justification: Economies of Worth.* Princeton, NJ: Princeton University Press.

Bowker, Geoffrey C., and Susan Leigh Starr. 1999. *Sorting Things Out: Classification and Its Consequences.* Cambridge, MA: MIT Press.

Cassell, Eric J. 2004. *The Nature of Suffering and the Goals of Modern Medicine.* Oxford: Oxford University Press.

Conrad, Peter, and Joseph W. Schneider. 1992. *Deviance and Medicalization: From Badness to Sickness.* Philadelphia: Temple University Press.

Fleck, Ludwig. 1935 (1979). *Genesis and Development of a Scientific Fact.* Chicago: University of Chicago Press.

Fox, Renée. 1997. *Experiment Perilous: Physicians and Patients Facing the Unknown.* Piscataway, NJ: Transaction.

Friedland, Roger, and Robert R. Alford. 1991. "Bringing Society Back in Symbols, Practices, and Institutional Contradictions." In *The New Institutionalism in Organizational Analysis*, edited by Walter W. Powell and Paul J. DiMaggio, 232–66. Chicago: University of Chicago Press.

Friedman, Asia, Jennifer Hemler, Elisa Rossetti, and Jeannie Ferrante. 2012. "Obese Women's Barriers to Mammography and Pap Smear: The Role of Conscientiousness." *Obesity* 20(8): 1611–17.

Gerrity, Martha S., Jo Anne L. Earp, Robert F. DeVillis, and Donald W. Light. 1992. "Uncertainty and Professional Work: Perceptions of Physicians in Clinical Practice." *American Journal of Sociology* 97(4): 1022–51.

Goodwin, Charles. 1994. "Professional Vision." *American Anthropologist* 96(3): 606–33.

Groopman, Jerome. 2008. *How Doctors Think.* New York: Mariner.

Haeckel, Ernst. 1897. *The Evolution of Man: A Popular Exposition of the Principal Points of Human Ontogeny and Phylogeny.* New York: Appleton, esp. plate xv.

Horwitz, Allan V. 2002. *Creating Mental Illness.* Chicago: University of Chicago Press.

Horwitz, Allan V., and Jerome C. Wakefield. 2006. "Is There an Epidemic of Mental Illness?" *Contexts* 5: 19–23.

Howard, Judith A. 1995. "Social Cognition." In *Sociological Perspectives on Social. Psychology*, edited by Karen Cook, Gary Alan Fine, and James House, 90–117. Needham Heights, MA: Allyn and Bacon.

Hudson, Shawna V., Suzanne Miller-Halegoua, Jennifer Hemler, Jeannie Ferrante, Jennifer Lyle, Kevin C. Oeffinger, and Robert S. DiPaola. 2012. "'Not What I Want, but Maybe What I Need': Adult Cancer Survivors Discuss Follow-Up in Primary Care." *Annals of Family Medicine* 10(5): 418–27.

Jutel, Annemarie G. 2011. *Putting a Name to It: Diagnosis in Contemporary Society.* Baltimore: Johns Hopkins University Press.

Jutel, Annemarie G., Michael G. Baker, James Stanley, Q. Sue Huang, and Don Bandaranayake. 2011. "Self-Diagnosis of Influenza during a Pandemic: A Cross-Sectional Survey." *BMJ Open* 1(2): e000234, doi:10.1136/bmjopen-2011-000234.

Kirk, Stewart A., and Herb Kutchins. 1992. *The Selling of DSM: The Rhetoric of Science in Psychiatry.* New York: Hawthorne.

Klitzman, Robert. 1995. *In a House of Dreams and Glass: Becoming a Psychiatrist.* New York: Simon and Schuster.

Lavater, J. C. 1855. *Essays on Physiognomy: Designed to Promote Knowledge and Harmony Among Mankind.* 15th ed., translated by T. Holcroft. London: William Tegg.

Light, Donald. 1980. *Becoming Psychiatrists: The Professional Transformation of Self.* New York: W. W. Norton.

Luhrmann, Tanya M. 2001. *Of Two Minds: An Anthropologist Looks at American Psychiatry*. New York: Vintage Books.

Mullaney, Jamie L. 2006. *Everyone Is Not Doing It: Abstinence and Personal Identity*. Chicago: University of Chicago Press.

Rosenhan, David L. 1973. "On Being Sane in Insane Places." *Science* 179: 250–58.

Schuman, Howard. 1995. "Attitudes, Belief, and Behavior." In *Sociological Perspectives on Social. Psychology*, edited by Karen Cook, Gary Alan Fine, and James House, 68–89. Needham Heights, MA: Allyn and Bacon.

Simon, Gregory E., Michael VonKorff, Marco Piccinelli, Claudi Fullerton, and John Ormel. 1999. "An International Study of the Relation between Somatic Symptoms and Depression." *New England Journal of Medicine* 341(18): 1329–35.

Smith, Dena T. 2011. "From Meaning-Making to Medicalization: The Art of Talk Therapy, the Science of the Biological Model and the Boundaries in Between." PhD diss., Rutgers University.

Sydenham, Thomas. 1769. *The Entire Works of Dr Thomas Sydenham, Newly Made English from the Originals:. . . To Which Are Added, Explanatory and Practical Notes, from the Best Medicinal Writers. By John Swan, M.D.* London: Edward Cave.

Thomas, William I., and Dorothy S. Thomas. 1928. *The Child in America: Behavior Problems and Programs*. New York: Knopf.

Timmermans, Stephan, and Marc Berg. 2003. *The Gold Standard: The Challenge of Evidence-Based Medicine and Standardization in Health Care*. Philadelphia: Temple University Press.

Vega, William A., William M. Shribney, Sergio Aguilar-Gaxiola, and Bohdan Kolody. 2004. "12-Month Prevalence of DSM-III-R Psychiatric Disorders among Mexican Americans: Nativity, Social Assimilation, and Age Determinants." *Journal of Nervous and Mental Disease* 192(8): 532–42.

Waza, Kazuhiro, Antonnette V. Graham, Stephen J. Zyzanski, and Kazuo Inoue. 1999. "Comparison of Symptoms in Japanese and American Depressed Primary Care Patients." *Family Practice* 16(5): 528–33.

Zerubavel, Eviatar. 1997. *Social Mindscapes: An Invitation to Cognitive Sociology*. Cambridge, MA: Harvard University Press.

Diagnostic Work
A Disorderly Process

Dawn Goodwin and Thomas McConnell

STARTING POINTS

- Making a diagnosis is a cognitive process involving evaluation and assimilation of information gathered from history, examination, and investigations.
- We often think of diagnosis as being performed by an individual doctor, rather than by the health-care team involved with that patient.
- The patient should be fully assessed before a diagnosis is made, and a diagnosis should be made before the treatment is given.

Cognitive psychology has provided the most established perspective on diagnosis, framing it as essentially an activity of problem solving or decision making conducted by individual doctors in isolation. But such cognitive framing erases or mystifies important parts of the process. First, that diagnosis is a process rather than a moment of cognition. Second, the practical and technical steps involved in making a diagnosis—examining, questioning, conversing, and testing—are a process of work that is interwoven with the cognitive process of "sense making." Third, diagnostic work is essentially collaborative; apart from an individual doctor, other doctors, nurses, **patients**, laboratory technicians, and radiographers, to name a few, are also intrinsically involved. Finally, although diagnoses have significant consequences in some respects (e.g., in organizing care and informing patient identities), in practice there is often an ambivalence about making a definitive diagnosis where managing the patient—working out what to do—is inseparable from working out what is wrong. In this chapter we discuss each of these points in turn.

DIAGNOSIS: NOT A MOMENT BUT A PROCESS

We often think of (and make reference to elsewhere in this book) diagnosis as a moment of cognition, a single episode in which the disorder is named, and this signals a clear dividing line for patients between knowing and not knowing they have a disease. This perception is ubiquitous. In popular culture, diagnosis is often portrayed as cunning detective work that culminates in a "eureka" moment. If you watch *House, M.D.*, you see this in every episode; diagnosis is a moment of inspiration in which everything changes for the patient. Even within social science, this "momentary" emphasis is central to many theorists' accounts. Jutel (2011, 1), for example, points to the way that "the **diagnostic moment** is simultaneously transformative and contingent" and indeed the verbal confirmation of a disease or disorder marks an irrevocable before/after boundary. But the moment is not as discrete as it would appear. While it might be metaphorically and heuristically useful to think of diagnosis in these terms, behind the moment is an important process, often extended over time. Thinking about diagnosis as a process opens up a different view on what is happening: one that sheds light on the practical and social elements of diagnosis.

Research by Schaepe (2011) highlights that patients often experience diagnosis as a practice distributed over time; not just what happens but when it happens assumes central importance. She explains how, when asked to recall the day they were told of their cancer diagnosis, patients included detailed descriptions of the path leading up to the diagnosis—including visits to clinics, conversations with different physicians, and listing all the diagnostic tests performed—before concluding with a typically brief paraphrasing of what the doctor said when confirming the diagnosis. Moreover, patients and caregivers in Schaepe's study described the realization that they had cancer as a two-fold process that began with an intellectual understanding of the cancer news, with a deeper emotional acknowledgment only following much later, sometimes well after treatment had commenced. The implications that Schaepe (2011) draws from thinking about diagnosis as occurring over an extended time frame is that "while hearing the diagnosis and realizing the news were significant moments to participants, the ability to cope with the news was tied only tangentially to one well-executed disclosure" (918).

Schaepe's argument points to how the organization of medical care and its increasingly technological nature have reshaped diagnostic work in important ways, introducing periods where patients are between one state and another, something we refer to as **liminality**. These periods might encompass the preliminary assessment and the testing procedures. Such processes frame a period of diagnostic uncertainty in which patients and their relatives might imagine alternative futures. Organizational routines and the technological character of medical work can, intentionally or not, optimize this imaginary space. The diagnostic tests in particular serve to forecast potential bad news and convey a stepwise progression in certainty of the impending diagnosis. As Schaepe (2011) puts it, "the incremental release of information throughout the testing phase functioned to . . . *begin the process*, and prepare the patient and the family for a shocking new reality" (919). Schaepe's account of diagnosis, then, suggests a gradual progression from one reality to another; however, as Timmermans (1998) demonstrates, even in the event of sudden death and attempted resuscitation—when this shift is much more sudden—a period of liminality is still important. For relatives, the attempt at resuscitation introduces a period where death is not necessarily inevitable and there is still some hope of recovery. Even when resuscitation fails, however, this period of liminality remains important because it conveys to relatives that everything possible had been done. Timmermans (1998) suggests that, rather than thinking of resuscitation only as a medical intervention that might save life, we should think of it as a ritual that allows the family to understand death as imminent despite everything being done to avoid it. In his own words, "during the reviving attempt, the victim is not dead yet but in between life and death. The resuscitative effort sustains a period of liminality which allows the relatives and friends to prepare for the transition to death if the reviving attempt fails to restore life" (Timmermans 1998, 162).

This insight into the value of a period of liminality holds important implications for diagnostic work, which may lengthen this period by weeks or even months. The BBC documentary *Between Life and Death* explored the experience of patients following traumatic brain injuries. It showed the diagnosis of brain death happening slowly over a process of weeks and months. Families adjusted to the unfolding diagnosis over time, and interestingly also had input into the process by reporting what they felt the patient would have wanted and even their own desires for the outcome. The *diagnostic moment* is not thus a cognitive instant; rather, it marks a shift within the process where a patient and the medical team move from one reality to another. The salient point for clinical practice that this discussion highlights is the purpose of thinking about diagnosis as sometimes occurring over a much longer time frame; it allows the clinical team to seed information about the potential diagnosis, and gives the patient and their relatives the opportunity to prepare themselves for that eventuality.

> Between survival and death there is a slightly grey area . . . It's really important to think about death not as an event but as a process. That process can be strung out quite considerably and slowed down. It can also be interrupted. (Professor David Mennon, BBC documentary *Between Life and Death*)

THE PRACTICALITIES OF DIAGNOSTIC WORK

Diagnosis does not happen spontaneously, and looking closely at how diagnosis actually happens in practice can show us that although popular accounts of diagnosis tend to emphasize the cognition it involves and to neglect the practical skills, often the two are inseparable. When distinguishing between normal and abnormal on an ultrasound scan of a seventeen-week fetus, Sandall (2010) explains how producing the image and interpreting it are closely interwoven. When learning how to produce good images, trainee midwives have to learn that subtle tilts of the transducer are required as well as direct movements, and to do this, hands-on instruction is central. Trainee midwives find it difficult to assimilate their movements of the transducer with what they see on the screen; therefore the supervisor will manually manipulate the transducer while in the hands of the trainee. This practical form of knowledge that is required in the execution of a skill and on which comprehension depends has been termed "embodied knowledge." Sandall (2010) states: "Since what has to be learned is embodied, the supervisor evaluates the skill and comprehension of the trainee through watching her movements, and teaches through correcting and instructing hands-on in the scanning situation" (35). The difficulty trainees experience arises from seeing a two-dimensional image but having to think three-dimensionally to produce it, something that highlights how artificial it is to separate thinking from doing.

Not all learning can be supervised, though; repetitive practice has to be added, too. The number of scans that need to be performed in order to embed the recognition of what is normal is constantly stressed in training. But volume alone does not ensure automatic progression from not knowing to knowing; Sandall points out how recognizing normal is learned partly through constant discussions with colleagues about how to interpret the images in terms of where to locate the boundary between normal and abnormal, and through being told to look for specific things: where to look, what to see, and what to react to. Consequently, "Learning to perform an ultrasound scan thus at the same time entails being able to produce good images and to see specific markers in them; these two aspects are inseparable in practice" (Sandall 2010, 37). Cementing this connection between doing and knowing, Sandall comments on how even experienced midwives call on colleagues for reassurance in their identification of abnormal, and when they did, the colleague would always take the transducer in their own hands to produce the image and see for themselves: "what to see and how to produce the images are intimately linked. This learning is accomplished through constantly discussing where the boundary between the normal and the abnormal lies in interpreting images" (Sandall 2010, 41). Sandall therefore shows us that it is in the "doing" of diagnosis where much of the learning occurs, and that learning is thoroughly social and embodied.

The midwives in Sandall's study drew a boundary between their practice of distinguishing normal from abnormal and the obstetric practice diagnosing the various kinds of abnormalities that may be found. Yet even in other medical and apparently diagnostic settings such as "reading" mammograms, diagnosis is not a discrete event but a process, as the end point of much of this work is a recall decision for further investigations rather than a distinct diagnosis. Therefore, instead of radiologists doing diagnosis, Slack et al. (2010) suggest the term "suspicion." The practice of reading mammograms involves "perceptual skills to find what may be faint and small features in the complex visual environment of the mammogram, and interpretative skills to classify them appropriately, as benign or suspicious and thereby worthy of further investigation" (229). Rather than posit suspicion as a mental state, however, they too stress the social and embodied nature of an apparently individual and perceptual practice of reading mammograms. This work entails different techniques for reading scans: adopting consistent search patterns, orientating to certain danger areas where abnormalities are more likely to be malignant, using magnifying glasses or high-intensity light boxes for especially dense breast tissue. It requires getting to know what the computer-aided detection system is good and poor at identifying, something Slack et al. called "developing a biography for the machine," so that this can be compensated for. When the machine is too sensitive, its prompts can be dismissed, and where there are places or circumstances it tends to overlook, these can be the subjects of a focused search. But abnormalities must be individually assessed as artifact or, alternatively, as actual problem. In one view a feature might be equivocal, in another it might be more distinct, or it might be an artifact produced when making the image, as when overlapping breast tissue can often mimic the appearance of particular lesions. By exploring the intricacies of diagnostic practices in this way, we can see it makes no sense to prioritize knowing over doing because, as expressed by the term "embodied knowledge," the two are deeply interwoven.

DIAGNOSTIC WORK IS COLLABORATIVE WORK

How diagnostic work is framed is an important point for reflection because when framed as a cognitive activity, diagnosis is an individual activity. Even thinking is a collaborative process, particularly within the hospital setting. Consider the case study below, which describes an intensive care unit (ICU) team trying to diagnose the cause of a patient's deteriorating condition. It illustrates the fluidity of the boundaries between one person's thoughts and actions and another's.

The patient looks asleep, and he wears an oxygen mask. Alan (an experienced anesthetic trainee) briefs us, detailing the postoperative history and indicating there had been a need for respiratory support [CPAP, or continuous positive airway pressure, a noninvasive method of supporting respiration] yesterday but that today "volume good, air entry . . . course breath sounds, decreased air entry left base" and neurologically he was "rousable and responds to pain."

    Anne (a nurse) arrives: "Morphine . . . not using his PCA [patient-controlled morphine pump]"

Mark (the senior anesthetist): "What are his blood gases like?"

    Anne: "Worse"

    Alan: "New ones are here." He hands a piece of paper to the consultant, who then hands it to the medical students and looks at previous results.

    Mark: "What do you think we should do?"

    Alan: "Frusemide . . . predominantly failure . . . off-loading may help . . . CPAP mask . . . hypoxia . . . not oxygenating the brain"

    Mark turns to Anne: "Anything you want to say?"

    Anne: "No, Alan's covered it all."

    Alan: "How do you know? You weren't here."

    Anne: "He's not as responsive."

    Alan: "Options: CPAP or intubate with a view to early tracheostomy. Tidal volumes actually quite good. Morphine."

    While the senior anesthetist explains the blood gas results to the medical students, Henry (a surgical trainee) asks about the patient's pupil size. Alan shrugs his shoulders. They both look at the size of the patient's pupils. Alan suggests, "try a bit of Narcan [a drug that reverses the effects of opiates] . . . Narcan-Doxapram [Doxapram is a drug that stimulates breathing] mixture . . . wakes everyone up."

    Mark: "What do you want to do?"

    Henry (a junior surgical trainee): "I say back on CPAP."

    "Is he over narcotized?" [it's unclear who says this]

Mark: "You want to try Narcan?"

Alan: "Yeah, let's do it!" He leaves the bedside shouting, "Keys!"

Mark: "And if it doesn't work?"

Henry: "Intubate"

Alan returns and injects something into the patient, who almost immediately becomes more alert and begins talking to him . . . the consultant negotiates with the patient, trying to coax him into putting the "tight fitting" CPAP mask back on.

Alan (holding syringe): "Anne, this will wear off in half an hour."

Mark: "Maybe put him on Tramadol [a different analgesic]."

Alan: "We will put him on Tramadol."

The patient coughs, and Anne hands him a tissue. We move on to the next patient. (Scenario taken from Goodwin, forthcoming.)

In this scene the patient is not improving after an operation, and the team is trying to determine the problem and how they should manage it. At the outset the symptoms, signs, and investigation results are framed as a problem of fluid overload and subsequent lung compromise. But by the end of the scenario, the team has reached a different conclusion: that the patient is oversedated with morphine. How the team arrives at this diagnosis illustrates the collaborative nature of diagnosis.

There are at least six prompts by four participants on the way to diagnosis. Anne, a junior nurse in the ICU, makes only small observations, but these take the diagnostic reasoning in a totally different direction than that proposed by the doctors. The first prompt, that the patient may be oversedated, occurs when Anne directs attention to the underused morphine pump. Her second contribution reinforces the idea that the patient is oversedated, describing him as "not as responsive." On both these occasions, however, Mark (the senior anesthetist) and Alan (the senior anesthetic trainee) continue to propose fluid overload or respiratory failure as the diagnosis. Anne does not press the issue, but Henry (the junior surgical trainee) picks up her comments when he asks about the size of the patient's pupils, a potential sign of oversedation. Next is the fourth prompt, which is Alan's suggestion of trying Narcan (a drug that reverses the effects of opiates). The fifth prompt (without an identified speaker) is a direct question: "is he over narcotized?" And, finally, the sixth prompt is another direct question from the consultant: "you want to try Narcan?" Alan replies, "Yeah, let's do it!," acknowledging by the treatment choice that a working diagnosis has crystallized through this collaborative discussion.

When this discussion is recorded in the medical notes, it is likely that Alan would be the one responsible for the diagnosis, but it makes no sense to credit him alone. The decision develops initially from Anne's prompts, which are promoted by Henry and finally cemented by Alan. This scenario plainly illustrates how it is the interactions between participants—the collaboration—that generate the diagnosis.

Understanding that diagnosis is a collaborative process shared by a team is at odds with the emphasis on individual accountability articulated by professional organizations like the American Nurses Association (ANA). These bodies often frame decision-making processes as something for which the doctor or nurse has sole and individual responsibility. The ANA describes the nursing process as the foundation of nurses' decision making; each of the six steps begins with "the registered nurse" and in the case of step two, "diagnosis": "The registered nurse analyzes the assessment data to determine the diagnosis or the issues" (ANA 2010, 9). Decisions in this context are deliberate and purposeful, not, as in Anne's contribution, observations simply floated to see where they might lead.

In practice, it is difficult to determine the degree to which one practitioner's thoughts and actions are informed by another's. Nurses in particular have considerable influence over doctors' diagnoses and prescriptions, perhaps describing a patient's condition in such a way that the doctor's response is the one the nurse desired, or by making direct requests for a specific prescription (Hughes 1988; Jutel and Menkes 2010; Prowse and Allen 2002; Strauss 1975), but their sometimes-dominant position within diagnostic work is not always recognized (see chap. 7).

Professional guidance documents may also suggest that there is a linear progression from diagnosis to treatment, but Berg (1992) proposes that we can only arrive at this tidy linearity in retrospect. In practice, he suggests, diagnosis and treatment are constructed together. Furthermore, he argues that diagnostic decisions are distributed across a complex network of factors in the environment. The factors that contribute to the diagnosis include things such as protocols, hospital policies, guidelines, and the availability of equipment and tests. Diagnostic decisions for Berg (1997) are a collective achievement, where the contributors are not necessarily even human. Rapley (2008) echoes this argument for the distributed nature of decisions, and like Schaepe he showed how decisions evolve over multiple encounters and among multiple people: "they emerge, transform and solidify in and through *multiple interactions* with *multiple others*, significant or otherwise, *over a period of time*" (436).

Once diagnoses are achieved, however, the labels themselves can cause problems when they become a shorthand way of discussing the patient, obscuring the complexity of their condition, narrowing the practitioner's focus, and discouraging any search for an alternative diagnosis (Goodwin 2010). The blindness to the severity of a patient's condition and the possibility that there is an alternative or additional explanation are evident in the case study from anesthetic practice described below. A junior anesthetist recounts a critical incident that occurred during weekend emergency work. Despite the name, most operations undertaken during "emergency work" are still routine. The incident concerns a young man awaiting an appendectomy. The anesthetist's recollections indicate just how drawn out in time diagnostic work is, and how his understanding of what was wrong with the patient was rooted to the phrase "just an appendix" used by a senior colleague.

(Before the operation)

It was a Saturday and it had been very busy . . . I saw Harry (the surgeon) a bit later in the morning and asked him what the appendix was like, and it was: "Fine, nothing to worry about. Just an appendix." I didn't get to see him; I could of gone at lunchtime but I barely had any time for lunch. Harry said he was all right, so I wasn't too worried about it. I eventually got to see him about seven o'clock, I think, and he didn't look particularly well, but just as I was getting onto the ward I was beeped by a theater nurse to ask could they send for the next one [patient], so I didn't really assess him as much perhaps as I should have. I saw he was clammy, and I looked at his fluid balance, and he had spiked a temperature so I thought he was getting dry [dehydrated]. He wasn't particularly well, and I just opened the drip right up, and infused the fluids over an hour, two hours, can't remember. Thought nothing more of it, went up [to the theater] and I think we were planning to do it about nine and for some reason; just theaters being theaters, I think he got to theaters around eleven thirty.

(After the operation)

So basically started waking him up, put him on left lateral and what have you. Saturations had been fine. He was taking a long time to wake up, and by this time the next patient had arrived in the anesthetic room. So it was a good five or ten minutes, I can't remember how long, but we were still sitting there. Eventually he started showing signs of waking up—just moved his arm a bit—and so I pulled the tube out and put the mask back on, and then he started with what I thought was a laryngospasm. Sats started dropping and we did have a little problem with the saturation monitor throughout the operation; we changed it to an ear thing [probe], and it took a little while to get that sorted, but once we got that sorted, once it was on, it was working fine [during the operation]. So first of all I thought it was that, but it was obvious when I looked at the patient again and he had started to go blue.

The operating department practitioner* was in with the next patient, and the recovery nurse was with me. It was obvious he was going blue, so I tried to get a good seal [on the face mask] and do a bit of CPAP, thinking it was laryngospasm, to try and break it. It obviously wasn't working. At this point I think I asked for some help. I asked someone to get Suxamethonium and some Propofol. [I was] still trying to bag but it wasn't working. Meanwhile someone asked, "shall I go and get George?" [the consultant anesthetist on call], and I said "yeah." Got him head down, gave him the Propofol first then gave him Sux, then popped tube back in, then frantic ventilation. The sats came up a little but only to about 80, by which time George arrived and at which point I sat down and thought, "Shit!" Basically George took over and we went over what happened and explained it all. I think we took the gases straight after . . . CO_2 was about 60 odd, PO_2 was 50–60, his base excess was minus 10, which means he has actually been septic for, you know, for quite a while—well a fair few hours. So obviously he'd been a lot more ill than we'd thought, you know. So basically then he went to ICU. (Scenario taken from Goodwin [2010].)

The anesthetist begins his account with a comment from the surgeon, that the patient's problem is "just an appendix," implying the routine nature of this particular

*Operating department practitioners are health providers who assess, plan, and assist during surgical operations. They manage many aspects of patient care during surgery.

kind of emergency work. This perhaps highlights the different frame of reference the surgeon has and what information he has gathered for himself: the nature of the operation he will need to perform and how urgently. Partial stories about patients and their diagnoses, as in this case, circulate among the staff and significantly inform a doctor's mind-set. There are, however, opportunities for the anesthetist to reevaluate his understanding. In the preoperative visit some details were noted, but this assessment was cut short by a call from theater. In working with the patient during induction and surgery, the anesthetist again has occasion to reassess the patient's condition; signs are noted repeatedly—tachycardia, low blood pressure, clamminess, and the somewhat tacit "not looking particularly well"—but in each case the diagnostic process is derailed by some interruption, distraction, or competing demand. Finally, postoperatively, the delay in emerging from anesthesia was noted but, again, the arrival of the next patient hurried this assessment. Prentice (2007) notes how anesthetists are often subject to the characteristic time pressures of operating theater work and how junior staff are expected to limit the fumblings of the beginner. The anesthetist clearly experiences this time pressure in his mention of the day's heavy workload, the delay in getting this patient to theater, and in his reference to the arrival of another patient. Diagnostic work, therefore, is a process distributed over time place, and among people, but it is also fraught with distractions, competing demands, time pressures, expectations of other workers, and reliance on colleagues' assessments. Diagnostic work might in principle be an independent, linear process of decision making, but in real-world clinical situations, it tends to be collaborative, incomplete, often interrupted, and balanced against the other demands of work.

Working with a senior surgical colleague leads the anesthetist in different directions because of surgeon's priorities. Detecting and managing septicemia is of primary importance to the anesthetic management, while the surgeon focuses on surgical aspects of patient need, illustrating that diagnosis cannot be a one-dimensional label. The label "appendix" is used as a shorthand term that sums up all relevant information. In this case it conveys routine work, a common and easily resolved problem, one that most often occurs in young, otherwise fit and healthy adults. It conjures up expectations of straightforward anesthetics. In short, the label says nothing about the severity or complexity of the patient's condition. In this case it obscured the fact that the patient was becoming extremely unwell with septicemia. Furthermore, working within a framework of commonly encountered problems, and holding onto the routine nature of this type of emergency work, led the anesthetist to continue to misinterpret the signs—after extubation, the anesthetist suspects the difficulty in ventilating the patient is due to laryngospasm and uses continuous pressure in an attempt to alleviate it. Later in the interview, the anesthetist confirms that the patient did not have laryngospasm but had in fact aspirated—where the stomach contents backtrack up the esophagus and enter the lungs—as a consequence of the sepsis.

The point we want to emphasize is that viewing diagnosis as individual and cognitive disguises the collaboration it necessarily involves; this collaboration may be beneficial as with the nurse's input in the case from intensive care, or it may be detrimental, as demonstrated here by the surgeon misleading the anesthetist.

Raising awareness of the collaborative nature of diagnostic work has implications for improving patient safety. To say that someone has a diagnosis implies that the diagnosis is all there is to know about a patient, when in fact different specialties will prioritize certain aspects of the patient's condition differently. This in turn raises questions about whether diagnosis or patient management is the salient frame of reference for directing care.

DIAGNOSTIC AMBIVALENCE

We often think of diagnosis as an essential prerequisite to beginning treatment and that the diagnosis determines the treatment. How would you treat someone for a pulmonary embolus before you knew that they had one? This message is present throughout the medical world, and its clearest articulation can be seen in medical school. Students learn the linear process of taking a patient history in the correct order followed by examination and running tests before finally beginning treatment. This approach is consistent with the cognitive account and articulates diagnosis as a rational, linear progression of collecting and interpreting information to reach the diagnosis, which then determines treatment. But as Berg suggested, and as we have just seen in the clinical example above, in practice this linearity does not exist; treatment is often started before a firm diagnosis is made or can even be started as part of the diagnostic process itself. In the previous scenario from the ICU, only in giving the treatment (Narcan) is the diagnosis of oversedation from morphine confirmed. Blaxter (1978) provided another example that illustrated how diagnostic categories unaccompanied by an effective treatment regime were simply redundant. If categories are not selected for classification in favor of more prescriptive terms, they fall out of use and the treatment then begins to define the disease. It is also a point well made by Willems (1998), who described how a trial of treatment is a standard step in establishing a diagnosis of asthma, so much so that this principle—of giving a treatment to determine the problem—is even embedded in guidelines. For example, the guidelines published by the British Thoracic Society (BTS) situate trial treatment as a central part of the diagnostic process. In cases where response is not clearly due to the treatment, a trial removal of treatment is suggested.

It has been argued that diagnosis has traditionally been seen as central to the practice of medicine because it has the power to explain and predict phenomena and to separate the expert doctor from the lay public. The possibility that

---

Trial by Treatment with Review

The choice of treatment (for example, inhaled bronchodilators or corticosteroids) depends on the severity and frequency of symptoms. Although a trial of therapy with inhaled or oral corticosteroids is widely used to help make a diagnosis of asthma, there is little objective evidence to support this approach in children with recurrent wheeze.

It can be difficult to assess the response to treatment as an improvement in symptoms or lung function may be due to spontaneous remission. If it is unclear whether a child has improved, careful observation during a trial of withdrawing the treatment may clarify whether a response to asthma therapy has occurred. (British Thoracic Society/Scottish Intercollegiate Guidelines Network 2011)

diagnosis may not be so significant in organizing care therefore sits uneasily in a rational framework that places diagnosis as an end point of assessment and the beginning of treatment. But the contemporary sociological theorizing we have drawn upon here has tended to emphasize how both disease and the appropriate treatment are constructed together. This is to say that a disease entity does not preexist and determine the disease; rather, what the disease is becomes defined in the process of working out how to treat it.

Both the nonlinearity of the diagnostic process and the collaborative nature of knowledge construction challenge conventional cognitive accounts of diagnostic work, the ramifications of which can be felt when working with administrative procedures that demand a definitive diagnosis. The problem is keenly felt in psychiatry, where the *Diagnostic and Statistical Manual of Mental Disorders* (DSM) has become institutionalized in administrative procedures for hospital admission, discharge, and, in the United States, for reimbursement by insurance companies. Taking the DSM literally, insurers expect a discrete diagnosis to be determined prior to treatment (Whooley 2010). By exploring how the DSM works in practice, and how the tensions it creates are overcome, Whooley describes the "workarounds" that psychiatrists employ. Workarounds are the ad hoc temporary solutions to problems arising when the official policies are perceived as hindering the task at hand; for example, although the DSM consists of over three hundred distinct diagnostic categories, psychiatrists routinely use only seven of them. Whooley (2010) explains that "diagnosis is not determined by an objective assessment of symptoms, but rather through the psychiatrist exercising professional discretion as to the type of treatment the patient may need . . . The label is applied after the fact . . . to justify a treatment based on the psychiatrist's individual normative assessment of the patient's need" (459). Particularly in the United States, where insurance reimbursement is contingent upon diagnostic category, psychiatrists may intentionally embellish a patient's condition if they are concerned that the patient will not be financially reimbursed for the cost of their care. Mitigating worries about overdiagnosis are concerns about **stigma**. Often in explicit consultation with the patient, diagnostic codes are "fudged," with the most benign diagnosis still meeting the desired ends being selected. In such cases patients have the opportunity to collaborate in how they are labeled and potentially elude some of the stigma associated with psychiatric diagnoses (Whooley 2010), as well as to satisfy insurers or other particular administrative requirements (see chap. 11). In his descriptions of diagnostic practices, Whooley captures the ambivalence psychiatrists feel toward diagnostic labels; they are necessary for administrative and bureaucratic reasons, but they are not necessarily helpful and sometimes even have pernicious consequences when they signpost stigmatizing conditions. For these reasons psychiatrists may adopt pragmatic, even utilitarian, approaches to diagnosis, superficially conforming to the organizational requirements for distinct diagnoses but "upcoding," or adopting whatever arbitrary category will best facilitate the desired outcome (which in some cases could be financial gain for the physician, or in others, better outcomes for the patient; Whooley 2010).

The focus on formulating an understanding of the individual patient's personal circumstances, personality, and presentation, as well as an approach of ongoing assessment, is something that psychiatry shares with many specialties dealing largely with chronic disorders. The complexity of care in these cases contrasts with the nature of a diagnostic label (which trends toward **reductionism**) and may explain in part the marginalization of diagnosis. The reductionist nature of a diagnostic label is not only unhelpful but in some circumstances may even have the potential to cause harm when factors like severity are rendered invisible, as in the case study from anesthesia described above. It is not that diagnosis is irrelevant, but reframing it as diagnostic work allows appreciation of the many smaller, more mundane assessments and the role these assessments play in protecting patient safety. In effect, the diagnostic label is less significant because, in practice, diagnostic work is always happening.

WORKING THROUGH DIAGNOSIS

Looking at diagnosis through the work it entails allows us to understand the factors that shape and constrain it, opening a window for consideration of where there may be scope for modification. Errors in diagnosis are relatively common, but sometimes they have devastating consequences. A recent survey of pediatricians asked them to report confidentially how many diagnostic errors they made and how many they believed resulted in harm to the patient. The results showed that errors were being made by about half of those surveyed at least once or twice a month and that these rates were higher in trainees (Singh et al. 2010). Although this study relies on self-reported estimations, it is consistent with the wider patient safety literature. At autopsy, Sakai et al. (2010) found that a number of outpatients had been allowed to return home with fatal conditions such as ischemic heart disease or ileus after physicians assessed them as nonurgent, suggesting that diagnostic errors are associated with more significant consequences than other types of medical errors, a finding supported by Sevdalis et al. (2010).

When a diagnostic error occurs, we tend to think of it as the fault of an individual doctor. But, as we have shown here, diagnosis is not a distinct event but a dynamic and ongoing process. In the example of the junior anesthetist who missed the diagnosis of septicemia, the diagnostic process spanned almost a full day. The multiple disruptions to the diagnostic process point to a "systems failure," an influential perspective in patient safety research. Systems failure usefully points to the organizational aspects of diagnostic error, but it can obscure the essentially human and social nature of diagnostic work. Earlier in the chapter we also saw how the diagnostic process is essentially collaborative, so perhaps we should think also about whether failures to work well collaboratively have resulted in the error. Lastly, understanding that factors in the working environment of health-care professionals can disrupt and constrain diagnostic process can help reduce error and detect when a decision may be becoming constrained. Being able to recognize when decisions are becoming constrained is an important part of being able to mitigate and change the constraints. Making these changes in your practice might involve small steps, like recognizing that when you make a diagnosis you may be responding to time pressures. Or we may aim to make sweeping changes, such as attempting to change professional guidance documents to take into consideration the shared nature of diagnosis.

TAKEAWAY POINTS

- Diagnosis is not an instantaneous event but a process that often occurs over an extended period of time.
- The whole health-care team contributes to forming a diagnosis.
- Diagnosis is not exclusively intellectual but involves "embodied knowledge" in making sense of signs, symptoms, and investigations.
- A diagnosis does not always precede and determine treatment, potentially resulting in ambivalence toward the diagnosis.
- Not recognizing these features of the diagnostic process can compromise patient safety.

DISCUSSION QUESTIONS

1. Can you recall a time when a nurse or health professional other than a physician has redirected, challenged, or questioned the prevailing explanation of a patient's condition? How was this decision talked about, recorded, and accounted for?
2. In your experience, once a patient has been diagnosed, how frequently are alternative or additional diagnoses considered? What are the circumstances in which alternative or additional diagnoses are sought?
3. How might the need for a diagnosis vary across different medical specialties? Why is this so?
4. Can you recall a patient whose diagnosis was unknown? How was the patient's treatment decided upon, and how was care organized?

REFERENCES

ANA. American Nurses Association. 2010. *Nursing: Scope and Standards of Practice.* 2nd ed. Silver Spring, MD: American Nurses Association.

Berg, Marc. 1992. "The Construction of Medical Disposals: Medical Sociology and Medical Problem Solving in Clinical Practice." *Sociology of Health and Illness* 14(2): 151–80.

———. 1997. *Rationalizing Medical Work: Decision-Support Techniques and Medical Practices.* Cambridge, MA: MIT Press.

Blaxter, Mildred. 1978. "Diagnosis as Category and Process: The Case of Alcoholism." *Social Science and Medicine* 12: 9–17.

British Thoracic Society/Scottish Intercollegiate Guidelines Network. 2011. *British Guideline on the Management of Asthma.* London: British Thoracic Society/Scottish Intercollegiate Guidelines Network, 2011.

Goodwin, Dawn. 2010. "Sensing the Way: Embodied Dimensions of Diagnostic Work." In *Ethnographies of Diagnostic Work: Dimensions of Transformative Practice*, edited by M. Buscher, D. Goodwin, and J. Mesman, 73–92. Basingstoke: Palgrave Macmillan.

————. Forthcoming. "Decision-Making and Accountability: Differences of Distribution." *Sociology of Health and Illness.*

Hughes, David. 1988. "When Nurse Knows Best: Some Aspects of Nurse/Doctor Interaction in a Casualty Department." *Sociology of Health and Illness* 10(1): 1–22.

Jutel, Annemarie. 2011. *Putting a Name to It: Diagnosis in Contemporary Society.* Baltimore: John Hopkins University Press.

Jutel, Annemarie, and David B. Menkes. 2010. "Nurses' Reported Influence on the Prescription and Use of Medication." *International Nursing Review* 57: 92–97.

Prentice, Rachel. 2007. "The Social Lessons of Embodied Surgical Learning." *Science, Technology and Human Values* 32(5): 534–53.

Prowse, Morag, and Davina Allen. 2002. "'Routine' and 'Emergency in the Pacu': The Shifting Contexts of Nurse-Doctor Interaction." In *Nursing and the Division of Labour in Healthcare*, edited by D. Allen and D. Hughes, 75–97. Basingstoke: Palgrave Macmillan.

Rapley, Tim. 2008. "Distributed Decision Making: The Anatomy of Decisions-in-Action." *Sociology of Health and Illness* 30(3): 429–44.

Sakai, Kentaro, Akihiro Takatsu, Akio Shigeta, Kenji Fukui, Kyoko Maebashi, Shuntaro Abe, and Kimiharu Iwadate. 2010. "Potential Medical Adverse Events Associated with Death: A Forensic Pathology Perspective." *International Journal for Quality in Health Care* 22(1): 9–15.

Sandall, Kerstin. 2010. "Learning to Produce, See and Say the (Ab)Normal: Professional Vision in Ultrasound Scanning during Pregnancy." In *Technology in Medical Practice: Blood, Guts and Machines*, edited by E. Johnson and B. Berner, 29–50. Farnham: Ashgate.

Schaepe, Karen Sue. 2011. "Bad News and First Impressions: Patient and Family Caregiver Accounts of Learning the Cancer Diagnosis." *Social Science and Medicine* 73: 912–21.

Sevdalis, Nick, Rosamond Jacklin, Sonal Arora, Charles A. Vincent, and Richard G. Thomson. 2010. "Diagnostic Error in a National Incident Reporting System in the Uk." *Journal of Evaluation in Clinical Practice* 16: 1276–81.

Singh, H., E. J. Thomas, L. Wilson, P. A. Kelly, K. Pietz, D. Elkeeb, and G. Singhal. 2010. "Errors of Diagnosis in Pediatric Practice: A Multisite Survey." *Pediatrics* 126(1): 70–79.

Slack, Roger S., Rob Proctor, Mark Hartswood, Alexander Voss, and Mark Rouncefield. 2010. "Suspicious Minds?" In *Ethnographies of Diagnostic Work: Dimensions of Transformative Practice*, edited by M. Buscher, D. Goodwin and J. Mesman, 227–44. Basingstoke: Palgrave Macmillan.

Strauss, Anselm L. 1975. *Professions, Work and Careers.* New Brunswick, NJ: Transaction.

Timmermans, Stefan. 1998. "Resuscitation Technology in the Emergency Department: Towards a Dignified Death." *Sociology of Health and Illness* 20(2): 144–67.

Whooley, Owen. 2010. "Diagnostic Ambivalence: Psychiatric Workarounds and the Diagnostic and Statistical Manual of Mental Disorders." *Sociology of Health and Illness* 32(3): 452–69.

Willems, Dick. 1998. "Inhaling Drugs and Making Worlds: The Proliferation of Lungs and Asthmas." In *Differences in Medicine: Unraveling Practices, Techniques, and Bodies*, edited by M. Berg and A. Mol, 105–18. Durham, NC: Duke University Press.

None of the Above
Uncertainty and Diagnosis

Rebecca Olson and Sudeepa Abeysinghe

STARTING POINTS

- A successful diagnosis is supposed to manage uncertainty and provide guidelines for treatment.
- Resolving uncertainty is a key reason why patients seek diagnosis.
- Medical professionals are trained to be certain, but they often deal with uncertain situations.

When something is amiss, **patients** seek professional advice to give meaning and order to their symptoms and define a path of action. Diagnosis can be a complex process, however, and is often far from certain, leading to important consequences for both patients and medical practitioners. This chapter illustrates the various sources of uncertainty within the diagnostic process and explores the tensions between medical training for certainty and the reality of an uncertain world. We investigate variations in health professionals' tolerance of uncertainty and some of the impacts that uncertainty has on patients and their caregivers. Despite these tensions, awareness of diagnostic uncertainty does not undermine medical practice; it can actually enhance the effectiveness of the consultation.

In some instances, obtaining a diagnosis is a straightforward process for both clinician and patient—a skier comes in for an X-ray of his arm to confirm that it is broken, or an adult goes to the sexual health clinic for an HIV blood test after having unprotected sex. In other instances, the diagnosis is not as clear-cut. Take influenza, for example. Influenza symptoms are nonspecific: the runny nose, headache, sore throat, fatigue, nausea, vomiting, and diarrhea of influenza can be symptoms of a benign and short-lived upper respiratory disease, but they could also be signs of serious sepsis and meningococcal meningitis. Can we be sure that a person has influenza and not one of these other conditions? A nasopharyngeal swab can confirm whether the patient has influenza, but they are costly, and during the flu season (especially during an epidemic or pandemic outbreak) public health officials advise people to stay home and seek medical help only if complications occur, to avoid spreading the infectious disease further.

So, instead of taking a blood sample to confirm the diagnosis, patients can be asked to self-diagnose or seek confirmation over a phone helpline. Yet Jutel et al. (2011) found that health-care workers and laypeople are often incorrect in

> Medical knowledge is engulfed and infiltrated by uncertainty. (Katz 1984, 35)

Health professionals, we assume, have the skill to make sense of confusion, shed light where there is darkness, and give hope where there is despair . . . Like all health professionals, I am trained to chase after an explanation, to look for a needle in every haystack, to try to find the one conclusion that will make all of the pieces fall into place. (Hodges 2010, 154–55)

their self-diagnoses of influenza. Only 33% of the health-care workers and 23% of adults not working in health care who had diagnosed themselves as having had influenza tested positive for the disease. Similarly, 25% of the health-care workers and 21% of adults not working in health care who reported that they had not had influenza also tested positive! The same symptoms can often be linked to many different diagnoses, and definitive tests can be unavailable or inaccurate.

When a diagnosis is not straightforward, health professionals run the risk of either being too hasty or too cautious, either of which can have lasting emotional and material consequences for the patient. If the health professional is too hasty, he might dismiss the patient's concerns as inflated and inconsequential when something more sinister is actually progressing and worsening. Take Lyme disease as an example. Lyme disease is a vector-borne disease that is prevalent in the northeastern and midwestern parts of the United States. Tiny deer ticks infected with the bacteria bite and infect humans (and pets), often causing headache, fever, fatigue, joint pain, and a circular "bull's-eye" rash around the tick bite in the short term (Halperin 2011). Diagnosis is most often made based on the appearance of the bull's-eye rash and accompanying fever. But in some cases the bull's-eye rash is delayed, hidden by hair, or poorly visible, or multiple rashes appear. Lyme disease can also cause facial paralysis; left untreated, it can cause permanent joint and nervous system damage. In the absence of a visible rash, a health professional might dismiss the illness as a passing virus.

Health professionals also run the risk of being too cautious: doing too much and causing patients to suffer unnecessary treatments. Prostate cancer is a good example. The third most common cause of death from cancer in men in developed countries (Damber and Aus 2008), prostate cancer can be local, slow growing, and not life threatening, or advanced. Medical professionals now use both digital rectal examination and prostate-specific antigen testing to screen for prostate cancer. Screening allows for early detection, before symptoms arise, and early intervention. Intuitively, the idea of screening and early intervention would logically improve a patient's chance of survival. But Djulbegovic et al. (2010) performed a meta-analysis of existing studies on the statistical relationship between prostate cancer screening and both disease-specific and overall mortality. They found that for men with no history of prostate cancer, screening made no difference to mortality. Instead, early detection and overtreatment may have an adverse impact

The Mayo Lung Project, which compared intensive screening for lung cancer to a standard nonscreening approach, found that mortality from lung cancer was higher in the screened group. This determination suggests that the abnormal nodules revealed through intensive screening and subsequent treatment may have had a greater and more detrimental effect (Marcus et al. 2006).

on a patient's quality of life, as prostate cancer treatments commonly have uncomfortable side effects such as incontinence and impotence.

UNCERTAINTY IN DIAGNOSIS

Despite the pursuit of certainty being a driving force behind seeking a diagnosis, uncertainty affects most aspects of diagnostic work. As Groopman (2007) declares in his book *How Doctors Think*, "medicine is, at its core, an uncertain science" (7). Uncertainty permeates medicine—and the act of diagnosis—in several ways.

In a seminal study that is still discussed and referred to frequently today, Renée Fox (1957), a major figure in the development of medical sociology in the United States, articulated three sources of uncertainty in diagnosis and medicine: the limitations of individual knowledge; the limitations of knowledge in the field; and the challenge of distinguishing between the two. These three factors are important considerations for the practitioner.

To what extent can you be certain that you are up to date with, and correctly apply, the latest medical knowledge? How can you be certain that this knowledge is actually correct, given that medical science is always changing and adapting? Within your clinical interactions, how do you know if your uncertainty is the result of gaps in the field of knowledge, or in your own inadequate knowledge? These are poignant questions for a diagnostician in cases where diagnosis is not straightforward, particularly if outcomes are bad or actions need to be later reviewed.

Other sources of uncertainty result from the nature of the medical encounter. The way the patient describes her symptoms, for example, can lead to uncertainty in the mind of the medical practitioner. Patients may talk about symptoms in ways that are hard to translate medically. Or they may fail to perceive the significance of some symptoms that are nonetheless key to diagnosis. Many more sources of uncertainty arise out of the medical system itself, including problems with the sensitivity and accuracy of laboratory tests or other diagnostic tools (Lingard et al. 2003). There may be insufficient evidence to make the correct diagnosis or any diagnosis at all. More generally, the idea that there is limitless possibility (though distinct probabilities) also creates uncertainty in diagnosis (Hall 2002). Going back to the case above, a presentation of fever and "flu-like" symptoms looks like seasonal influenza or the common cold, but it might be malaria if a patient recently traveled to a malaria-endemic area. The number of possibilities created by this presentation is almost limitless, if all potential explanations are considered, even though some options are more unlikely.

These sources of uncertainty are evident in everyday medical practice. Many diagnoses cannot be adequately evidenced. Alzheimer disease, for example, cannot be confirmed until an autopsy is performed (Hodges 2010). Unreliable tests and "imperfect" symptoms impose further uncertainty on the diagnostic process. Biopsies, for instance, may need to be repeated. Groopman (2007) explains: "in my field of hematology, more than one bone marrow examination may be needed to find a

Diseases do not come into the hospital in Little Red Wagons: they come in human beings, with all of their marvellous and challenging complexity, their infinite variability of presentations and responses to treatments, and their always unique selves. (O'Connor 2010, xiv)

malignancy like a lymphoma, because tumors are not uniformly present in the bones, and I may have placed the biopsy needle in an area of the marrow that did not contain the tumor. After review or repetition, the tests still may not give the answer" (262).

Pathology results can also be inaccurate. The pathology test for Lyme disease may result in a false negative if taken sooner than a few weeks after infection (Halperin 2011). Symptoms may also appear imperfect because more than one disease is affecting the patient, and symptoms can vary from person to person.

From a critical sociological perspective, other sources of uncertainty manifest in diagnostic practice. These include the boundaries of scientific knowledge and the limits on how much can really be definitively known with respect to illness. Another site of uncertainty (particularly from the patient's perspective) comes from the limits of professional agreement. Within a hospital setting particularly, a further key point of uncertainty arises from the structure of medical practice: moving a patient between wards of the hospital results in the need for doctors and nurses to interpret one another's notes. There can be uncertainty over why a procedure was performed, whether anything has been inadvertently left out of the notes, and how descriptions should be analyzed. Communication problems associated with patient handovers can produce similar concerns (Randell et al. 2011).

The results of this diagnostic uncertainty can be seen definitively in its culmination—through autopsy. Medical practitioners and social scientists of medicine have noted the decline of the autopsy in the last few decades (Horsley 2010; Vance 1990), reinforced by the shift toward the understanding of medicine through increasingly cellular, molecular, and genetic means. But one important function of an autopsy is to resolve, and some would argue also to illustrate, the presence of diagnostic uncertainty. Prior to its decline, autopsies were a regular event after hospital deaths. Around 50% (up to as high as 80%) of deaths in hospitals resulted in autopsy in the 1950s (Horsley 2010), partly because autopsies were seen as a teaching exercise and were not necessarily performed to resolve disputed causes of death. During these commonplace investigations, there was a surprisingly high rate of inconsistency between diagnoses made premortem by clinicians and those made postmortem by pathologists.

Autopsies too often fail to definitively identify the cause of death, however, which for medical students can be unsettling. They report being disquieted or disappointed with the fact that even autopsies can fail to reach a diagnosis, or that postmortem diagnoses are often not specific. Despite the decline of autopsies, the rates of discrepancy have not decreased. In a study by Anderson et al. (1990) involving thirty-two community hospital and academic medical centers, 33% of premortem diagnoses did not match the postmortem diagnoses. Long-term studies on the effect of increasing medical technology similarly show that while there are changes in the accuracy of diagnosing certain conditions, the overall rate of diagnostic inaccuracy remains consistent.

Perhaps the starkest example of the effect of uncertainty within diagnosis is the case of medically unexplained symptoms, where patients experience illness but doctors cannot explain the cause. In such events, patients enter what Corbin and Strauss (1985) refer to as **diagnostic limbo**, which can be problematic for doctor and patient alike. In some cases, symptomology may be categorized and defined as broad syndromes, such as irritable bowel syndrome, chronic fatigue syndrome, or Gulf War syndrome (Nettleton 2006; Zavestoski et al. 2004). Despite the label, a significant portion of the symptoms suffered by the patient cannot be adequately medically explained (or even treated in some cases), as the disease etiology has not been definitively established.

Even where symptoms are recognized as legitimately somatic, patients experience guilt, shame, and anxiety when placed in diagnostic limbo (Nettleton 2006; Zavestoski et al. 2004). For the medical profession, the presence of medically unexplained symptoms and syndromes highlights uncertainty about what symptoms mean and how disorders can be best identified (Nettleton et al. 2004; Pickersgill 2011).

TRAINING FOR CERTAINTY IN AN UNCERTAIN WORLD

Though uncertainty is part of making a diagnosis, most medical schools teach students to expect certainty and organization. "Medical students are taught that the evaluation of a patient should proceed in a discrete, linear way: you first take the patient's history, then perform a physical examination, order tests, and analyse results. Only after all the data are compiled should you formulate hypotheses about what might be wrong" (Groopman 2007, 11). Students participate in practice-based learning activities on actors with standardized cases and on mannequins with textbook symptoms. Fostering certainty may be done to instill confidence in these future clinicians and to help them take action (Katz 1984). But it can lead clinicians to ignore contradictory evidence, lacking sensitivity to variation and intolerant of ambiguity. This is called making a representative error: when "your thinking is guided by a prototype, so you fail to consider possibilities that contradict the prototype and thus attribute the symptoms to the wrong cause" (Groopman 2007, 44). Physical symptoms often result from psychological causes (Kroenke 2003), but this fact can lead practitioners to favor psychological over physical explanations when symptoms are imperfect, varied, or ambiguous.

Atkins (2010), in her book *My Imaginary Illness*, describes her physical, psychological, emotional, and financial losses from having her paralysis attributed to "functional" (psychological) and not "organic" (physical) causes because her myasthenia gravis (an autoimmune disorder where antibodies attack neural pathways so that muscle cells do not receive messages from nerve cells) was undiagnosed for over a decade. "Confronted by a difficult and ambiguous

It is inaccurate to equate physical symptoms with physical (i.e., medical) disorders since many patients with stable medical disorders are asymptomatic, and many patients with physical symptoms do not have a medical disorder that accounts for the presence and/or severity of their physical symptoms. (Kroenke 2003, 11) case, most doctors and nurses routinely grasped for certainty rather than attempting to tolerate any ambivalence. It was easier to categorize me as a 'head case' than to accept that I was suffering from an atypical and life-threatening illness about which they had very limited understanding and control" (Atkins 2010, 149). Another extreme but illustrative example of uncertainty being labeled psychosomatic is the misdiagnosis Munchausen syndrome by proxy (MSBP). The parents of children who have severe illnesses of an indeterminate cause are sometimes falsely accused of having MSBP, a psychiatric disorder where caregivers harm their loved ones in an attempt to gain attention (Rand and Feldman 1999).

> We carve out order by leaving the disorderly parts out. (William James as cited by Groopman [2007])

Part of this drive for certainty and the belief that we can achieve it has led to the development of **evidence-based medicine** (EBM), where truth is believed to be realizable through objective observation and scientific testing with a large number of research participants (experiments). EBM emerged in the 1990s out of a concern that policymakers and practitioners were not basing their diagnoses and treatment decisions on the best available evidence (Evidence-Based Medicine Working Group 1992). EBM supporters argue that all diagnoses and treatments should be based on evidence and, more specifically, evidence derived from randomized control trials (RCTs) and meta-analyses (systematic reviews of RCT studies that combine data sets for greater generalizability) of these experiments.

EBM has become the subject of much debate. Some argue that EBM is too reductionist, that it excludes or discounts what it cannot see (or does not yet have the technology or understanding to see and measure). Similarly, another limit to certainty stemming from EBM and biomedical research is the limit of applying epidemiological data such as population health statistics to one individual, even though in principle the evidence should be combined with information from the individual patient and clinician. Atkins (2010) explains that basing clinical practice on substantive evidence of efficacy is a good idea, but it has limitations: "EBM means that patients who are statistical outliers, or who do not meet diagnostically normative models, are potentially overlooked and cannot have their needs met because there is no evidence to back up nonstandard therapies. They do not fit in within a statistical or conceptual framework and thus a clinician cannot back up treatment options with proper scientific evidence" (145).

> In biomedical research, "any phenomenon, process or experience that one literally cannot 'put their fingers on' simply does not exist . . . This orthodoxy leaves no room for other modes of knowing that construct other realities" (Hollenberg and Muzzin 2010, 39).

Many statistics are collected about the probability that a symptom is associated with a diagnosis and the probability of survival associated with certain treatments. A specialist might say, "35% of adults who undergo this radiation treatment for bladder cancer survive five years postdiagnosis." But this approach harbors its own sources of problematic clinical uncertainty (Griffiths et al. 2005) in applying population level evidence to individuals. As Stephen J. Gould (1995) so famously explained, "the median isn't the message." How is a physician to know if their patient is in the 35% basket or the 65% basket? This is where the art of science becomes so relevant. A big part of managing the uncertainty in giving a diagnosis and prognosis is using experience, knowing the patient, reflecting on emotional responses to the patient and his condition, and knowing the population. As Groopman (2007) writes, "statistics cannot substitute for the human being before you; statistics embody averages, not individuals" (6).

Those who argue that truths are relative and that they depend on the observations of culturally shaped observers and the researcher's current hypothesis have also challenged claims to a certain truth. All peptic ulcers, for instance, were originally thought to be the result of stress. In the 1950s, patients with this diagnosis were advised to change their diet and to relax (Centers for Disease Control and Prevention 2006). In 1984, Australian researchers Marshall and Warren (1984) discovered that most people with stomach ulcers had helicobacter pylori in their digestive system. As a result of this research, physicians began treating peptic ulcers not with counseling, but with antibiotics and antacids (Donaldson et al. 2009). More recently, researchers made the discovery that more than 50% of the world's population has helicobacter pylori in their digestive system. But the percentage of the world suffering from peptic ulcers is much smaller than 50%. Researchers are now reexamining stress as a cause of peptic ulcers, in addition to helicobacter pylori (Wachirawat et al. 2003). At the least, it is clear that the presence of bacterial colonization must combine with other factors (some of which may be still unknown) in causing ill health. So, instead of an absolute truth, it is safer to say that biomedical research lends us temporary truths: evidence-based ways of knowing that are accepted and acted upon in the present, until challenged by future evidence and replaced by the next temporary truth.

A further challenge to biomedical certainty comes from within. The whole system of biomedical research has been scrutinized in recent years because of emerging awareness of conflicts of interest present from pharmaceutical industry–sponsored research. The pharmaceutical industry's role in shaping the evidence that underpins clinical practice has shaken the certainty around clinical foundations. RCTs used to prove the efficacy and safety of medications may not be objective at all; they may only provide a selective representation undermining the certainty attached to the results. Ebeling explores this in greater depth in chapter 9.

Nonetheless, medical education generally emphasizes certainty and decisiveness. There is good reason why, as it is important for practitioners to be confident about their decision making. Although uncertainty is unavoidable within medicine, contemporary medical schools emphasize the correctness of medical knowledge and foster faith in the power of medicine. Due to the **socialization** of confidence, medical students tend to approach uncertainty as something to be avoided. Where unavoidable, they understand that the best way to handle uncertainty is to disguise, deny, or deflect it (Lingard et al. 2003). These actions help to impose a perception of mastery and control over the uncertain situation (Hall 2002). Students feel caught out by the experience of uncertain diagnosis. Some even argue that an important facet of medical education involves training students how to be confident despite their uncertainty, how to adopt rhetorical techniques that help frame uncertainty within clinical encounters with both colleagues and patients (Atkinson 1984; Hall 2002).

Diagnostic and other clinical uncertainty is a considerable source of stress and concern for doctors. Having been trained in the biomedical frame, diagnostic uncertainty can feel like a personal failure. As a response to diagnostic uncertainty, both experienced doctors and medical students experience guilt, denial, and other defensive and protective emotions (Christakis 2003; Lingard et al. 2003).

One of the ways in which this stress can be alleviated is through an appreciation of the causes and role of uncertainty within diagnosis, and through a greater awareness of the boundaries of medical knowledge. This understanding tends to develop over time. While new medical students are deeply defensive regarding uncertainty (often attributing it to personal deficits), as medical training continues, it becomes easier to handle. Likewise, it has been found that as the experience of physicians increases, the likelihood of disclosing uncertainty does, too, at least to oneself and colleagues (though not necessarily to patients; Christakis 2003; Lingard et al. 2003). With experience, practitioners become more accepting of the reality of uncertainty, and more aware of ways in which it can be dealt with, both personally and with others. This includes understanding ways in which uncertainty can be managed clinically, being comfortable in reporting uncertainty, and being able to understand uncertain events as opportunities for further learning and improvement.

UNCERTAINTY AND SOCIAL LOCATION

While uncertainty is present throughout medicine, it is more apparent in some types of medical practice. Pimlott (2007) called managing uncertainty the "specialty" of general practice or family medicine. Specialists, on the other hand, are perceived to be more likely to attain certainty because patients typically first seek advice from their primary care physician. In this first encounter with the medical profession, the "breadth of possibilities" can appear endless (Brill 2010, 471). As the starting point, it is the doctor's job to suggest possible or probable diagnoses and to refer patients to specialists who confirm or refute the hypothesis of the general practitioner (GP). In their qualitative research with New Zealand GPs, Dew et al. (2005) found that GPs were rarely certain. One interviewee explained that GPs will only describe a diagnosis as definite or certain when "there's bones sticking out through the skin." More often, GPs "actually risk manage and live in this glorious twilight zone of uncertainty" (1194). Communicating these uncertainties in verbal or written form takes more time (Mayor et al. 2012) and requires the use of "hedging" terms within clinical documentation: ambiguous expressions such as "possible" or "might" related to unclear probability, frequency, or presentation (Hanauer et al. 2012; Kassirer 1989).

Specialists, in contrast, are said to be certain in their diagnoses (Dew et al. 2005). But variation in diagnosis across specialists suggests that uncertainty is pervasive in secondary care, as well, though not so often acknowledged. In many cases, different branches of medicine disagree about the meaning of the presentation of identical symptoms, or at least which symptoms and problems are most important. One example of this is the diagnosis of community-acquired pneumonia. Pneumonia is diagnosed through both the clinical evaluation (history and physical evaluation) and through chest X-ray. Isolating the infectious agent is the most definitive diagnostic option, but the tests to obtain this diagnosis are not frequently performed. There is professional disagreement over the interpretation of chest X-rays. Novack et al. (2006) found that an important aspect of the diagnosis was facilitating professional agreement between different specialist branches. Within any given case, this collaborative agreement might include radiologists, pulmonologists, infectious disease specialists, and internal medicine staff. The study found that there was a low agreement rate between these specialist groups, meaning that final diagnoses (following negotiation) differed significantly from the diagnosis that any one of these specialists would have provided on their own. While the low agreement rate was not related to the final clinical outcome, such variations result in a shift in narrative surrounding an individual case, and highlight variation within professional perspectives. In respect to other illness, lack of professional agreement about "what is" can be prominent, especially where illness categories themselves are contested. An example of this is the case of multiple chemical sensitivities, which is recognized and legitimated by some medical professionals, but not others (Phillips 2010).

Despite uncertainty being pervasive in both primary and secondary care, the differences in the perception and acknowledgment of uncertainty across these two social locations can have real consequences for medical students and practitioners. Medical students who are more tolerant of uncertainty are more likely to go into family medicine (Brill 2010). Some students and practitioners experience frustration and anxiety when faced with uncertainty, which can ultimately lead to burnout (Luther and Crandall 2011). These practitioners tend to use more resources and order more diagnostic tests (Luther and Crandall 2011, 800; Schneider et al. 2010). Students who identify themselves as intolerant of uncertainty are more likely to become specialists (Luther and Crandall 2011).

THE EFFECT OF DIAGNOSTIC UNCERTAINTY ON MEDICAL CARE

Uncertainty affects diagnosis at every level. At the individual level, symptoms and responses to treatments vary from person to person, making it difficult to apply (presumably objective) statistical data. In the laboratory, tests—such as biopsies and pathology results—are also fallible. Faced with all this uncertainty, doctors turn to their experience and subjective understanding of the patient for assurance. They relay this assurance in their communications with patients and family, which can often inspire hope in patients, but it can be much more. It can involve shaping a patient's and his family's perceptions of the present and the future, and shaping what they are hopeful about.

In a recent study, Olson (2011) found that caregivers of cancer patients described hearing a diagnosis as an interaction where medical professionals not only provide patients and families with information, but also shape their orientation in time. The diagnosis itself may cause patients to experience **biographical disruption**, where their sense of who they are comes into question (Bury 1982). For the spouses of these cancer patients the diagnosis caused a sense of temporal anomie: a sense of normlessness in time and an inability to plan for the future (Olson 2011). What medical practitioners do in delivering a cancer prognosis (in translating population-based statistics to a singular patient) is (1) communicate this prediction and (2) shape patients' and caregivers' perceptions of the future and their orientation in time. These prognoses can come in many forms: "You are/aren't likely to survive," "You are/aren't likely to regain the use of your face muscles," "You have a 10% chance of surviving the next five years." Caregivers whose spouses had uncertain futures were given this information and directed to enjoy "the now," to become present oriented, and to celebrate the time they had left with their spouse. Caregivers whose spouses had more certain futures (such as a 95% chance of surviving five years or more) were directed to carry on as usual and to continue to be future oriented. One caregiver said the surgeon told her that cancer "should be a thing of the past" after they had successfully removed her husband's cancerous bladder. These messages show that health professionals do not just deliver a diagnosis or inspire hope, they encourage patients and caregivers to manage their fears and emotions about their diagnosis and uncertain future. They guide caregivers and patients to focus on the present or the future, and they tell patients and caregivers what they can be "positive" about.

Diagnostic uncertainty therefore presents important consequences for practitioners, patients, caregivers, and even the broader public health. Decisions and diagnoses made within individual clinical interactions cumulatively influence the statistical measures that underpin public health decisions. Again drawing upon the example of influenza, diagnostic uncertainty can have interesting effects. As discussed above, there is a high level of uncertainty and discrepancy in the diagnosis of influenza. When taken to the population level, statistical uncertainty is high. During the recent H1N1 pandemic, the high degree of statistical uncertainty resulted in clear consequences for the managing global public health institution, the World Health Organization (WHO).

> We doctors and nurses must recognize our tendency to feel powerless in the face of uncertainty. However, a shared feeling of impotence will not help the patient. Instead, we must find something to ally with the patient against. That something, however, does not necessarily have to be a clear-cut, codified diagnosis from the *International Classification of Diseases*. (Hodges 2010, 180)

Globally, many health-care systems simply did not have the means or capacity to conduct expensive and time-consuming testing of individual patients to determine H1N1 infection. Even within developed systems, as Jutel et al. (2011) demonstrated, accurate diagnosis is difficult. Owing to the potentially catastrophic nature of a severe pandemic event, however, during the 2009 H1N1 scare, the WHO needed to act despite the statistical inaccuracy. Epidemiological statistics were needed to help predict and manage the event, but in a global context they did not necessarily exist (because the data were not always collected) or were haphazard in nature (because collection methods and reliability varied across WHO member regions). As a result, the WHO made major decisions, including deciding when to declare that the spread of H1N1 constituted a pandemic and when to advise mass vaccination campaigns, based upon uncertain statistics (Ben Embarek 2009; Fukuda 2009). In this case, diagnostic uncertainty even led to the public criticism of the WHO's response. The Council of Europe suggested that the WHO's actions were unjustified, in part because surveillance did not adequately distinguish H1N1 from other influenza-like illnesses (Flynn 2010).

This example shows that individual instances of diagnostic uncertainty can potentially have large follow-on effects. It also demonstrates a dilemma when dealing with uncertainty and possible severe consequences at a population level. Public health authorities would no doubt have been equally criticized if they were reticent in the face of a 1918-style influenza epidemic.

> Uncertainty is an opportunity for growth. Its acceptance shows respect for the opacity and integrity of other subjectivities. (Wellberry 2010, 1687)

PRACTICE IMPLICATIONS

Uncertainty is an inescapable aspect of medicine. As such, it is important for medical professionals to balance the art and science of diagnosis, to be as thorough as possible where symptoms do not allow for a straightforward diagnosis, and to be aware of the impact of diagnostic uncertainty upon their patients. In some sense, doctors may need to adapt the way in which they think about uncertainty. One important way of adapting is by recognizing, rather than denying, the role of uncertainty in clinical practice. By doing so, doctors can increase their effectiveness in terms of engagement with their patients and in recognizing and reacting to the reality of the situation (Groopman 2007). Part of being more effective as a clinician is recognizing that diagnostic uncertainty is a result of medical structures, not individual inadequacy. The view that there is one correct way of comprehending the world must also be challenged in accepting that there might not be a truth to be found, or it might not be achievable or measurable. Keeping uncertainty in perspective, especially in cases where diagnosis is not straightforward, is an important aspect of effective medical practice.

TAKEAWAY POINTS

- Professional socialization is crucial to a practitioner's orientation toward uncertainty.
- Medicine exhibits an aura of certainty, but it is fundamentally uncertain. Uncertainty is why the "art" of medicine can be so important.
- Certainty or uncertainty in diagnosis orients a patient's emotions, illness management, and lifestyle decisions.
- Medical students and professionals exhibit different reactions to uncertainty depending upon their career stage, specialization, and role.

DISCUSSION QUESTIONS

1. Consider an experience of diagnostic limbo or uncertainty to which you have been a witness or participant. How was that uncertainty (or how might it have been) experienced by the patient? By the medical practitioner?
2. Imagine a patient who presents with complaints for which you can find no diagnostic explanation. How might you speak to him about his illness? What ways can you support him in getting better?
3. This chapter identifies some sources of diagnostic uncertainty. What other sources of uncertainty can you think of?
4. Will diagnoses ever be completely certain? Why or why not?
5. What are the benefits of acknowledging and embracing uncertainty?

REFERENCES

Anderson, Robert E., Renée Fox, and Rolla B. Hill. 1990. "Medical Uncertainty and the Autopsy: Occult Benefits for Students." *Human Pathology* 21(2): 128–35.

Atkins, Chloe. 2010. *My Imaginary Illness: A Journey into Uncertainty and Prejudice in Medical Diagnosis.* Ithaca, NY: Cornell University Press.

Atkinson, Paul. 1984. "Training for Certainty." *Social Science and Medicine* 19(9): 949–56.

Ben Embarek, Peter. 2009. "WHO Press Briefing 04/05/09." http://www.who.int/media centre/multimedia/swineflupressbriefings/en/index.html.

Brill, John. 2010. "Handling Uncertainty." *Family Medicine* 42(7): 471–72.

Bury, Michael. 1982. "Chronic Illness as Biographical Disruption." *Sociology of Health and Illness* 4(2): 167–82.

Centers for Disease Control and Prevention. 2006. "History of Ulcer Diagnosis and Treatment." www.cdc.gov/ulcer/history.htm.

Christakis, Nicholas A. 2003. "On the Sociological Anxiety of Physicians." In *Essays in Honor of Renée C. Fox: Society and Medicine*, edited by C. Messikomer, J. Swazey, and D. Glicksman, 135–44. New Brunswick, NJ: Transaction.

Corbin, Juliet, and Anselm Strauss. 1985. "Managing Chronic Illness at Home." *Qualitative Sociology* 8(3): 224–47.

Damber, Jan-Eric, and Gunnar Aus. 2008. "Prostate Cancer." *Lancet* 371: 1710–21.

Dew, Kevin, Anthony Dowell, Deborah McLeod, Sunny Collings, and John Bushnell. 2005. "'This Glorious Twilight Zone of Uncertainty': Mental Health Consultations in General Practice in New Zealand." *Social Science and Medicine* 61: 1189–200.

Djulbegovic, Mia, Rebecca J. Beyth, Molly M. Neuberger, Taryn L. Stoffs, Johannes Vieweg, Benjamin Djulbegovic, and Phillip Dahm. 2010. "Screening for Prostate Cancer: Systematic Review and Meta-Analysis of Randomised Controlled Trials." *BMJ* 341: 4543–51.

Donaldson, Liam J., Gabriel Scally, and Raymond J. Donaldson. 2009. *Donaldsons' Essential Public Health.* 3rd ed. Oxford: Radcliffe.

Evidence-Based Medicine Working Group. 1992. "Evidence-Based Medicine: A New Approach to Teaching the Practice of Medicine." *JAMA* 268(17): 2420–25.

Flynn, Paul. 2010. "The Handling of the H1N1 Pandemic: More Transparency Needed." Council of Europe, Strasbourg. http://assembly.coe.int/CommitteeDocs/2010/20100604 _H1n1pandemic_E.pdf.

Fox, Renée. 1957. "Training for Uncertainty." In *The Student-Physician*, edited by R. Merton, G. Reader, and P. Kendall, 207–41. Cambridge, MA: Harvard University Press.

Fukuda, Keiji. 2009. "WHO Press Briefing 22/05/09." http://www.who.int/mediacentre/multimedia/swinefupressbriefings/en/index.html.

Gould, Stephen. J. 1995. *Adam's Navel and Other Essays*. London: Penguin.

Griffiths, Francis, Eileen Green, and Maria Tsouroufli. 2005. "The Nature of Medical Evidence and Its Inherent Uncertainty for the Clinical Consultation: Qualitative Study." *BMJ* 330(7490): 511–18.

Groopman, Jerome. 2007. *How Doctors Think*. Boston: Houghton Mifflin.

Hall, Katherine H. 2002. "Reviewing Intuitive Decision-Making and Uncertainty: The Implications for Medical Education." *Medical Education* 36: 216–24.

Halperin, John J., ed. 2011. *Lyme Disease: An Evidence Based Approach*. Wallingford: CABI.

Hanauer, David, Yang Liu, Qiaozhu Mei, Frank Manion, Ulysses Balis, and Kai Zheng. 2012. "Hedging Their Mets: The Use of Uncertainty Terms in Clinical Documents and Its Potential Implications when Sharing the Documents with Patients." *AMIA Annual Symposium Proceedings Archive* 2012: 321–30.

Hodges, Brian D. 2010. "Clinical Commentary." In *My Imaginary Illness: A Journey into Uncertainty and Prejudice in Medical Diagnosis*. Ithaca, NY: Cornell University Press.

Hollenberg, Daniel, and Linda Muzzin. 2010. "Epistemological Challenges to Integrative Medicine: An Anti-Colonial Perspective on the Combination of Complementary/Alternative Medicine with Biomedicine." *Health Sociology Review* 19(1): 34–56.

Horsley, Philomena. 2010. "Teaching the Anatomy of Death: A Dying Art?" *Medicine Studies* 2(1): 1–19.

Jutel, Annemarie, Michael G. Baker, James Stanley, Q. Sue Huang, and Don Bandaranayake. 2011. "Self-Diagnosis of Influenza during a Pandemic: A Cross-Sectional Survey." *BMJ Open* 1(2): e000234, doi:10.1136/bmjopen-2011-000234.

Kassirer, Jerome. 1989. "Diagnostic Reasoning." *Annals of Internal Medicine* 110: 893–900.

Katz, Jay. 1984. "Why Doctors Don't Disclose Uncertainty." *Hastings Center Report* 14(1): 35–44.

Kroenke, Kurt. 2003. "The Interface between Physical and Psychological Symptoms," supplement, *Primary Care Companion Journal of Clinical Psychiatry* 5(7): 11–18.

Lingard, Lorelei, Kim Garwood, Catherine F. Schryer, and Marlee M. Spafford. 2003. "A Certain Art of Uncertainty: Case Presentation and the Development of Professional Identity." *Social Science and Medicine* 56: 603–16.

Luther, Vera, and Sonia Crandall. 2011. "Commentary: Ambiguity and Uncertainty. Neglected Elements of Medical Education Curricula?" *Academic Medicine* 86(7): 799–800.

Marcus, Pamela M., Eric J. Bergstralh, Mark H. Zweig, Ann Harris, Kenneth P. Offord, and Robert S. Fontana. 2006. "Extended Lung Cancer Incidence Follow-Up in the Mayo Lung Project and Overdiagnosis." *Journal of the National Cancer Institute* 98 (11): 748–56.

Marshall, Barry J., and J. Robin Warren. 1984. "Unidentified Curved Bacilli in the Stomach of Patients with Gastritis and Peptic Ulceration." *Lancet* 1(8390): 1311–15.

Mayor, Eric, Adrian Bangerter, and Myriam Aribot. 2012. "Task Uncertainty and Communication during Nursing Shift Handover." *Journal of Advanced Nursing* 68(9): 1956–66.

Nettleton, Sarah. 2006. "'I Just Want Permission to Be Ill': Towards a Sociology of Medically Unexplained Symptoms." *Social Science and Medicine* 62(5): 1167–78.

Nettleton, Sarah, Lisa O'Malley, and Philip Duffey. 2004. "Enigmatic Illness: Narratives of Patients Who Live with Medically Unexplained Symptoms." *Social Theory and Health* 2(1): 47–66.

Novack, Victor, Lane S. Avon, Alexander Smolyakov, Rachel Barnea, Ann Jotkowitz, and Francisc Schaeffer. 2006. "Disagreement in the Interpretation of Chest Radiographs among Specialists and Clinical Outcomes of Patients Hospitalized with Suspected Pneumonia." *European Journal of Internal Medicine* 17: 43–47.

O'Connor, Bonnie B. 2010. "Foreword." In *My Imaginary Illness: A Journey into Uncertainty and Prejudice in Medical Diagnosis*, xi–xvi. Ithaca, NY: Cornell University Press.

Olson, Rebecca. 2011. "Managing Hope, Denial or Temporal Anomie? Informal Cancer Caregivers' Accounts of Spouses' Cancer Diagnoses." *Social Science and Medicine* 73(6): 904–11.

Phillips, Tarryn. 2010. "Debating the Legitimacy of a Contested Environmental Illness: A Case Study of Multiple Chemical Sensitivities (MCS)." *Sociology of Health and Illness* 32(7): 1026–40.

Pickersgill, Martyn. 2011. "Ordering Disorder: Knowledge Production and Uncertainty in Neuroscience Research." *Science as Culture* 20(1): 71–87.

Pimlott, Nicholas. 2007. "Letters: Managing Uncertainty." *Canadian Family Physician* 53: 1000.

Rand, Deirdre C., and Marc D. Feldman. 1999. "Misdiagnosis of Munchausen Syndrome by Proxy: A Literature Review and Four New Cases." *Harvard Review of Psychiatry* 7(2): 94–101.

Randell, Rebecca, Stephanie Wilson, and Peter Woodward. 2011. "The Importance of the Verbal Shift Handover Report: A Multi-Site Case Study." *International Journal of Medical Informatics* 80(11): 803–12.

Schneider, Antonius, Bernd Löwe, Stefan Barie, Stefanie Joos, Peter Engeser, and Joachim Szecsenyi. 2010. "How Do Primary Care Doctors Deal with Uncertainty in Making Diagnostic Decisions? The Development of the 'Dealing with Uncertainty Questionnaire.'" *Journal of Evaluation of Clinical Practice* 16: 431–37.

Vance, Richard. P. 1990. "An Unintentional Irony: The Autopsy in Modern Medicine and Society." *Human Pathology* 21(1): 136–44.

Wachirawat, Wariya, Paibul Suriyawongpaisal, Susan Levenstein, Kanit Atisook, Cherdsak Theerabutr, Somchit Hanucharurnkul, Sasiprapa Boontapisit, Juree Jearanaisilavong, and Tassana Bootong. 2003. "Stress, but Not Helicobacter Pylori, Is Associated with Peptic Ulcer Disease in a Thai Population." *Journal of the Medical Association of Thailand* 86(7): 672–85.

Wellberry, Caroline. 2010. "The Art of Medicine: The Value of Medical Uncertainty?" *The Lancet* 375: 1686–87.

Zavestoski, Stephen, Phil Brown, Sabrina McCormick, Brian Mayer, Maryhelen D'Ottavi, and Jaime C. Lucove. 2004. "Patient Activism and the Struggle for Diagnosis: Gulf War Illness and Other Medically Unexplained Physical Symptoms in the US." *Social Science and Medicine* 58(1): 161–75.

I Am Not a Doctor, but . . .
The Lay-Professional Relationship in Diagnosis

Kevin Dew and Annemarie Goldstein Jutel

STARTING POINTS

- A traditional view of the doctor-patient relationship is one where the doctor knows best.
- In this view a good patient is compliant and does not challenge diagnoses.
- An important reason why patients often did not challenge their diagnoses is that doctors had access to information that patients did not.

Hippocrates wrote that "if [the doctor] is able to tell his **patients** when he visits them not only about their past and present symptoms, but also to tell them what is going to happen, as well as to fill in the details they have omitted, he will increase his reputation as a medical practitioner and people will have no qualms in putting themselves under his care" (Chadwick and Mann 1983, 170). His words underline the importance of diagnosis. Diagnosis lies at the heart of medical practice, not only in confirming the professional status of the doctor, but also in delineating the lay-professional relationship. It provides a rationale for the consultation. It confirms the authority and prestige of the medical profession. It delegates responsibility for labeling an illness.

Diagnosis is interactional. Layperson and professional come together to discuss what ails the former, and what remedy the latter can provide. It is ultimately social: two individuals, or more, with different roles, sometimes in one space (often in several). What happens next—negotiation, explanation, understanding, and follow-up—all depends on relationships, communications, beliefs, culture, education, and social status.

> The natural authority of the doctor, the confidence the patient feels in his professional knowledge, his unselfish, disinterested respect for intimate communications, the tradition, so long accepted, that the relationship between doctor and patient is confidential and the sentiment of the patient that the more the doctor knows about him, the more helpful he can be, all these attitudes and assumptions establish a basis for free and unbiased communication that is possible in few other human situations. (Robinson 1939, 2)
>
> *A historic description of a traditional medical doctor.*

This chapter focuses on the social implications of the lay-professional relationship. It delineates the roles of the participants in the diagnostic process and identifies potential points of conflict, tension, and alignment.

WHY NOT "PATIENT"?

You may wonder why this chapter is not titled "The Doctor-Patient Relationship" and be surprised by the panoply of terms that refer to people who seek support from a health practitioner. Where is the patient? Patient is the traditional word for the nonmedical partner in the diagnostic relationship. The labels we use to refer to this or that participant in a particular interaction also imply the role we expect that participant to fulfill. "The words used to describe those who use our services are, at one level, metaphors that indicate how we conceive them. At another level such labels operate discursively, constructing both the relationship and attendant identities of people participating in the relationships, inducing very practical and material outcomes" (McDonald in McLaughlin 2009, 115).

The word "patient" appears early in English. In the fourteenth century, Chaucer made reference to the "pacient" in the prologue to the *Canterbury Tales*, whose Doctour of phisyk "kepte . . . a ful greet deel In houres by his magik naturel" (lines 417–18). Etymologically, the word comes from the Latin verb *pati* "to suffer." The adjectival form of the word implies forbearance, tolerance, perseverance, and passivity.

The term "patient" fits a traditionally paternalistic mode of interaction. In this model the doctor assumes a parental, authoritative role, determining what is best for the sick person, and placing more value on health outcomes than on patient autonomy. Bailey (1764) defined this relationship in his eighteenth-century dictionary, describing the patient as "one under the *direction* of a physician or surgeon in order to be cured of some distemper" (622; emphasis added). The patient (in this type of relationship, it is the appropriate word) is passive and accepts medical authority. A "good" patient here is "compliant," follows medical "orders," and defers to, rather than challenges, the doctor on matters of diagnosis, disease treatment, and management.

Historically this good patient would have been found in the early hospitals, which were places reserved for the poor. From the Middle Ages to the eighteenth century, "bedside medicine," in which the individualized personalities of the doctor and patient were paramount, dominated (Jewson 1976). Before the invention of stethoscopes, electrocardiograms, laboratory tests, and the whole plethora of diagnostic instruments that exist today, patients would have available to them the same signs of the condition that a doctor had. Doctors would reach a diagnosis by asking patients questions and looking at such physical signs as the color of the skin and palate as well as the color, smell, and taste of urine. With the invention of the stethoscope, the doctor had available to him (rarely her) an instrument that delivered signs (sounds from the chest) that were

---

The family doctor would come to the bed of the child who was ill . . . He would take blood pressure, temperature, generally, you know, a gentle hands-on approach, and he was actually very comforting. His nature was a very comforting nature. I suppose we all revered him in a way because it was the general feeling in that period that the family doctor was someone you really listened to and respected. (Lupton 1997a)

The traditional paternalistic doctor-patient relationship.

not available to the patient. Now the doctor could diagnose on the basis of the unseen. From this point on, doctors could exercise more control over information than the patients and could decide whether to make information available to them, providing more power over diagnosis.

But even with this increasing control over the medical diagnosis, the home continued to be an important site of therapeutic practice (including diagnosis) away from the direct oversight of medical practitioners (Dew et al. forthcoming). In seventeenth-century England, "Well-stocked homes had kitchen-physic: bottles of homebrewed or shop-bought purges, vomits, pain-killers, cordials, febrifuges (medicines to reduce fever) and the like," and people were "less doctor dependent than today" (Porter 1987, 29).

Today homes are similarly stocked with medications, supplements, salves, and lotions that laypeople self-administer without seeking medical attention. Similarly, the ever-increasing availability of information online and elsewhere allows the individual to draw on a wider range of views and provides a smattering (or perhaps even a wealth) of medical knowledge. The individual may be an active participant in decision making about her treatment and may even expect to direct treatment choices.

It is difficult, however, to reject the word "patient," because the alternatives are also fraught with shortcomings. The words "client," "service user," or "consumer" are often used instead. These terms imply a relationship that is metaphorically and discursively contractual, framed by a market relationship in a commodity culture. They place the individual in the role of customer, engaging as a rational individual aware of her choices irrespective of educational, social, and personal circumstances (McLaughlin 2009). It places a heavy burden on the layperson and the professional because the former is both entitled and responsible. On the doctor's part, a failure to cure becomes an unpaid debt; on the client's side the failure to heal becomes a moral shortcoming. To see the patient in this light also effaces what many health professionals consider critical to the diagnostic encounter—that it is a relationship based not on business but on caring and human interaction.

Throughout this book, we attempt to think critically about the labels we apply to the individual in the diagnostic encounter. We generally opt for the terms "individual" and "layperson," both of which are reasonably nonjudgmental. But they are not unproblematic. To be a layperson is to have common knowledge, but being sick is not only the lot of "simple folk." Doctors, too, can become ill. When they do, they assume a new role in the consulting room. Despite their advanced medical knowledge, doctors find themselves wedged somewhere between the role of patient, service user, consumer, and layperson. This position of doctor-as-patient can be helpful in understanding and practicing medicine more effectively. Medical journals publish articles by doctors who have found themselves unexpectedly on the other side of the lay-professional relationship.

THE DIAGNOSTICIAN

The word "doctor" is not open to dispute as easily as the word "patient." To be a doctor is to possess particular professional qualifications. It usually involves having completed a required course of study, applied to an organizational body with regulatory authority, complied with registration requirements, and adhered to a set of practices, deviance from which may be punishable by the regulatory organization and even the state. There is collective agreement about what it is to be a doctor, despite variations in conditions of practice from state to state. An important aspect of this definition is the autonomy it affords the practitioner. Preserving autonomy is one characteristic of a profession. Thus, while the state retains ultimate authority, it delegates important components of its authority to the medical profession. For example, the state will not arbitrate whether an individual is well enough to work, or determine a cause of death; it asks doctors to do so. Not just anyone can have the authority to make a definitive diagnosis; this responsibility falls predominantly under the jurisdiction of medicine. Diagnosis, therefore, is an important aspect of how the medical profession defines itself.

Sometimes you'd just feel like all they wanted to do was measure you. Before you're even asked how you're feeling, there's this thermometer in your mouth, you've been weighed and had your blood pressure taken. And all this without them even asking why you were there in the first place.

Objective data can trump both the patient account and the clinical examination.

Because of the prestige and autonomy afforded to the profession that has jurisdiction over medical diagnosis, a number of other **professions** have sought an increased role in this diagnostic arena. Medicine has (sometimes reluctantly, sometimes gracefully) relinquished its control over making certain diagnoses or influence in certain settings. Today the nurse practitioner, the clinical psychologist, and the physiotherapist also have specific diagnostic realms. And their roles are agreed upon and legislated, too. Consequently, they are also part of the diagnostic encounter, which we discuss below. For the sake of convenience, we use the term "doctor" with regard to one who makes a diagnosis.

DIAGNOSTIC ENCOUNTER

Feeling unwell is the usual prompt for seeking medical attention. The individual has assessed this unwellness and has attributed its source to disease rather than to any one of a range of other possible causative factors. But the sick person needs the explanatory power of diagnosis in order to access treatment, which the doctor has the authority to deliver.

The layperson's desire to understand the discomfort—cough, rash, swelling, or cramp—gives her reasons to see her doctor. In turn, the doctor directs the story of illness, asking questions about personal and family history as well as the presentation of symptoms. The doctor then undertakes a physical assessment, palpating, auscultating, and measuring the body to create a narrative that explains the patient's complaint. And frequently both layperson and professional acquiesce to external findings contained in such tests as X-rays, scans, blood counts or manometers, privileging such measurements over the subjective history or clinical presentation (Leder 1990; see chap. 10 for more on the role and practice of diagnostic technology).

The process by which the illness is described and contextualized in the consultation is the first step in "organizing" an illness. Balint (1964) described the diagnostic encounter as an organizational task where deciding what is wrong directs the approach to the illness. He explains that the process of offering a diagnosis involves some negotiation, as the layperson and doctor both try out various labels. This model remains relevant to contemporary lay-professional relations and may be even more pertinent in today's era of increasing patient autonomy and knowledge. The individual consults the doctor to present an organizing explanation of his ailments for confirmation. In a sense, the doctor "proposes" a diagnosis.

Not only may the individual's opening story suggest a possible candidate diagnosis, but it may well outline a number of possible diagnoses that have been considered and dismissed, with evidence provided to justify the conclusions. In addition, the individual may describe the condition in such a way as to convince the doctor that the condition is not trivial and that they are not wasting the doctor's time. So at an early stage of the consultation a great deal of diagnostic work undertaken by the patient may be revealed.

After justifying the need for the consultation, the most pressing and immediate problem for the patient is "*the request for the name of the illness, for a diagnosis*. It is only in the second instance that the patient asks for therapy" (Balint 1964, 25). The diagnosis to which Balint refers is a medical diagnosis, one that carries a particular authority. The illness proposal must be recognized by—and negotiated with—the doctor. The form this interaction might take could be the presentation of a set of symptoms. Already the first step in organization has taken place. A statement such as "I have a headache; do you think it might be a tumor?" enables the doctor to organize the information gathering. She might go on to ask her patient, "Why do you think it might be a tumor?" "What is the nature of the pain?" "Have you any changes in your vision?" "Any tingling in your fingers?" The doctor ideally proceeds to a sequence of steps that rule in or out (in order of seriousness) the possible explanatory diagnoses, from brain tumor to migraine to stress to benign headache. In the ideal encounter, or series of encounters, the doctor responds to the illness as offered, exploring the patient's organizational strategy, testing its pathophysiological coherence, and offering alternative diagnoses until such time as both patient and doctor can agree, at least during the time of the consultation, upon the fundamental diagnosis underpinning the patient complaint. Leana Wen (2013), author of *When Doctors Don't Listen: How to Avoid Misdiagnoses and Unnecessary Tests*, has written that the patient story and human connection tell us much more about the probable cause of illness in a patient than tests and investigations. Listening (and also, for patients, practicing telling their stories), writes Wen, is the key to robust diagnosis.

THE ILLNESS-DISEASE DICHOTOMY

The **illness-disease dichotomy** is an important aspect of the lay-professional inter-action. We could call illness the personal experience of sickness (Kleinman et al. 1978). Illness is an undesirable change in the way a person feels or interacts, which is explained by the person as originating from a sickness. It is interesting to note the cultural variation in illness definitions. Different cultures may differently value changes in function, for example. Illness in one culture may not be seen as such in another. Gastrointestinal disease in developing countries may be such a common experience that it is not seen as requiring particular action, whereas in developed countries it is likely to lead to a medical consultation (Fanany and Fanany 2012).

Disease, in contrast, is codified. Western medicine identifies, labels, and cements the definition of disease through diagnostic systems of classification. Fleischman (1999) refers to diseases as conceptual entities, or "categories of clinical taxonomy . . . extrapolated from an aggregate of similar illnesses on the basis of what is thought to be common to the illnesses so classified" (7). Disease is diagnosed. Illness is not; rather, it is presented to a clinician as *presumed* disease. The transformation from illness to disease takes place during the diagnostic encounter.

While not all illnesses can be diagnosed, their narratives are the starting point for diagnosis. Note that there is more than one narrative: for a diagnosis to materi-alize, the patient's and the doctor's stories must first juxtapose and then merge. The patient's stories, emerging from his own experience, culture, and consideration of the role of the doctor, are transformed into medical accounts after their telling. The doctor interrogates, interprets, and retells the story, establishing the "plot" and a diagnostic organization (Hunter 1991). In Leder's model, the patient has already determined that the explanation for his discomfort is medical in nature, and a doc-tor (rather than a different social authority such as a rabbi or lawyer) will confer meaning to the narrative. Illness is the story that results when an individual sees the interpretation in terms of health and medicine. In contrast, diagnosis is the story of medicine, told in the language of disease. "In the narrow biological terms of the biomedical model," says Kleinman (1988), "this means that disease is reconfig-ured *only* as an alteration in biological structure or functioning" (5–6).

Arthur Frank (1995) claims that a social expectation of being ill is not just seek-ing care, it is "a narrative surrender" in which the patient must relinquish her story to the doctor to retell it through diagnosis. The new story is "the one against which others are ultimately judged true or false, useful or not" (5–6). Kleinman main-tains that doctors are taught to be skeptical of patients' narratives about illness, a view shared by Foucault (1963), who wrote that clinical medicine sought to silence the patient's story unequivocally. "In order to know the truth of the pathology, the doctor must abstract the patient . . . who, by trying to show things, ends up con-cealing them" (8; translation ours).

The diagnosis thus confers legitimacy to illness, yet it does not necessarily align with the patient's narrative for a number of reasons, not the least of which is the position from which the stories are recounted. Illness narratives "reveal what life is like for the narrator . . . [including] the practical consequences of managing symptoms, reduced mobility and so on. In telling their story, individuals also reveal, or indeed may assert, their self and social identity" (Nettleton et al. 2004, 49). Medical narratives are constructed around the diagnosis, which conveys power as a result of its institutionalization. The diagnosis has presumed objectivity as it emerges from a scientifically agreed-upon taxonomy. It brings with it an authority that can trump the lived experience of the sick person.

Yet the experience of living through disease represents the more tangible reality for most individuals (Frank 1995). The paradox of relinquishing the personal narrative to the professional one is not without consequence. It begins, writes Frank (1995), "when popular experience is overtaken by technical expertise, including complex organizations of treatment. Folk no longer go to bed and die, cared for by family members . . . [they] go to paid professionals who reinterpret their pains as symptoms, using a specialized language that is unfamiliar and overwhelming" (5).

The languages of disease and illness may be peculiarly discordant. A "transformed and medicalized narrative may be alien to the patient: strange depersonalized, unlived and unliveable. Returned to the patient in this alien form the medical narrative is all but unrecognizable as a version of the patient's story—and all but useless as an explanation of the patient's experience" (Hunter 1991, 13). Such alienation occurs when the medical model takes inadequate account of the illness problems (such as how the patient has actually lived, explained, and accounted for her dysfunction) and is unable to incorporate this in its own narrative through the diagnostic label.

Mildred Blaxter, a medical sociologist, has movingly described her personal trajectory of illness and the means by which the process of diagnosis effaced her lived experience of disease (Blaxter 2009). Diagnostic technology replaced her own voice as the focus of medical attention. Symptoms and patient history were subordinated to scan results; patient knowledge and information, even clinical examination, took a back seat. In Blaxter's experience, the abnormal scan result could have been explained as a "shadow" from her youth, possibly a vestige of a childhood tuberculosis. Her lung specialist rather hastily refuted this explanation.

When personal and professional narratives align, health outcomes may improve. The Polynesian man suffering from gout who attributes his pain to an incompletely healed rugby injury and the British-trained rheumatologist who explains the mechanics of purine metabolism may seem to be poles apart.

> I went to the doctor because I had this bad-tasting cough. He gave me some antibiotics for an anaerobic infection, because the bad taste is supposed to be a sign of an anaerobic infection. But I didn't get better. So he tested me for all kinds of things, and found out I'd been exposed to some pneumonia germ. But I knew I didn't have pneumonia and I told him so. And so I took the meds that come with that kind of pneumonia and it wasn't any better. So, finally, I went to see someone else, and he said I had reactive airways, and that made sense, because I have always been a cougher, especially after a cold. He gave me a puffer, and I used it religiously. I got better straight away.
>
> *Diagnosis involves the patient account, clinical assessment, tests, and, ultimately, negotiation between the layperson and the clinician.*

But talking, testing, listening, and acknowledging are the starting points for treating the person and reducing the burden of disease. Enabling a patient's story—its plot, characters, setting, and description (rather than inserting the patient's words into a clinical picture)—acknowledges the patient's expertise in the construction of illness. It allows "joint authorship" by doctor and patient of the explanatory framework, the therapeutic decision, and the clinical outcomes (Clark and Mishler 1992).

This common project is not compatible with the paternalistic model of care to which we referred in the opening pages of this chapter. And it is one that shifts the locus of authority in the lay-professional relationship.

CHANGING ROLES

Diagnoses and their classificatory systems define and enable the influence of professional medicine. Similarly, at an individual level, the ability to diagnose confers authority to the doctor as allocator of resources (De Swaan 1989). When a doctor deems a patient's condition to be medical, the latter receives previously unauthorized privileges, such as permission to be absent from work, priority parking, insurance benefits, reimbursement for treatment, or access to services. The doctor certifies the medical nature of the complaint and "medical advice" informs administrative and policy decisions.

Authority in medicine comes from its officially approved monopoly over the right to define health and to treat illness (more on this in chap. 7). This monopoly confers high public esteem (Freidson 1972). The doctor, as the agent of medicine, is accorded a prominent position on the hierarchy of expertise and a mandate to exercise her authority over other health professionals, in addition to over laypeople (Freidson 1972).

The medical dominance articulated by Freidson is not immutable, however. The power of the medical profession has declined in many ways, first evidenced perhaps by the introduction of malpractice lawsuits, profit-driven administration of physician performance, and cost-management strategies in medicine (Light and Levine 1988). More recent evidence of change in the status of doctors shows increasing patient complaints, use of alternative therapies, and critical media portrayals of doctors as well as a lack of financial autonomy (Lupton 1997b). Finally, wider access to information has led to changes in the doctor-patient relationship, with patients more willing to challenge their doctor, to dispute findings, or to seek advice outside of the doctor-patient relationship (Lupton 1997a; Nettleton 2004).

Lay movements advocate for conditions to be recognized as diseases despite widespread medical skepticism (Brown and Zavestoski 2004). Commercial forces are eager to tap the modern patient's increased access to previously privileged medical information, seeing in self-diagnosis an excellent means by which to promote particular conditions (and by extension their concordant therapies; Healy 2006). But health policies, too, have encouraged a transformation of traditional relationships in health care, emphasizing a more active role by the layperson, whose expertise is derived from experience rather than knowledge (Wilson 2001).

So, what seems to be the problem?

I have a sore stomach.

Where is it sore?

Down here. [circular hand-sweep from belly button towards pubis then back up again]

What kind of pain do you have?

I'm not sure you'd call it "pain"—it's like sore, or just uncomfortable.

How would you describe it?

Um, it's not all the time, but then when it comes, it's sore, and I feel like bending over. And when I wake up in the morning, too.

Do you think it's related to your bladder being full? Does it feel like your bladder is irritated?

Well, I feel bad when I need to pee, but I also feel gassy other times. And if you touch it here, it's sore, too.

But you wouldn't call it pain?

That depends what you call pain. I think of pain being like a knife or something. And it doesn't feel like a knife. But it doesn't feel good either.

If you were to put it on a scale, of say zero to ten, with ten being the worst pain you've ever had and zero being no pain, how would you rate this pain?

Huh?

The languages of disease and illness may be peculiarly discordant.

Seeking other avenues for diagnosis is not a new phenomenon, for just as Hippocrates described the importance of the medical diagnosis, so too did he describe the unruly patient, reluctant to submit to medical care. He questioned their resolve: "Although they have no wish to die, they have not the courage to be patient . . . [is] it not more likely that they will disobey their doctors rather than that the doctors . . . will prescribe the wrong remedies?" (Chadwick and Mann 1983, 142). Hippocrates also emphasized the knowledge gap between layperson and doctor: "the symptoms which patients with internal diseases describe to their physicians are based on guesses about a possible cause rather than knowledge about it. If they knew what caused their sickness, they would know how to prevent it" (Chadwick and Mann 1983, 145).

But we know that laypeople today, more so than ever before, have better access to specialized information about what causes their illness. According to Nettleton (2004), medical knowledge has escaped (or "e-scaped") from books and libraries, flowing as information through myriad electronic networks and Internet sources, enabling the patient greater access to information about disease before the encounter with the doctor.* Data from the Health Information National Trends Survey in the United States confirmed that only 10.9% of American adults go to their

---

*Although not necessarily to "good" information, nor to correct interpretation.

physicians first for health information, with almost half using Internet resources as their initial port of call (Hesse et al. 2005).

The availability of medical knowledge outside of the halls of learning reduces the power of the physician, creating an "informed consumer" rather than an acquiescent patient. Now educated consumers may consult the physician for support in making choices about information they already possess. Emanuel and Emanuel (1992) would refer to this as the "informative model," where the objective of the clinical encounter is for the physician to elucidate the options available to the patient, thus enabling her to make an autonomous choice.

Transforming the place of medical authority is not without challenges. Positioning patients as consumers opens the door for them to become the vulnerable prey of commercial interests. The ability to assess quality, reliability, and morality of health information is not necessarily within the grasp of most laypeople, presenting a difficulty on two fronts. On the one hand, any attempt to mediate access to information, or to recapture control of its delivery, will infringe upon lay autonomy. On the other, consuming information without adequate understanding puts the patient, the doctor, and the doctor-patient relationship at risk. This is most poignant in self-diagnosis: the turning on the head of traditional diagnostic responsibilities.

> I need a doctor's certificate because I had a bad headache yesterday and couldn't go to work. I am not allowed back if I don't have a certificate.
>
> *Medical authority certifies the legitimacy of health complaints.*

Self-diagnosis, or at least early lay recognition of diseases, serves an important tool in public health. During the H1N1 influenza pandemic of 2009, the Centers for Disease Control and Prevention sought to reduce the spread of the influenza virus by asking people to stay away from the doctor if they believed they had the flu. The principle is that self-isolation is linked with self-diagnosis; the germs can stay at home (Centers for Disease Control and Prevention 2009). Self-diagnosis is widely used by both commercial and lay disease awareness campaigns, encouraging individuals to self-identify with a particular disorder, thus bypassing the conventional diagnostic processes. In this case, the layperson is encouraged to recognize signs of particular disorders, which they then present to the doctor, asking if "X [substitute name of remedy] is right for you." Both forms of self-diagnosis present challenges to medicine as they redefine roles in the doctor-patient relationship.

Reviews of this trend toward self-diagnosis have focused on patient safety. A prominent theme in the medical literature is that patients (having inadequate training to consider differential diagnoses) might overlook other morbidities. Ferris et al. (2002) explain that the frequency and severity of misdiagnosis of vaginal yeast infections are concerning. Inaccurate diagnosis can lead to delays in the treatment of more serious disorders. The yeast infection example provides a useful heuristic. First, medical views are clearly divided as to whether yeast infections offer a suitable condition for self-diagnosis. Second, it is a common condition. And third, the doctor no longer needs to serve as gatekeeper to treatment in many countries, because antifungal medication for its treatment is readily available without prescription.

The first approval for an over-the-counter (OTC) antifungal was made in the United States in 1990. Many other countries followed suit. This approval led to a reduction in prescription costs and physician services (Gurwitz et al. 1995), but an increase in pharmaceutical sales (Ferris et al. 1996). The result of the switch from prescription to OTC remedy was more likely to have contributed to shifting the financial burden from insurance carriers to the health consumer (Harrington and Shepherd 2002).

Accompanying the switch to OTC status is the drive by the pharmaceutical industry to increase lay awareness of vaginal yeast infections, particularly in countries such as the United States and New Zealand, where **direct-to-consumer** advertising (DTCA) is legal. Self-screening tools are prevalent in this drive for disease recognition, and they frequently appeal to emotional, rather than clinical, imperatives. The Monistat website provides an excellent example (Monistat 2013). It provides symptom lists and a "treatment finder" as well as "questions for your doctor." A nurse practitioner is also available to answer questions submitted to the website. Research on DTCA indicates that, even where a woman ends up consulting her own doctor, advertising leads to more prescriptions for the advertised medicines regardless of what the doctor thinks about the treatment (Mintzes et al. 2002).

Self-diagnosis is not driven by the pharmaceutical industry alone. Online communities—some funded by the industry, others not—also promote disease awareness. The website of the CFIDS Association of America, which represents and advocates for people with chronic fatigue and immune dysfunction syndrome, provides an interactive screening tool to assess the probability of an individual having chronic fatigue syndrome (CFS) with the caution, "Only a doctor or qualified health professional can diagnose CFS. This assessment, however, can help you determine whether your symptoms may indicate CFS" (CFIDS Association of America 2009).

The contestable nature of diseases such as CFS helps to explain medical ambivalence, if not resentment, of lay prediagnosis. A number of conditions—some common, others idiosyncratic—find their recognition thwarted by medicine. They are not accepted by doctors, government, or insurance companies, yet are they experienced by the individual as illnesses. This uncomfortable clash of perceptions is at the base of what is referred to as contested, or disputed, diseases. These are conditions that medicine does not acknowledge but the laity—be it an individual

---

So, I went in and told the doctor about this rash. And he looked at me—well, he studied me really. He didn't make eye contact, and he didn't ask me any questions. He just looked at my hands, and turned them over, and looked at them again. I tried to talk for a moment, but he shushed me. Then after about 30 seconds, he said, "Well, Judy, you've got SLE." And I just said, "Hey back up!" He looked at me as if I was crazy. "Do you know what I DO?" I got a blank stare. "I am a research scientist and I am exposed to all sorts of toxic chemicals, usually on my hands, and usually right up to here (indicating the upper margin of the raised rash). Don't just tell me I have SLE without talking to me first! I declare!" I was so mad, I just left the room. I couldn't believe he'd be so ignorant. Now it may be that I've got SLE, but I don't buy it. In any case, I don't buy the fact that he'd just look at my body and tell me about it as if I didn't have anything to say. What in the world was he thinking?

Challenging the doctor's assessment and approach.

or a group of individuals with certain symptoms in common—considers to be disease (see chap. 11).

But self-diagnosis appears to be welcome in a certain number of well-defined circumstances. Already the emphasis on self-care and "concordance" (rather than compliance) seek to cast the layperson as a decision maker (Mullen 1997). Extending the autonomy of the individual beyond care to diagnosis, however, is more unusual. Outside of the discussion of vaginal yeast infection, self-diagnosis has its most robust supporters in those conditions where medical assistance is not available, is unreliable, or is a burden to the public health system.

The extreme examples of malaria and altitude sickness are conditions that tend to surface in geographic locations where doctors are rarely found. Self-diagnosis becomes an imperative, or at least an aspiration. But the closer-to-home example of H1N1 influenza virus is perhaps more pertinent. As mentioned above, self-diagnosis was a cornerstone of pandemic management. It falls under the category of "elimination of potential exposures," which is on the top level in the hierarchy of actions designed to minimize transmission of influenza (Centers for Disease Control and Prevention 2009). By minimizing outpatient visits for those with mild influenza-like illness, the self-diagnosed person is also self-isolated, concurrently reducing his opportunities to transmit the virus.

While the possibility of reducing the rate of transmission makes self-diagnosis of influenza highly desirable, it is not effective. A recent cross-sectional serosurvey of 1,141 individuals found that self-diagnosis of influenza was neither sensitive nor specific. Among adults, 23% of those who reported having had influenza were seropositive for H1N1, but among those reporting no influenza, 21% were also seropositive (Jutel et al. 2011).

This rush to self-diagnosis results in two potential liabilities. Researchers recently reported delays in treatment for potentially life-threatening illnesses that resulted from the incorrect diagnosis of influenza (Houlihan et al. 2010). Further, along with self-diagnosis comes self-treatment, and in many cases the rush to obtain certain treatments like oseltamivir (Tamiflu), which has been released in many countries as an OTC medication, creates the same commercial forces and potential conflicts as described above.

What makes this case interesting is that medicine, through the push for improved public health, has deemed that self-diagnosis is acceptable in this instance, but it vigorously refutes its utility in lay-led, contested conditions where the consequences of misdiagnosis are arguably no more severe (see, e.g., Brown 1995). This selective acceptance of self-diagnosis confirms the authoritative role of medicine, even while it enables individuals to decide for themselves what ails them. With respect to influenza infection, medicine remains the custodian of the diagnosis but determines who its delegates should be.

Self-diagnosis may present challenges not only to the doctor but also to the compliant "patient." While contemporary "consumers" may participate in their health care in new and autonomous ways, authorized self-diagnosis is nonetheless transformative and complex. As Henwood et al.'s (2003) research showed, many individuals do not wish to assume responsibility for medical information and decision making. They indicated that it was the "doctor's job" and that ignorance about such matters was a relief, rather than a source of disempowerment. The skills required to seek, source, and appraise information are not within the ability, or even the interest, of all people.

There are no clear binaries to guide the incorporation of self-diagnosis into contemporary health management. It is a complex matter because it is a relational one, tightly bound in the ways in which laypeople and doctors position themselves and interact relative to one another.

WHAT NEXT?

In spite of these changing dynamics, lay and expert knowledge each retain their traditional position in the layperson-doctor hierarchy. Medicine gets the last word in the consulting room. This inequitable balance can explain the contested diagnoses discussed in chapter 11. It also explains why doctors and laypeople alike experience the integration of new players previously external to the lay-professional relationship (such as technology and pharmaceutical firms, DTCA, disease advocacy groups, managed care, and others) as introducing both vulnerability and empowerment.

Diagnosis brings the layperson and professional together in a curiously intimate and consequential way, with the goal of achieving a better understanding of a problematic state of being. The ideal encounter is explanatory, predictive, and curative. But, as Blaxter (2009) asks, "What is the place of the patient in the co-production of a diagnosis?" In the presence of new technologies, must the patient vanish? Similarly, we should perhaps ask, "Where does the doctor go in this new era of the patient consumer-expert-advocate?"

New models for the doctor-patient relationship abound. They focus on partnerships (Williamson 1999), concordance (Mullen 1997), coprovision (Buetow 2005), interpretation (Leder 1990), negotiation, productive alliance (Filc 2006), and homogilisation (Buetow et al. 2008). The patient may be involved, expert, compliant, autonomous, or resourceful. But for the majority these models focus on transformation of the patient *identity* within the dominant biomedical model. Medicine is still the final authority and enables patient participation, albeit on a short leash. The "expert patients" manage their own care: monitoring symptoms, using the appropriate treatment, knowing how to optimize their well-being, and generally managing their illness independently from the doctor (Wilson 2001). This patient expertise implies compliance to the medical model, including acceptance of medicine's definition of disease. Yet, as Julia Neuberger has written, "active" and "patient" are contradictory terms (Wilson 2001, 135).

These models do not all take into account the constant diagnostic work done by nonmedical individuals outside of the consulting room and hospital setting: the self-monitoring to determine whether some action needs to be taken and whether that action requires the expert assistance of the medically trained, and the monitoring of others (e.g., parents overseeing their children) to note symptoms, name conditions, provide advice, and consider treatment options. The spheres of medical and lay diagnosis come together in the consulting room, and through that interaction a label is determined; the patient response to that label is often obscured to the doctor when the patient has left the room. Diagnosis does lie at the heart of medical practice, but it is worth bearing in mind that diagnosis is also a ubiquitous and everyday activity for us all.

TAKEAWAY POINTS

- In contrast to the traditional view, a diagnosis is a negotiated label.
- Patients may come to a doctor after already undertaking much diagnostic work.
- The patient experience of illness might not align with the disease categories used in diagnosis.
- Many factors, such as the rise in the use of alternative therapies and wider availability of health information, have challenged the doctor's diagnostic authority.

DISCUSSION QUESTIONS

1. Recall the last time you went to see a doctor. What were the factors that prompted you to seek medical intervention?
2. Of these factors, could any of them be considered (in another setting, or with a different combination of factors, perhaps) to belong to a jurisdiction other than medicine's? Which? Would you have preferred to have handled the problem on your own? What prevented you from doing so?
3. Reflecting on a lay-professional encounter you have experienced, either as clinician or as recipient of care, jot down the two perspectives as stories. Which is the lay story, and what is the professional story? Are they the same? At what points do they differ? How do the points of difference present challenges for each party?
4. How might you encourage a patient to tell her story and to speak on her own terms, rather than on yours? How might you reconcile such a story with the diagnostic task?

REFERENCES

Bailey, N. N. 1764. *An Universal Etymological English Dictionary: Comprehending the Derivations of the Generality of Words in the English Tongue, Either Ancient or Modern, from the Ancient British, Saxon, Danish, Norman and Modern French, Teutonic, Dutch, Spanish, Italian; as Also from the Latin, Greek and Hebrew Languages, Each in Their Proper Characters*. London.
Balint, M. 1964. *The Doctor, His Patient and the Illness*. 2nd ed. Kent: Pitman Medical.

Blaxter, M. 2009. "The Case of the Vanishing Patient? Image and Experience." *Sociology of Health and Illness* 31(5): 762–78.

Brown, P. 1995. "Naming and Framing: The Social Construction of Diagnosis and Illness." *Journal of Health and Social Behavior* 35: 34–52.

Brown, P., and S. Zavestoski. 2004. "Social Movements in Health: An Introduction." *Sociology of Health and Illness* 26(6): 679–94.

Buetow, S. 2005. "To Care Is to Coprovide." *Annals of Family Medicine* 3(6): 553–55.

Buetow, S., A. Jutel, and K. Hoare. 2008. "Shrinking Social Space in the Doctor-Modern Patient Relationship: A Review of Forces for, and Implications of, Homologisation." *Patient Education and Counseling* 74(10): 97–103.

Centers for Disease Control and Prevention. 2009. "Interim Guidance on Infection Control Measures for 2009 H1N1 Influenza in Healthcare Settings, Including Protection of Healthcare Personnel." http://www.cdc.gov/h1n1flu/guidelines_infection_control .htm.

CFIDS Association of America. 2009. "Diagnosis: Do I Have CFS?" http://www.cfids.org /about-cfids/do-i-have-cfids.asp.

Chadwick, J., and W. N. Mann, trans. 1983. *Hippocratic Writings*, edited by G. E. R. Lloyd. London: Penguin.

Chaucer, G. *Canterbury Tales*. Electronic Literature Foundation, http://www.canterbu rytales.org/canterbury_tales.html.

Clark, J. A., and E. G. Mishler. 1992. "Attending to Patients' Stories: Reframing the Clinical Task." *Sociology of Health and Illness* 14(3): 344–72.

De Swaan, A. 1989. "The Reluctant Imperialism of the Medical Profession." *Social Science and Medicine* 28(11): 1165–70.

Dew, K., K. Chamerblain, D. Hodgetts, P. Norris, A. Radley, and J. Gabe. Forthcoming. "Home as a Hybrid Centre of Medication Practice." *Sociology of Health and Illness* doi:10.1111/1467-9566.12041.

Emanuel, E. J., and L. L. Emanuel. 1992. "Four Models of the Physician-Patient Relationship." *JAMA* 267(16): 2221–26.

Fanany, R., and D. Fanany. 2012. *Health as a Social Experience*. South Yarra: Palgrave Macmillan.

Ferris, D. G., C. Dekle, and M. S. Litaker. 1996. "Women's Use of Over-the-Counter Antifungal Medications for Gynecologic Symptoms." *Journal of Family Practice* 42(6): 595–600.

Ferris, D. G., P. Nyirjesy, J. D. Sobel, D. Soper, A. Pavletic, and M. S. Litaker. 2002. "Over-the-Counter Antifungal Drug Misuse Associated with Patient-Diagnosed Vulvovaginal Candidiasis." *Obstetrics and Gynecology* 99(3): 419–25.

Filc, D. 2006. "Power in the Primary Care Medical Encounter: Domination, Resistance and Alliances." *Social Theory and Health* 4: 221–43.

Fleischman, S. 1999. "I Am . . . , I Have . . . , I Suffer from . . . : A Linguist Reflects on the Language of Illness and Disease." *Journal of Medical Humanities* 20(1): 3–32.

Foucault, M. 1963. *Naissance de la clinique*. Paris: Presses Universitaires de France.

Frank, A. W. 1995. *The Wounded Storyteller: Body, Illness and Ethics*. Chicago: University of Chicago Press.

Freidson, E. 1972. *Profession of Medicine: A Study of the Sociology of Applied Knowledge*. 4th ed. New York: Dodd, Mead.

Gurwitz, J. H., T. J. McLaughlin, and L. S. Fish. 1995. "The Effect of an R_x-to-OTC Switch on Medication Prescribing Patterns and Utilization of Physician Services: The Case of Vaginal Antifungal Products." *Health Services Research* 30(5): 672–85.

Harrington, P., and M. D. Shepherd. 2002. "Analysis of the Movement of Prescription Drugs to Over-the-Counter Status." *Journal of Managed Care Pharmacy* 8(6): 499–511.

Healy, D. 2006. "The Latest Mania: Selling Bipolar Disorder." *PLoS Medicine* 3(4): e185, doi:10.1371/journal.pmed.0030185.

Henwood, F., S. Wyatt, A. Hart, and J. Smith. 2003. "'Ignorance Is Bliss Sometimes': Constraints on the Emergence of the 'Informed Patient' in the Changing Landscapes of Health Information." *Sociology of Health and Illness* 25(6): 589–607.

Hesse, B. W., D. E. Nelson, G. L. Kreps, R. T. Croyle, N. K. Arora, B. K. Rimer, and K. Viswanath. 2005. "Trust and Sources of Health Information: The Impact of the Internet and Its Implications for Health Care Providers: Findings from the First Health Information National Trends Survey." *Archives of Internal Medicine* 165(22): 2618–24.

Houlihan, C. F., S. Patel, D. A. Price, M. Valappil, and U. Schwab. 2010. "Life Threatening Infections Labelled Swine Flu." *BMJ* 340: c137, doi:http://dx.doi.org/10.1136/bmj.c137.

Hunter, K. M. 1991. *Doctors' Stories*. Princeton, NJ: Princeton University Press.

Jewson, N. 1976. "Disappearance of the Sick-Man from Medical Cosmologies, 1770–1870." *Sociology* 10: 225–44.

Jutel, A., M. G. Baker, J. Stanley, Q. S. Huang, and D. Bandaranayake. 2011. "Self-Diagnosis of Influenza during a Pandemic: A Cross-Sectional Survey." *BMJ Open* 1: e000234, doi:10.1136/bmjopen-2011-000234.

Kleinman, A. 1988. *The Illness Narratives: Suffering, Healing, and the Human Condition*. New York: Basic.

Kleinman, A., L. Eisenberg, and B. Good. 1978. "Culture, Illness, and Care: Clinical Lessons from Anthropologic and Cross-Cultural Research." *Annals of Internal Medicine* 88(2): 251–58.

Leder, D. 1990. "Clinical Interpretation: The Hermeneutics of Medicine." *Theoretical Medicine* 11: 9–24.

Light, D., and S. Levine. 1988. "The Changing Character of the Medical Profession: A Theoretical Overview." *Milbank Quarterly* 66: 10–32.

Lupton, D. 1997a. "Consumerism, Reflexivity and the Medical Encounter." *Social Science and Medicine* 45(3): 373–81.

———. 1997b. "Doctors on the Medical Profession." *Sociology of Health and Illness* 19(4): 480–97.

Monistat. 2013. "Get the Cure. Get MONISTAT." July 24, http://www.monistat.com.

McLaughlin, H. 2009. "What's in a Name: 'Client,' 'Patient,' 'Customer,' 'Consumer,' 'Expert by Experience,' 'Service User'—What's Next?" *British Journal of Social Work* 39(6): 1101–17.

Mintzes, B., M. L. Barer, R. L. Kravitz, A. Kazanjian, K. Bassett, J. Lexchin, R. G. Evans, R. Pan, and S. A. Marion. 2002. "Influence of Direct to Consumer Pharmaceutical Advertising and Patients' Requests on Prescribing Decisions: Two Site Cross Sectional Survey." *BMJ* 324(7332): 278–79.

Mullen, P. D. 1997. "Compliance Becomes Concordance." *BMJ* 314(7082): 691–92.

Nettleton, S. 2004. "The Emergence of E-Scaped Medicine." *Sociology* 38(4): 661–79.

Nettleton, S., L. O'Malley, I. Watt, and P. Duffey. 2004. "Enigmatic Illness: Narratives of Patients Who Live with Medically Unexplained Symptoms." *Social Theory and Health* 2(1): 47–66.

Porter, R. 1987. *Disease, Medicine and Society in England, 1550–1860*. Basingstoke: Macmillan.

Robinson, G. C. 1939. *The Patient as Person: A Study of the Social Aspects of Illness*. New York: Commonwealth Fund.

Wen, Leana. 2013. "The Low-Tech Revolution to Health Care Reform." *Huffington Post*, July 22, http://www.huffingtonpost.com/leana-wen-md/doctor-mistakes_b_3628808.html?utm_hp_ref=tw.

Williamson, C. 1999. "The Challenge of Lay Partnership: It Provides a Different View of the World." *BMJ* 319(7212): 721–22.

Wilson, P. M. 2001. "A Policy Analysis of the Expert Patient in the United Kingdom: Self-Care as an Expression of Pastoral Power?" *Health and Social Care in the Community* 9(3): 134–42.

When the Penny Drops
Diagnosis and the Transformative Moment

Annemarie Goldstein Jutel

STARTING POINTS

- The moment of diagnostic disclosure, when the disease is serious, is difficult for patient and diagnostician alike.
- Strong communication skills and best-practice protocols may help a diagnostician communicate a serious diagnosis.
- Patients may not respond to a diagnosis in the way that a clinician expects.

We have discussed how important a diagnosis is in providing direction. Like a map, the diagnosis reveals the road ahead and suggests which way to turn. By labeling an illness, we are able to predict its outcome, suggest treatments, and explain its ins and outs. We can do so because treatment and prognosis are so closely linked to diagnosis. A diagnosis explains the relationship between symptoms and findings, and predicts what will happen next. It's hard for anyone to plan life around an illness without a diagnosis. Symptoms may be random or linked, incidental or pathognomonic, trivial or grave. In the absence of diagnosis, causation is obscure and treatment tentative at best. Naming the ailment is usually the doctor's first step in seeking a cure.

The process of diagnosis may be slow and progressive, a weighing-up of physical findings, laboratory results, working hypotheses, trial, and error. Or it may happen almost spontaneously, ushered in by an indisputable sign, an unequivocal profile. But regardless of how a diagnosis is arrived upon, once it is settled, for all but the most trivial of complaints, there is a shift in more than just treatment. Even if only temporarily, the way in which a life is lived and understood is disrupted.

The **diagnostic moment** may turn the world on its head, instantly transforming the individual's approach to life itself. With serious diagnosis may also come changes in **identity**. You went to the doctor thinking you had the flu and you left with leukemia. You had a blood test and became diabetic. But even if your diagnosis was only bronchitis, you were not the same as when you went in. Today is somehow different from yesterday. You have a newly organized sense of what your experiences mean. The more serious the diagnosis, the more significant the shift. Suzanne Fleischman (1999), in her poignant discussion of her own (ultimately fatal) disease, explained that "the verbal act of presenting a **patient** with a diagnosis is never a simple act of conveying value-neutral biomedical information. It is an act fraught with symbolism. If a person is told 'you have cancer' (or any life-threatening disease) *these words* irrevocably alter that person's consciousness, view of the future, relationships with family and friends, and so on. Moreover, the utterance marks a boundary. It serves to divide a life into 'before' and 'after,' and this division is henceforth superimposed onto every rewrite of the individual's life story" (10).

A number of practices in medicine acknowledge the power of this transformative moment. Think, for example, of HIV testing. In the early days of the disease, a positive diagnosis meant difficult treatment followed by certain death. The disclosure of results was surrounded by precaution. Standard protocol required that negative and positive results be delivered face to face. A return appointment was routinely booked at the time of the original blood test, which was the standard practice not only so the individual could be helped through the diagnostic moment in case of a positive test, but also so that a return visit wouldn't generate undue anxiety. Otherwise, being asked to come back to the clinic could suggest to the individual that they were in the grasp of a fatal illness with no exit.

Some cultures actually consider that the transformative power of diagnosis is too powerful for a layperson to endure. In France, historically and still to a certain extent today, *patients* did not necessarily receive a diagnosis if it was serious. Fearful of psychological fallout from a terminal diagnosis, doctors, and sometimes family, tended to keep bad diagnoses from the afflicted individual (Reich and Mekaoui 2003). Shifts in the approach to disclosure now have French oncologists following a carefully prescribed list of steps designed to "respect the weight of the diagnosis and the emotions which it may generate" (Institut National du Cancer 2005, 7).

An Italian study asked 675 doctors whether patients should be told if they had cancer. About 45% of participants believed, in principle, that they should be. But in practice, only 25% reported that they always disclosed the diagnosis (Grassi et al. 2000). This discrepancy underlines the difficulty of communicating bad news, the complexity of diagnostic disclosure, and the impact of diagnosis on the individual. Neither doctors nor families are always convinced that truth telling will be "good" for the patient.

A diagnosis can provide transformative relief as well as dread. To have an explanation for a persistent ailment may reduce its significance as much as it may confirm the worst. As one example, the convoluted pathway that leads to the diagnosis of epilepsy can appease one and shock another. Schneider and Conrad's (1983) work on people's experience of epilepsy demonstrated both outcomes. One of their interviewees commented: "it was a relief. I mean if you thought you had a brain tumor, wouldn't *you* be relieved to know that it was something as simple as epilepsy?" (74). Others were devastated by the same diagnosis. "I was kind of numb," said one woman. "It didn't really hit me until after I had gotten out of the hospital. What they said was just like so shocking to me that everything else just didn't register" (72).

IDENTITY: WHAT DOES IT MEAN TO BE ME?

To say that diagnosis is transformative is to recognize the impact that a medical diagnosis can have on an individual's identity. Identity is not a simple concept. It is experienced from within, but it is also shaped from the outside. It is an assemblage of all the elements that make each one of us who we are. Some of our identity comes from our relationships within groups and social networks. We can identify as straight or queer, black or white, Jewish or atheist. But identity also comes from the notion of a self, one with persistent characteristics, and a more or less cohesive collection of stories, intentions, and dreams. In the paragraphs that follow, we review some theories of identity and then explore the role of identity in the diagnostic moment. We conclude with some lay and professional perspectives on the tasks of diagnosis, and consider how we might minimize the negative impacts of diagnostic disclosure.

The story of our life captures our identity. This is not the story as told by someone else; rather, it's the story we tell as we highlight meaningful events, explain our reactions, pick out a plot, and order characters and narrative. What we select to tell, and how we decide to tell it, is revealing of our sense of self. As Mathieson and Stam (1995) write, "constructions of narrative order are essential in providing one's life with meaning and a sense of direction for the future." Our identity is part of an ever-shifting interweaving of possibility and realization: a mix of what we think we can be, and what we end up doing (Frank 1993). These two threads may fluctuate in importance over a lifetime. The thread of possibility is based on the sometimes-stable sense of a life course, of what the social dynamic is likely to be, and of how we will interact with our environment.

Social interaction both depends on and changes who we are. We are never solely responsible for our social roles. To be a "doting grandmother," for example, involves being part of a social network with a particular set of normative expectations including support and reciprocity. It probably also involves being able to pick up and speak to one's grandchild, a possibility that is restricted by a debilitating stroke or motor neuron disease. Not being able to fulfill the expectations of the network turns relationships on their head and submits its members to new kinds of connections involving different protagonists. It involves recognizing "the worlds of pain and suffering, possibly even of death, which are normally only seen as distant possibilities or the plight of others" (Bury 1982, 169).

Identity studies straddle the disciplines of psychology and sociology because identity is couched in the personal (internal) and the social (relational). Erik Erikson, whose theories of identity underpin numerous theories of developmental psychology, described identity as "the awareness of self-sameness . . . and continuity . . . [and] the style of one's individuality [that] coincides with the sameness and continuity of one's meaning for others in the immediate community" (quoted in Schwartz 2001, 8). Erikson speaks about "identity synthesis," which is the way an individual positions and directs features of her personality toward a set of self-determined ideals. This is what Erikson calls a "present with an anticipated future." His theories, as well as those of others who followed him (see, e.g., Berzonsky and Adams 1999; Marcia 1988; van Hoof 1999), focus on the work involved in identity construction, both conscious and subconscious. One isn't born with an identity. Rather, through various life stages, one gathers information about one's self, adheres to goals and values, and develops a sense of purpose and continuity (Marcia 1980).

Identity is thus anchored in plans and expectations, in stability over one's life course, and in those activities that are central to how we narrate or describe ourselves. Disease can shake these foundations and alter life plans, however. Opportunities are narrowed by the potential physical, social, and emotional constraints of the illness. Activities must be adjusted to declining physical capacity. Where a nondiagnosed individual has relative autonomy over life directions, the sense of autonomy is compromised as a new actor enters the scene. The diagnosis brings its own identity, creating an overlay with new configurations of the present and the future.

Sociologist Pierre Bourdieu (1984) speaks of a concept he calls **habitus**, which is helpful for understanding our response to a shift in identity. Habitus is a set of skills and dispositions that are formed by processes of **socialization**, our experiences, and the particular social and cultural setting in which these processes take place.

> It used to be I was just me. Now, I am me and the cancer. I've got all the rest of my life, but it always has a shadow that comes with it and even crowds the rest out. It's never not there.
>
> *Diagnosis creates an overlay that may displace other parts of identity.*

This habitus is shaped by, and in turn facilitates access to, different forms of economic, cultural, and social capital or resources that help us negotiate this change. In brief, economic capital refers to material resources. **Cultural capital,** on the other hand, is a product of education and upbringing, including the values and habits that are passed on to us. Our cultural capital provides us with status in particular spheres, from our capacity to savor fine wine to the credentials we carry as diagnosticians. Cultural capital could include health literacy. And social capital refers to the network of relations that can provide various forms of support (but also obligation). Being connected to particular social groups or individuals may enhance our capacity to learn about our diagnosis, to find out what other people do, and to access therapeutic practices.

So our identity and social position shape our habitus and provide us with different capacities to negotiate the social world. The ways in which diagnoses transform us, the possibilities of transformation, are enhanced and constrained by our habitus. With higher levels of certain forms of capital, we may have more opportunities to experience a positive transformation in the face of a serious diagnosis. Accumulated capital carried by individuals facilitates the successful negotiation of different **institutions** and arenas, or of what Bourdieu refers to as **fields**. In this sense, our habitus and its related cultural resources influence opportunities for health gains (Abel 2007).

IDENTITY, ILLNESS, AND DISEASE

"Being sick" interferes with many of the elements that construct an individual's identity. So does "being diagnosed," but in a different (albeit sometimes overlapping) way. We return for a moment to the **illness-disease dichotomy** to clarify this point. Recall that making a distinction between illness and disease is helpful from a sociological perspective.

Illness is the physical dysfunction identified by an individual as being medical in nature and as worthy of presentation to the diagnostician. The patient consults the doctor to develop an organizing explanation of his ailments for confirmation and perhaps—in the current era of increasing patient autonomy and knowledge—to propose the diagnosis (see Balint's [1964] model of doctor-patient interaction). But patients' proposed diagnoses are often unacknowledged or not responded to by the expert diagnostician (the reasons why are complicated and are, at least in part, a result of patients presenting their diagnoses during the history-taking phase of a consultation, a phase during which diagnostic decisions are not usually voiced; Gill and Maynard 2006).

Illness, or being sick, implies an alteration in physical capacity, experience, or perception. This in and of itself may affect an individual's sense of identity, as changes in functional status interfere with both individual and social expectations. As in the grandmothering example above, not being able to pick up a grandchild alters one's role, which in turn may have an impact on identity. The physical consequences of illness often diminish personal autonomy, limiting, for example, what one can eat or drink, the hobbies in which one can engage, and the place one assumes at work or in the family.

Diagnosis, on the other hand, is a social transaction in which a particular illness (or, in some cases, the threat of an illness) receives an agreed-upon label that in turn has its own set of impacts upon identity. According to Englehardt (1992), one of the important functions of diagnosis is to give a sense of direction to the person so diagnosed: "One invests labor in making a diagnosis not simply in order to know truly, but because one would hope to be able to avoid or mitigate some unpleasant state of affairs. In the case of prognosis, one wants at least to be able to plan for likely unpleasant future developments" (73).

With diagnosis comes organization of the physical symptoms around an explanatory framework. Treatment can now be prescribed, and a prognosis made. Prognosis has a potentially powerful impact on identity. Like identity, prognosis sets a blueprint for the future competing with, challenging, and shifting one's life story, personal values, and intention. Future direction is modified, compromised, or even nonexistent. We have all probably imagined what it would be like to have cancer, Alzheimer disease, or leukemia, and our make-believe scenarios test how we would find ourselves with a new, shaky sense of direction.

The diagnostic moment may be punctual and discrete, or part of a buildup toward a finalizing instant. Fleischman (1999) described it as a critical turning point. "Out of the blue," she wrote, "my life plan was radically altered, my future thrown into question" (3). Others have described the diagnosis as a culmination of a slow process, progressively shedding light on the soon to be obvious. Precursor symptoms, multistaged testing, numerous experts, and consultations progressively prepare the individual for the diagnosis (Schaepe 2011). But even where the buildup has been more progressive, the diagnostic moment is nonetheless significant.

> I felt this cold feeling come through me, and I was frozen. I couldn't talk or even react to the news the doctor just gave me. I just sat there—numb.
>
> *Learning a serious diagnosis can be devastating.*

The way in which serious diagnoses are disclosed may be more or less identity preserving. Who tells the news? How and where do they tell it? The significance of the diagnosis to the sense of self will vary by individual, by culture, and by disease. What might sound trivial to one person may be devastating to another. Imagine the variable impact of a diagnosis of allergic chronic laryngitis on a data-entry operator, or an opera singer. Now imagine these same people hearing a diagnosis of peripheral neuropathy.

Diagnosis can also wreak havoc with identity even when a person is not sick. Genetic mapping and other forms of screening can reveal information about disease potential ahead of the appearance of any symptoms. An individual can be notified of pending disease or of the potential to transmit disease. For example, genetic mutations of BRCA1 or 2 indicate a high potential for malignant breast cancer, mutations in the HTT gene denote Huntington disease, and H8 and H9 genetic mutations are associated with hemophilia. With ever-increasing exploration of the human genome, more links between genetic makeup and diagnoses are being made, and genetic testing has wedged itself into regular clinical practice.* A bout with iritis

> The doctor came in to my room. My friend was visiting from work. And there was a nurse aid just tidying up my table. He pulled the curtain part way, but it didn't close. I know that because I could still see the lady in the other bed, so I suppose she could see me too. Anyway, those curtains aren't soundproof. And just like that, he told me my cancer had come back.
>
> *How a diagnosis is disclosed matters.*

might be followed by a blood test for HLAB27 (a common genetic finding in patients with iritis), a harbinger of other conditions such as ankylosing spondylitis, psoriasis, and Crohn disease.

Because it is so revelatory, genetic diagnosis may profoundly alter the perception of one's identity. Its composite picture of an individual's chromosomal makeup presents a certain kind of "truth" about the nature of the individual. Couched in terms of empirical **positivism**, this "truth" can be at odds with subjective† experience.

---

*Even though many of the diseases that worry us the most—such as heart disease or cancer—are multigenetic and the presence or absence of single genes has little to no predictive value.
†The word "subjective" has different meanings in science and philosophy. From a scientific perspective (perhaps more familiar to readers of this text), **subjectivity** is likely linked with the idea of nonneutrality and has a negative connotation in empirical research. A subjective perspective is linked to an individual's perception rather than to externally measurable data. Here, in the case of subjective experience, we refer to those feelings that are unique to the individual person. Subjectivity is a mark of personhood and individuality. It is subjectivity

As David Armstrong et al. (1998) have written, exploring the genetic map may spoil the sense of self, delivering a stigmatizing label that extends beyond the individual to her relatives. The identity of the individual self then becomes interlinked with a wider web of identities. Here the relational nature is based on genetic and social factors. These authors argue that geneticization causes this identity shift to be something other than a "new" identity; rather, it is a disclosure of one's previously concealed "real" identity.

Genetic screening describes the supposed social risk presented by a particular profile, giving individuals the potential to respond to their future and to plan for healthy offspring. But the genetic movement has difficulty shifting its eugenic roots (Kerr and Cunningham-Burley 2000). The potential to detect genetic predispositions for disease may lead to discriminatory practices reminiscent of eugenic practices such as selective breeding and "racial hygiene." This potential is notable in insurance coverage, where genetic testing and future technologies offer a new range of risk profiles that insurers may be loath to assume.

DESCRIBING IDENTITY

Mildred Blaxter presents identity as plot, which makes sense in the context of our discussion above. A plot, like identity, is temporal in nature and includes a past, present, and future. Yet diagnosis shifts the future expectation, and even, as Blaxter expounds, the past. When people tell illness narratives, they may give new meanings to past events as a way of connecting the dots. A personal story starts to take a different form. The new story line requires an adjustment: the childhood rugby injury, the frequent respiratory infections, or the exposure to garden chemicals may now be part of today's gout, chronic obstructive pulmonary disease, or aplastic anemia. A different story emerges out of, or explains, an illness identity.

Rewriting the past is common after a life-changing diagnosis. In order to make sense of a series of previously unconnected events, a certain reorganization is imperative. It enables us to see our lives as logical continuums, which in turn allows us to assert our identity (Blaxter 2004).

What Blaxter makes clear is that health and identity are inextricably linked. She sees a circular relationship between the two in the construction of the personal narrative. An individual can be poked and prodded by disease in ways beyond her control. Yet self-identity is determined by the stories we tell about our responses to, or even responsibility for, these ailments.

According to Arthur Frank (1993), diagnosis offers an opportunity for redemption and personal reorganization. Many people write about surviving serious diseases. They publicly share their experience of illness to make sense of what they have experienced, or perhaps to propose a model for survival. Frank focuses on how the illness provides an opportunity for redemption. As mentioned above, the

---

that we must respect, and indeed pursue (rather than control), because the individual subject is the focus of medical care.

disease alters the meaning and direction of life. As it does, though, it provides an epiphany from which the individual can emerge, phoenix-like, from the ashes. Disease lays bare the nature of the self, providing an opportunity to reconstruct oneself afresh and to create a new existence. The illness narrative, says Frank, contains a memory of the past, but also defines what one has become.

Michael Bury (1982) wrote about how the experience of illness changed people's lives and direction, referring to it as **biographical disruption**. Illness is a major event, one that disrupts and unsettles. It radically interrupts daily routines and introduces worlds previously only imagined. Bury's notion of biographical disruption highlights the fact that chronic illness disturbs the structures upon which daily life is anchored. We then require new forms of knowledge to make sense of life and to negotiate social interactions. One useful example for understanding this biographical disruption is described in the work of Daniele Carricaburu and Janine Pierret (1995), who describe how HIV-positive men respond to their diagnosis.

Receiving a diagnosis of HIV infection led the men they interviewed to make significant organizational changes in their daily lives. First, because of the stigmatizing nature of their diagnosis, maintaining (or not) secrecy was a central issue. Deciding whether to tell, and if so, who to tell, changed the nature of their relationships. There was often a redefinition of "closeness." Second, they reviewed their personal situations, mobilizing resources as a result. Some attempted to maintain their lives using the resources they had always known, while others pursued new avenues, including medicine, activist networks, and relationships. Finally, all fought uncertainty. Some of these men did so, ironically, by taking risks, others by taking extreme care (Carricaburu and Pierret 1995). The point here is that the biographical disruption of diagnosis may require a complete redirection of personal life or, alternatively, significant effort in order to keep on the same track.

> The radiographer came out and her face was white. She said: "He [the radiologist] wants me to look at this more carefully." I went white too, and it was like my heart stopped. I said, "what'd you see?" She said: "There's this big white spot. See?" and she pointed to this, yeah, big white spot on the picture of my breasts. I said OK, and she took another series of scans, and then "he" said he wanted an ultrasound too. So we did that, and then I had to wait. While I was waiting, I went outside, and smoked like four cigarettes, so that I could just keep breathing. And in the end, it wasn't a tumor, and I was so relieved. On my way home, I went straight to the drug store and bought some nicotine gum, and I haven't smoked since. The threat of breast cancer, even if cigarettes don't cause it, just made me rethink how I was living.
>
> *From a diagnosis may emerge the opportunity for redemption and reconstruction of self.*

COLLECTIVE HEALTH IDENTITIES

A serious diagnosis with future- or function-altering impact can, in some cases, provide a new sense of identity. Particularly in today's Internet era, diagnosis serves as a focal point for collective identity and political action. With a diagnosis, one can seek others with similar conditions for support, ideas, activism, and community.

Klawiter's (1999) work on cultures of breast cancer provides a model for understanding the collective impact of diagnosis. Having breast cancer can be experienced beyond the individual and in different ways, according to particular agendas within what could be called a breast cancer movement. This cancer activism, argued Klawiter, revolves around distinct cultures representing different collective perspectives. Her description of the breast cancer movement in the 1990s includes different threads of activism, including the victorious cancer sufferer participant in medicine's battle and the sufferer suspicious of the pharmaceutical industry and corporate pollution and collusion. They are all embodied health movements linked to the diagnosis of breast cancer, but each has its own specific political and collective frames of action.

An embodied health movement hinges on the experience of individuals with a particular disease who are seeking to challenge, often in cahoots with scientists and health professionals, existing medical and scientific knowledge and practice (see also chap. 7 on authority; Brown et al. 2004). These movements are a form of collective action that is directly linked to diagnosis. Examples of embodied health movements include tobacco control, Gulf War veteran groups, and the AIDS movement. These movements have sought recognition of causal links (tobacco and lung disease), of disease entities (posttraumatic stress disorder, or PTSD), and of the urgency for developing treatments for life-threatening illnesses (AIDS).

The breast cancer activism described by Klawiter provides a useful example of the various identities that women with breast cancer assume. Identities can shift, in the same individual, around chronologically distinct diagnoses of breast cancer (Klawiter 2004). The agendas, identities, social relations, policies, and emotional vocabularies at various times transform how a person might understand breast cancer, and in turn can transform the personal narrative of someone with the disease. Klawiter's research included interviewing a woman who was diagnosed with breast cancer at two different points in time. She reconceptualized her identity in response to the different public discourses on breast cancer during each episode.

There are a number of distinct cultures that formed around breast cancer in the mid-1990s. The Race for the Cure, established by a breast cancer foundation in memory of a woman who died from breast cancer, typifies one of these cultures. The goal of Race for the Cure was to improve awareness of the disease and to raise funds for breast cancer research. The race became a symbol of breast cancer advocacy. In this movement, women who have had breast cancer are identified as survivors, provided with pink visors, lauded for their courage, and celebrated for their willingness to be visible and to reject any sense of shame or **stigma** associated with the disease (Klawiter 1999).

There are alternative constructions of collective identity among people with breast cancer. Klawiter described Breast Cancer Action (BCA), which, like Race for the Cure, is still active fifteen years after her original publication. Unlike Race for the Cure, however, BCA challenges the rationale, treatment, and screening of breast cancer. BCA (2011) says that "the cancer industry consists of corporations, organizations, and agencies that diminish or mask the extent of the cancer problem, fail to protect our health, or divert attention away from the importance of funding and working to prevent the disease." The highly politicized movement does not kow-tow to the powerful medical establishment. Rather, they question conflicts of interest in what Adele Clarke et al. (2003) refer to as the "Biomedical TechnoService Complex, Inc.," the ever-expanding sector of politicoeconomic and sociocultural biomedicine. The alliance between the commercial interests of the pharmaceutical industry and medical research results in a fuzzy boundary with which BCA is dissatisfied. Even as the pharmaceutical industry markets a cure for a cancer, for example, BCA argues that the same industry is causing cancer through its manufacture of highly toxic pesticides and insecticides (Klawiter 1999). The point here is not that there is a good or bad way to identify with breast cancer, rather that there are ways in which breast cancer becomes identified, and all of these ways affect how a woman will see herself: a victim, a survivor, or an activist.

Because of what Nettleton (2004) has referred to as the "e-scaping" of medicine, a growing number of diagnosis-focused communities have emerged on the Internet. Web pages assemble individuals around both existing and emerging diseases. Dumit (2006) explains that Internet communities offer a means of survival for sufferers of medically unexplained symptoms. They provide an alternative support structure when the absence of a diagnosis impugns the medical legitimacy of the individual's complaint. These communities "create their own separate and distinct medical culture, a culture that gives primary importance to the role of subjective experience" (Goldstein 2004, 127). An example of a virtual community serving to create an alternative culture are pro-anorexia sites that seek to redefine anorexia nervosa outside medical discourse, instead casting it as a sanctuary, a "place where control and purity [can] be found" (Fox et al. 2005, 958). Health providers have also launched Internet communities as site where patients can be transformed from consumers into a "community of practice" with potentially improved health outcomes (Winkelman and Choo 2003).

PRACTICE IMPLICATIONS

Robert Klitzman (2009) interviewed sixty-four individuals who according to genetic testing either had or were at risk of serious, life-changing diagnoses (Huntington disease, breast cancer, or alpha-1 antitrypsin deficiency). While his findings clearly indicated that diagnostic status had an impact on his research participants' sense of self, he also noted that some individuals constrained the space they would afford diagnosis in their individual identity. This reaction of some of the participants in Klitzman's study group provides a glimmer of hope for identity preservation in the presence of serious illness. There are also examples of people who refuse to take treatments in order to prevent the diagnosis from affecting their lives. While the diagnosis has a transformative impact, there are also protective reactions that both individuals and clinicians can foster. Klitzman underlines how the clinician should fully consider decisions about testing, disclosure, and treatment.

As other chapters in this book describe, the diagnosis both frames and is framed by the lay-professional relationship. The pursuit of diagnosis usually drives the

I am who I am. I had breast cancer. I beat it. I may get it again. I'll deal with it when I get it again, if I get it again.

Diagnosis is only one part of identity.

individual to the doctor for help; the ability to diagnose confers power and status to the diagnostician. It is on the doctor's word that resources are allocated, and, in the case of the transformation that this chapter describes, that identity shifts on diagnosis. Awareness of this relationship and the revolving power positions it contains (see chap. 7) should give the clinician pause. Considering who the patient is and how she perceives herself matters greatly. We can see how the patient in the second box on page 83 responded to being given a diagnosis by someone he didn't know. He was angry and defensive. Knowing him might have made a difference to the diagnostician and to the patient.

Anatole Broyard (1995), an American literary critic and essayist who wrote about his experience of prostate cancer, likely would have agreed. He described his ideal doctor as one who would know him: "I wouldn't demand a lot of my doctor's time; I just wish he would *brood* on my situation for perhaps five minutes . . . I would like to think of him as going through my character, as he goes through my flesh, to get at my illness, for each man is ill in his own way . . . just as he orders blood tests and bone scans . . . I'd like my doctor to scan *me* to grope for my spirit as well as my prostate" (179). Broyard's point is that he identifies himself as more than a mere medical project or a prostate. It is not uncommon, however, for medicine to reduce individuals to their diagnoses, using the diagnosis as synecdoches for the person ("You'll have a busy shift. You've got an infarct on the ward, and a V-tach on the unit"). Conversely, for some patients, personal disclosure is not something readily given because it can lead to a sense of losing control. By divulging our concerns we make ourselves vulnerable, so to do so requires either a high level of trust, a desperate need, or a sense of still being able to retain control (Dew et al. 2007).

Something that's really difficult is that I used to be a pianist. I've got a baby grand in my living room, and I played for weddings all around the town. But the terrible thing is that I can't feel my fingertips any more. It was both a combination of having disease in my nerves and the drugs they used to kill it. So, I am alive now. Right. But my fingers are all thick and clunky, and I can't play any better than my five-year-old grandson. I can't feel the keys any more. Yeah. I can't really call myself a pianist anymore.

The impact that diagnosis makes on how individuals see themselves may vary significantly from one person to another.

Knowing the individual includes a consideration of how the diagnosis may affect her. Is she physically active? What does she do for a living? What kind of social relationships and support structures does she have? What are her plans and values? It may seem as if a doctor has to know her patient for a lifetime to be able to answer such questions, but there are many opportunities for doctors to make these connections. Eric Cassell's words of a quarter century ago describe eloquently still today that the job of the doctor is more than treating diseases—it is treating patients who have diseases (Cassell 1976). Getting close to the patient's fears and concerns is as important as understanding the disease at the root of these worries. Every encounter with a patient provides a chance for rapprochement and personal exchange between the clinician and the layperson or, as Broyard suggests, a means of groping for the person's spirit.

Recognizing the challenges of communicating difficult diagnoses to patients, there are protocols that can serve as guides to clinicians. The SPIKES protocol (Baile et al. 2000) is one such tool, which presents a set of goals that are focused on improving communication by "gather[ing] information from the patient . . . provid[ing] intelligible information in accordance with the patient's needs and desires . . . support[ing] the patient by employing skills to reduce the emotional impact and isolation experienced by the recipient of bad news . . . [and] develop[ing] a strategy in the form of a treatment plan with the input and cooperation of the patient" (305). The protocol specifies a number of steps that a physician might use to put an individual at ease and to help them determine what treatment plan they would like to follow. Such protocols can usefully highlight issues of communication for diagnosticians, but they must also be used cautiously. Using them in a linear fashion can disrupt the intricate interactional work that is required to communicate delicate or sensitive issues to patients (Dew et al. 2010).

This particular protocol recognizes that diagnoses may be upsetting, and strives to help clinicians become empathetic, but it does not articulate the impact disease labels can have on the idea of the self. The focus is clearly on treatment and assisting the individual to identify the appropriate treatment regimen. We can safely say that whatever this may be will depend on the individual's sense of self, future priorities, and enduring values.

Diagnosis does more, as we said in the opening paragraphs, than explain a physical ailment and propose its treatment; it reorganizes how the diagnosed person sees herself and explains her life. This is a powerful feature, one that clinicians must consider with care. The discussion questions below offer ways to ask questions about identity at a personal level.

TAKEAWAY POINTS

- Diagnosis can introduce a shift in both the sense of identity and meaning an individual attributes to particular physical and social experiences.
- Identity is linked to social relationships and anchored in plans and expectations.
- Diagnosis may come as a relief when it clarifies or makes sense of dysfunction and links to a future management (or even elimination) of the problematic state.
- Understanding the impact of diagnosis is linked to understanding the social identity of the individual and the alteration the diagnosis will bring to a person's previous directions.

DISCUSSION QUESTIONS

1. Is the truth always necessary? What are some circumstances under which you might not tell a person their diagnosis?
2. Complete the following sentence below and explain how it helps define your identity: "I hope one day, I'll be able to ___ ."

3. Make a list of the roles you play in your life (woman, daughter, employee, activist, pet owner, etc.). How do these roles interact and intersect? Around which role do you organize most of your time and energy? What expectations do you and others link to each of these roles?

4. Name one physical and one psychiatric diagnosis that could interfere with the aspirations or sense of self you have identified above. Describe what steps you might take in the presence of either diagnosis to preserve your sense of who you are. What support structures or actions could help you maintain this identity? What additional actions might you need to take to preserve these roles? What aspects of your identity might shift or change?

5. What steps could you take to minimize the personal destabilization that comes from a life-altering diagnosis you are about to disclose?

REFERENCES

Abel, Thomas. 2007. "Cultural Capital in Health Promotion." In *Health and Modernity*, edited by D. McQueen, I. Kickbusch, J. M. Pelikan, L. Balbo, and T. Abel, 43–73. New York: Springer.

Armstrong, David, Susan Michie, and Theresa Marteau. 1998. "Revealed Identity: A Study of the Process of Genetic Counselling." *Social Science and Medicine* 47(11): 1653–58.

Baile, Walter F., Robert Buckman, Renato Lenzi, Gary Glober, Estela A. Beale, and Andrzej P. Kudelka. 2000. "SPIKES—A Six-Step Protocol for Delivering Bad News: Application to the Patient with Cancer." *Oncologist* 5(4): 302–11.

Balint, Michael. 1964. *The Doctor, His Patient and the Illness*. 2nd ed. Kent: Pitman Medical.

BCA. Breast Cancer Action. 2011. "Whose Interests Are Being Served?" http://bcaction .org.

Berzonsky, Michael D., and Gerald R. Adams. 1999. "Reevaluating the Identity Status Paradigm: Still Useful after 35 Years." *Developmental Review* 19(4): 557–90.

Blaxter, Mildred. 2004. "Life Narratives, Health and Identity." In *Identity and Health*, edited by David Kelleher and Gerard Leavey, xii. London: Routledge.

Bourdieu, Pierre. 1984. *Distinction: A Social Critique of the Judgement of Taste*. Cambridge, MA: Harvard University Press.

Brown, Phil, Stephen Zavestoski, Sabrina McCormick, Brian Mayer, Rachel Morello-Frosch, and Rebecca Gasior Altman. 2004. "Embodied Health Movements: New Approaches to Social Movements in Health." *Sociology of Health and Illness* 26(1): 50–80.

Broyard, Anatole. 1995. "Doctor, Talk to Me." In *On Doctoring*, edited by Richard Reynolds and John Stone, 175–81. New York: Simon and Schuster.

Bury, Michael. 1982. "Chronic Illness as Biographical Disruption." *Sociology of Health and Illness* 4(2): 167–82.

Carricaburu, Danièle, and Janine Pierret. 1995. "From Biographical Disruption to Biographical Reinforcement: The Case of HIV-Positive Men." *Sociology of Health and Illness* 17(1): 65–88.

Cassell, Eric J. 1976. *The Healer's Art: A New Approach to the Doctor-Patient Relationship*. Philadelphia: J. B. Lippincott.

Clarke, Adele E., Janet K. Shim, Laura Mamo, Jennifer Ruth Fosket, and Jennifer R. Fishman. 2003. "Biomedicalization: Technoscientific Transformations of Health, Illness, and U.S. Biomedicine." *American Sociological Review* 68(2): 161–94.

Dew, Kevin, Sonya Morgan, Anthony Dowell, Deborah McLeod, John Bushnell, and Sunny Collings. 2007. "'It Puts Things out of Your Control': Fear of Consequences as a Barrier to Patient Disclosure of Mental Health Issues to General Practitioners." *Sociology of Health and Illness* 29(7): 1059–74.

Dew, Kevin, Maria Stubbe, Lindsay Macdonald, Anthony Dowell, and Elizabeth Plumridge. 2010. "The (Non)Use of Prioritisation Protocols by Surgeons." *Sociology of Health and Illness* 32(4): 545–62.

Dumit, Joseph. 2006. "Illnesses You Have to Fight to Get: Facts as Forces in Uncertain, Emergent Illnesses." *Social Science and Medicine* 62(3): 577–90.

Engelhardt, H. Tristram. 1992. "The Body as a Field of Meaning: Implications for the Ethics of Diagnosis." In *The Ethics of Diagnosis*, edited by J. L. Peset and D Gracia, 75–77. Dortrecht: Springer.

Fleischman, Suzanne. 1999. "I Am . . . , I Have . . . , I Suffer From . . . : A Linguist Reflects on the Language of Illness and Disease." *Journal of Medical Humanities* 20(1): 3–32.

Fox, N., K. Ward, and A. O'Rourke. 2005. "Pro-Anorexia, Weight-Loss Drugs and the Internet: An 'Anti-Recovery' Explanatory Model of Anorexia." *Sociology of Health and Illness* 27(7): 944–71.

Frank, Arthur W. 1993. "The Rhetoric of Self-Change: Illness Experience as Narrative." *Sociological Quarterly* 34(1): 39–52.

Gill, V. T., and D. Maynard. 2006. "Explaining Illness: Patients' Proposals and Physicians' Responses." In *Communication in Medical Care: Interaction between Primary Care Physicians and Patients*, edited by J. Heritage and D. Maynard, 115–50. New York: Cambridge University Press.

Goldstein, D. E. 2004. "Communities of Suffering and the Internet." In *Emerging Illnesses and Society: Negotiating the Public Health Agenda*, edited by R. M. Packard, P. J. Brown, R. L. Berkelman, and H. Frumkin, 121–38. Baltimore: Johns Hopkins University Press.

Grassi, Luigi, Tullio Giraldi, E. G. Messina, K. Magnani, E. Valle, and G. Cartei. 2000. "Physicians' Attitudes to and Problems with Truth-Telling to Cancer Patients." *Supportive Care in Cancer* 8(1): 40–45.

Institut National du Cancer. 2005. "Recommandations nationales pour la mise en oeuvre du dispositif d'annonce du cancer dans les etablissements de sante." Paris : Institut National du Cancer.

Kerr, A., and S. Cunningham-Burley. 2000. "On Ambivalence and Risk: Reflexive Modernity and the New Human Genetics." *Sociology* 34(2): 283–304.

Klawiter, Maren. 1999. "Racing for the Cure, Walking Women, and Toxic Touring: Mapping Cultures of Action within the Bay Area Terrain of Breast Cancer." *Social Problems* 46(1): 104–26.

———. 2004. "Breast Cancer in Two Regimes: The Impact of Social Movements on Illness Experience." *Sociology of Health and Illness* 26(6): 845–74.

Klitzman, Robert. 2009. "'Am I My Genes?': Questions of Identity among Individuals Confronting Genetic Disease." *Genetics in Medicine* 11(12): 880–89.

Marcia, James E. 1980. "Identity in Adolescence." In *Handbook of Adolescent Psychology*, edited by J. Adelson, 159–87. New York: Wiley.

———. 1988. "Common Processes Underlying Ego Identity, Cognitive/Moral Development, and Individuation." In *Self, Ego, and Identity: Integrative Approaches*, edited by D. K. Lapsley and F. C. Power, 211–66. New York: Springer-Verlag.

Mathieson, Cynthia M., and Henderikus J. Stam. 1995. "Renegotiating Identity: Cancer Narratives." *Sociology of Health and Illness* 17(3): 283–306.

Nettleton, Sarah. 2004. "The Emergence of E-Scaped Medicine." *Sociology* 38(4): 661–79.

Reich, Michel, and L. Mekaoui. 2003. "La Conspiration du Silence en Cancérologie: Une Situation a ne pas Négliger." *Bulletin du cancer* 90(2): 181–84.

Schaepe, Karen S. 2011. "Bad News and First Impressions: Patient and Family Caregiver Accounts of Learning the Cancer Diagnosis." *Social Science and Medicine* 73(6): 912–21.

Schneider, Joseph W., and Peter Conrad. 1983. *Having Epilepsy: The Experience and Control of Illness*. Philadelphia: Temple University Press.

Schwartz, Seth J. 2001. "The Evolution of Eriksonian and Neo-Eriksonian Identity Theory and Research: A Review and Integration." *Identity* 7(1): 7–58.

van Hoof, Anne. 1999. "The Identity Status Approach: In Need of Fundamental Revision and Qualitative Change." *Developmental Review* 19(4): 622–47.

Winkelman, W. J., and C. W. Choo. 2003. "Provider-Sponsored Virtual Communities for Chronic Patients: Improving Health Outcomes through Organizational Patient-Centred Knowledge Management." *Health Expectations* 6(4): 352–58.

Patient-Centered Care or Discrimination?
Diagnosis among Diverse Populations

Kevin Dew

STARTING POINTS

- Health professionals want to treat their patients fairly.
- The ethnic, cultural, or social situation of a patient should not influence our diagnostic processes.
- Research shows that the level of diagnostic testing and the diagnoses made differ according to gender and racial classification.

If you ask a clinician whether she treats her **patients** differently, the chances are she will say she treats them all the same. By making such a claim, the clinician puts forward an ideal that we can treat people in a manner that is not influenced by our own values, experiences, or understandings and that we are not influenced by the characteristics of the people with whom we are interacting. But this ideal is beyond the capacity of human beings. The claim is also based on an assumption that to treat people differently is inherently negative. This chapter suggests that while there are many negative aspects to treating people in dissimilar ways, doing so is not only inevitable, it is not necessarily bad.

To illustrate differences in diagnosis and treatment (in an example taken from **empirical** research), we can consider three men with similar upper respiratory symptoms, all visiting the same clinician. For one, the doctor goes through the standard stages of a consultation, asking the patient to present his symptoms, posing questions to clarify certain points, and then examining him physically. He then prescribes antibiotics. For the second patient, the clinician decides on antibiotics after the patient presents his symptoms but before he undertakes a history or an examination. And finally for the

> For me as a practitioner, as a surgeon, I don't look at what color they are, where they come from, or what their religion is, none whatsoever. If somebody's got a condition that needs treatment, we give it, and I can vouch for all other surgeons in this hospital, or any other hospitals. (Dew et al. 2008)

third, after a full examination and history, the doctor simply recommends the patient "take it easy," drink lots of fluids, and take acetaminophen (paracetamol) if necessary (Dew et al. 2008).

Why would the same doctor make such divergent decisions with patients ostensibly suffering from the same condition? While it is not possible to completely discount clinical reasons, there are other factors at play here. What we can't see in the short descriptions above is that the first patient was a twenty-two-year-old Chinese exchange student with an upcoming exam, the second a sixty-six-year-old self-employed white man, and the third an adult male who was about to go on vacation. Such differences in social context can have an effect on medical decision making.

The doctor's response depended on things like the patient's need to be fit and well for the exam or for work, the presence or lack of social resource surrounding the individual, and maybe even the order in which the appointments occurred. It could be that a fear of overprescribing could have made the doctor reluctant to prescribe antibiotics when he had twice dispensed them already, which could explain why patient number three didn't get any. But whatever the reason, we can clearly see differences in decision-making outcomes, including variations in diagnosis. In the case above, for the doctor to have prescribed antibiotics, he needed to consider the symptoms to be the result of secondary bacterial infection. For him to have advised rest and acetaminophen (as with the third patient), he must have presumed the disorder to be viral, where the prescription of antibiotics would have been futile.

In this example a few things have been held constant. The clinician is the same person, and the three patients are all male. But even when patients seem similar superficially, there are many variables that can lead a clinician to treat his patients differently. We can consider gender, ethnicity, social class, age, education, religion, and body shape, to name a few. The term "hyperdiversity" has been used to describe the "increasingly diverse nature of patient populations in contemporary American healthcare settings" (Delvecchio Good et al. 2011), the term also alluding to diversity within particular social groups. This chapter provides evidence of and explanations why social groups may have varying diagnoses and then considers the consequences for health-care outcomes.

EVIDENCE OF DIFFERENT DIAGNOSES

Time and again, research has shown that there is a strong social gradient in health outcomes. The poor, the less educated, and those living in deprived neighborhoods have a lower life expectancy and are more likely to be sicker than their more fortunate neighbors. In addition, persistent disparities in health outcomes by ethnicity have been shown in just about every diagnosed condition: heart disease, diabetes, cancer, injury, and so on. Some of this disparity can be explained by such things as comorbidities, health behavior (conditioned by the environment in which the individual has been raised), the impact of the environment (e.g., dangerous workplaces or hazardous neighborhoods), and lack of access to resources and services. But epidemiologists also tell us that some of this disparity is associated with the delivery of health services. People of varying social backgrounds seem to get different services and different results.

It has been clearly demonstrated that there can be contrasting health outcomes for people with the same condition. In the United States, there is a vast literature showing that whites use different levels of health resources than African Americans and Latinos, with minorities receiving inferior health care even at the same level of need (Balsa and McGuire 2001). Blue-collar workers in Finland have lower rates of coronary bypass operations than their white-collar colleagues even though the mortality rate for coronary heart disease (CHD) is twice as high among blue-collar workers (Keskimaki et al. 1997). The indigenous Māori population in New Zealand also has lower rates of bypass grafts than the settlers, who have much lower rates of CHD mortality (Robson 2008). This sort of discrepancy has been named the inverse care law, which stipulates that the availability of medical care varies inversely with the need for medical care in the population (Tudor Hart 2000). This law means that the poor, who suffer a higher burden of illness, use fewer health-care and medical resources than those who are more advantaged. The inverse care law also suggests, as evidenced by the various levels of intervention, the possibility of different diagnoses depending on the population group. In short, a patient who does not receive a diagnosis of CHD won't receive treatment for it.

So is there evidence that diagnosis plays a part in bringing about disparities in health outcomes? Are there particular diagnoses or diagnostic interventions that are assigned differently depending on the social group? The answer is yes. The clearest and most consistent variations in diagnosis by race relate to cardiac care, but there are racial disparities in the receipt of cancer diagnostic tests. African Americans receive fewer diagnostic evaluations and less effective ones than other Americans. They are also less likely to receive posttreatment surveillance (Smedley et al. 2003). Research also shows that African Americans with cerebrovascular disease receive fewer diagnostic procedures. In relation to the process of diagnosing diabetes, African Americans are less likely to have lipid testing or to undergo measurement of glycosylated hemoglobin (Institute of Medicine 2003). An Institute of Medicine report on unequal treatment concluded that "racial and ethnic minority patients are found to receive a lower quality and intensity of healthcare and diagnostic services across a wide range of procedures and disease areas. This finding is remarkably consistent and robust" (Smedley et al. 2003). Another well-researched area that demonstrates differences in outcomes from encounters with the health-care system is gender. Epidemiologists have demonstrated that women get sicker, but men die quicker (Lorber 1997). And while life expectancy is longer for women, they suffer from more illness and disability. Men and women also deal with illness in different ways. Men tend to use primary health services less frequently than women and are more likely to delay seeking help when they are ill. It has been argued that men are also more likely to adopt health-damaging behaviors such as excessive alcohol consumption, violence, and unsafe sex (Cameron and Bernades 1998; Farrimond 2012) and to be in occupations with higher rates of workplace deaths (Feyer et al. 2001).

But men and women are also diagnosed differently. Under particular scrutiny in recent years is the relationship between medical practitioners and women. It has been suggested that the medical encounter reinforces patriarchal domination and is frequently based on assumptions of stereotypical male and female role models. Women run a higher risk of being labeled deviant, and possibly mentally disordered as well, if they fail to conform to stereotypical roles of mothers and housewives.

In fact, women face a greater risk of depression, especially following crises involving housing, reproduction, and children (but women are at no greater risk of depression than men following other crises, such as financial or marital relationship ones). This difference is primarily the result of the different roles that men and women have in the gendered division of labor and the stresses associated with those roles (Nazroo et al. 1998).

It may be no surprise that as women are diagnosed with depression more frequently than men, so they also consume psychotropic drugs in larger quantities. In cases where men and women both have mental distress symptoms, women consume more antidepressants and hypnotics or anxiolytics (Huasken et al. 2007). Critics see this trend as a medicalized response to personal troubles and potentially as a form of social control of women where social problems are reconceptualized as individual problems and psychotropic medications used as a form of constraint (Norris et al. 2011). But it is not just differences in the life experiences of men and women that account for the higher rate of depression diagnoses for women. Sexism in medicine is evident in how doctors sometimes ignore women's accounts of their own symptoms (Broom 2009). In a study of people who had been diagnosed with chronic fatigue syndrome, a contested condition in medicine, 85% of the women received, at some stage in their illness, a psychiatric diagnosis, but only 30% of men did. Men's accounts of their physical symptoms were more likely to be given credence than women's accounts (Broom and Woodward 1996).

In contrast, research across nations, including the United States, has found that women are underdiagnosed for coronary artery disease (Weisz et al. 2004), with men more likely to receive a correct diagnosis of heart disease (Curry and O'Brien 2006). In the case of ischemic heart disease, women are less likely to receive medically proven secondary prevention therapies such as beta blockers, aspirin, and angiotensin-converting enzyme inhibitors than men but are more likely to be prescribed anxiolytic benzodiazepines (Williams et al. 2003). This disparity suggests that physicians are more likely to attribute the symptom of angina in women to something other than ischemic heart disease—in particular, to anxiety.

Men are less likely to be diagnosed as having depression than women, but men are more likely to be labeled as alcoholics. Research has also shown that women who are hospitalized for strokes are less likely to receive interventions, like carotid endarterectomies, than men (Ramani et al. 2000). So what applies to heart disease applies to cerebrovascular disease. And chronic diseases are not alone. Women are also more likely to die from hospital-acquired pneumonia than men (Crabtree et al. 1999).

There are many other examples of differences in diagnosis and treatment outcomes, but the examples outlined above are sufficient to make the point. People are often treated differently in the health system depending on the social group with which they are identified. Why?

WHY DO WE TREAT PEOPLE DIFFERENTLY?

There are many reasons why the same clinician might vary her approach to diagnosis depending on the patient. Outlined below are some of the numerous explanations for disparate diagnoses by social group. None of these explanations rules out another, and for any one individual, several reasons may be at play in relation to a specific medical encounter.

Categorizing and Stereotyping

As described in chapter 1, on classification, all individuals deploy mechanisms to cope with social life. In order to deal with the massive amount and complexity of information we confront in our daily lives we all categorize, classify, typify, and **stereotype** (van Ryn and Burke 2000). When we meet people, we assign them to a particular group, and we associate particular groups with certain characteristics—that is, we anticipate and expect people to behave in particular ways. We use what some sociologists have called membership categorization devices (MCDs). When we use MCDs, we are assigning people to a particular category, and for each category we apply some rules. One rule is that there are certain activities associated with those categories, or category-bound activities. So, to take an everyday example, when we see a baby crying and we see an adult woman respond by picking the child up, we are likely to assign them the categories of mother and child, and with the category of mother we probably view the activity of picking up the crying child as one of caring. Caring for her children is a category-bound activity of mothers, and that is how we "read" the interaction (Housley and Fitzgerald 2009).

Categorizing people is an everyday activity, but it is also an activity that occurs in institutional settings and in medical encounters (diagnosing is categorization *par excellence*). It may be even more pressing for clinicians to categorize patients given the complexity of the task, and to make quick judgments about situations (van Ryn and Burke 2000). So perhaps it is not surprising that we categorize and stereotype. But there are consequences. Jerome Groopman has described how even experienced physicians may be fooled by their stereotypes. He recounts how Pat Croskerry, a specialist in diagnostic decision making, missed diagnosing a heart attack when he saw a healthy-looking, active young man with chest pain (Groopman 2007). Just because we can categorize someone does not mean that the activities associated with that category always apply. The rules can be—and are frequently—broken. So it can become a problem in the medical encounter if our capacity to categorize overrides our attention to the individual before us. Doing so may lead to different diagnoses and treatment plans for whole groups of people when diagnoses and treatment plans should be specific to the particular individual.

There is a great deal of evidence to suggest that clinicians categorize in ways that may be inappropriate. Research undertaken at New York State hospitals revealed that clinicians were more likely to perceive African American patients with coronary artery disease as "at risk for noncompliance with cardiac rehabilitation, substance abuse, and having inadequate social support" and were more likely to be rated by clinicians "as less intelligent than white patients, even when patient sex, age, income and education were controlled for." Clinicians reported "less affiliative feelings toward African-American patients" (van Ryn and Burke 2000). African Americans were perceived as being less rational, less intelligent, and less pleasant than whites and were rated as less educated than whites even at the same levels of educational attainment. Similarly, clinicians were more likely to view patients with lower socioeconomic status as having responsibility for the care of family members than patients with higher socioeconomic status. This attitude persisted even when the researchers controlled for dependent family members (van Ryn and Burke 2000). Overall, the research found that clinicians had more positive perceptions of white and higher-class groups than African American and lower-class groups, and associated different activities with them.

Another study surveyed emergency room patients presenting with chest pain to ascertain what questions they were asked by clinicians. The responses of the 308 participants indicated that nonwhite patients were more likely to be asked about alcohol, smoking, and cocaine use than white patients (James et al. 2006). In other words, nonwhites were more likely than whites to be asked questions about their personal behavior. Changing the method of interrogation depending on the ethnicity of the patient could, paradoxically, result in lower levels of care for whites—for example, cocaine can be a trigger for acute myocardial infarction (James et al. 2006).

Assumptions about Risk

Clinicians often make assumptions about risk on the basis of social group. In vignette studies of primary care doctors' diagnosis of CHD, women patients were asked fewer questions than men (Arber et al. 2004), were less likely to receive components of a physical examination than men (McKinlay et al. 2007), and physicians were more certain of a CHD diagnosis for men compared to women (Lutfey et al. 2010). So in this research physicians treated a demographic variable—gender—as a diagnostic feature that lowered the risk of CHD. This occurred in a situation where the presentation of symptoms by the men and women actors in the vignettes was the same (Lutfey et al. 2010), with one explanation being that physicians had prior assumptions about risk that overrode presenting symptoms in the determination of the diagnosis.

An interesting way of thinking about assumptions about risk is the concept of **statistical discrimination**. In medicine, statistical discrimination is where a doctor applies a "reasonable decision making rule" that leads to unequal treatments between different groups (Balsa and McGuire 2001). Here physicians draw on statistical averages or their previous experience of a set of symptoms with people from a particular group (gender, ethnicity, and age being obvious groupings; Lutfey et al. 2010). It may be that research indicates that people with a particular characteristic are less likely to comply with a particular drug regime and so the prescription is not given (Balsa and McGuire 2001). Or it might apply in situations where there is uncertainty about a diagnosis, and if "the underlying prevalence of the illness is associated with race, the doctor might take race into account in deciding about the diagnosis and treatment of a particular patient" (Balsa et al. 2005). So if a doctor believes that the prevalence of a disease is more or less likely for a particular group, that belief may influence their diagnostic decision making.

The reliance on disease statistics in diagnosis may become more prominent if the patient is difficult to understand. In this instance the "noise" of the miscommunication may sharpen the focus on the "signal" provided by prior research on probabilities and risk profiles (Balsa et al. 2005). It has been found, for example, that U.S. physicians behave in this statistical fashion for hypertension and diabetes when diagnosing African American and white patients. By contrast, when it comes to depression, the diagnosis is based on what the patient says, how she describes her condition, and how she presents herself. So in the case of depression, how patients communicate symptoms is likely to play more of a role in diagnosis than the clinician's understanding of the prevalence of a condition in a particular social group, which might explain why clinicians are less likely to diagnose depression in African Americans (Balsa et al. 2005).

In the vignette study on CHD discussed above, there was no evidence of the social class of the patient being associated with differences in decision making or treatment (Arber et al. 2006). Given that individuals from a lower social class have a higher probability of suffering from CHD, the authors of the study suggest that primary care practitioners treat their lower-class patients as if they had the same risk profile as their middle-class patients (Arber et al. 2006). Working-class patients, however, were more likely to be given advice about diet and exercise than middle-class patients, suggesting an alignment of physicians' views with evidence about differences in diet and exercise across classes (Arber et al. 2004).

Cultural Representations and Social Impacts

We can understand categorizing and stereotyping through the cultural representations that are available to us, which tell us something about the social **norms** that influence us and how those social norms are reinforced. To illustrate, research on medical advertising has shown that the majority of patients portrayed in advertisements in medical journals for cardiovascular medications are male, whereas in advertisements for antidepressants, most patients are portrayed as female (Curry and O'Brien 2006). The advertisements aimed at clinicians are drawing on stereotypes and, in doing so, reinforcing those stereotypes.

Some differences in diagnosis may be the result of the frequency of contact with the health system. Individuals who are more likely to go to a doctor are more likely to receive a diagnosis, because diagnosing is what doctors do. Women are more likely to be diagnosed with conditions because they have more frequent encounters with health services (an outcome of, among other things, being primarily responsible for the health care of children and contraception and being the target of screening programs for cervical and breast cancer). Women's higher rates of diagnosis could also be because of the historical tradition of medicalizing women's and children's health. As one example, menstruation was considered a serious explanation for ill health among middle-class women during the Victorian era, a practice that still echoes in our contemporary era. It has set a precedent for ready recourse to the doctor for matters that arguably are not medical in nature (Vertinsky 1994).

The social backgrounds of individuals clearly influence access to and use of health-care services (Boulton et al. 1986; Davies and Elwyn 2008). There are numerous reasons for this influence. The social distance between the physician and the patient can have a bearing; the more educated are able to take advantage of opportunities (Davies and Elwyn 2008). Evidence for this social division is seen in research on physicians finding that they tend to perceive working-class patients as not seeking a role in decision making and as having a limited capacity to understand health information (Davies and Elwyn 2008).

It has also been suggested that clinicians treat patients differently as a result of **aversive racism**. Aversive racism occurs when dominant groups avoid interactions with subordinate groups (Smedley et al. 2003), and it may occur among individuals who hold on to liberal values, including wanting to overcome and combat racism, but at the same time are uncomfortable or uneasy around members of a different ethnic group. If we apply this finding to the health setting, it may mean being ill at ease with the social chitchat that provides important opportunities for the clinician to establish trust and communication lines, and to informally assess the patient's condition.

There are also differences in health knowledge and health beliefs between physicians and patients of various backgrounds that can affect diagnosis. This may be the case particularly where patients come from another cultural background than the physician and therefore may hold contrasting ideas about disease causation and treatment, but such differences can be present within the same culture when patients may have low levels of education (Boulton et al. 1986).

I'm quite ignorant of the different cultures. I'd go in to a person of ethnic minority not as relaxed, generally more uptight . . . You're on edge . . . because you're thinking I don't want to put my foot in this, so that can make them uneasy with you. (Kai et al. 2007)

The problem is not just about laypeople misunderstanding what doctors communicate; medical staff may also have a poor understanding and appreciation of the needs of different social groups and their communities.

One's cultural group may, as already noted, influence the level of comfort within the consultation. Middle-class patients with higher levels of education may deal better with bureaucratic organizations and be more assertive in consultations, which may lead to more diagnostic testing and different diagnoses from their lower-class counterparts (Arber et al. 2006). The capacity of middle-class patients to better negotiate the health-care system relates to their level of **cultural capital**. Cultural capital is a kind of resource that accrues to people in the early stages of **socialization**. It provides individuals with the skills and knowledge that they draw on, but they do not have to be conscious of them (Bourdieu 1986). Patients with more privileged backgrounds accrue

[The] Chinese don't have a word for cancer and it's absolutely considered taboo to actually talk to somebody with cancer and say they've got it . . . so how do you start to talk to them about giving them chemotherapy if you're not actually allowed to use the word cancer? (Kai et al. 2007)

more cultural capital and so are more likely to get their views across in the consultation. But it is not necessarily the case that more testing will have positive outcomes, as additional tests may also lead to overdiagnosis.

There is evidence that there are differences in diagnosis as a result of patient expectations. A study of pediatric practices in Los Angeles found that Latino and Asian parents of children with cold symptoms were more likely to expect that their sick child needed antibiotics than other parents, and that the higher parental expectation was associated with higher levels of bacterial diagnoses and antibiotic prescribing from the clinicians (Mangione-Smith et al. 2004). This study shows how clinicians respond differently to their perceptions of patient expectations in their diagnoses, and as there is ethnic variation in expectations, patients are treated differently by their ethnicity.

SO WHAT SHOULD A CLINICIAN DO?

We can see a bit of a conundrum for physicians when it comes to the ideal of treating everyone the same. If they treat all patients the same way, they run the risk of not attending to the risk profiles of different populations groups and being less thorough than they should with higher-risk patients. From this perspective, treating people differently might be a good thing. But if they treat people differently as a result of the patient's particular characteristics—race, gender, class, age, religious persuasion, or any number of other factors—physicians run the risk of discriminating on the basis of nonclinical characteristics. But part of this conundrum arises from the attempt to artificially separate the clinical from the social. The two are intensely intertwined. As the chapters in this book emphasize, there are ways that social factors contribute to how we frame and respond to diagnoses, and how clinicians diagnose. This is one more example of how social forces shape the diagnostic process for better or for worse.

More importantly, we all must recognize that the ideal of treating everyone the same is not humanly possible. Life is too complicated and time is too short. What we can do is to reflect on how we treat people, and to do the best we can to treat all patients with compassion and dignity. We can work to overcome such obstacles as aversive racism and to be aware of our responses to patient characteristics and demands so that we make the best possible diagnoses and provide the optimal treatment plan.

TAKEAWAY POINTS

- In order to deal with the complexity of social life, we all categorize.
- We make assumptions about behaviors, activities, and risk on the basis of the categories we use.
- Clinicians' perceptions of patient expectations also shape their diagnostic activities, and the way we categorize people influences these perceptions.
- Aspiring to treat everyone with dignity may be a better goal than aspiring to treat everyone the same.

DISCUSSION QUESTIONS

1. Recall the last time you interacted with a new patient who was at some social distance from you (distance in education, social class, age, or ethnic background). How did this interaction go? Were there any difficulties? How did you make yourself and your patient comfortable?
2. What strategies could be developed to overcome aversive racism? Are there any particular processes you could incorporate into your everyday practice to try and limit it?
3. Have you ever felt discriminated against? Why do you think this was the case? How did you react to it? Did the experience affect how you responded to similar situations afterward?

REFERENCES

Arber, S., J. McKinlay, A. Adams, L. Marceau, C. Link, and A. O'Donnell. 2004. "Influence of Patient Characteristics on Doctors' Questioning and Lifestyle Advice for Coronary Heart Disease: A UK/US Video Experiment." *British Journal of General Practice* 54(506): 673–78.

———. 2006. "Patient Characteristics and Inequalities in Doctors' Diagnostic and Management Strategies Relating to CHD: A Video-Simulation Experiment." *Social Science and Medicine* 62(1): 103–15.

Balsa, A. I., and T. G. McGuire. 2001. "Statistical Discrimination in Health Care." *Journal of Health Economics* 20(6): 881–907.

Balsa, A. I., T. G. McGuire, and L. S. Meredith. 2005. "Testing for Statistical Discrimination in Health Care." *Health Services Research* 40(1): 227–52.

Boulton, M., D. Tuckett, C. Olson, and A. Williams. 1986. "Social-Class and the General-Practice Consultation." *Sociology of Health and Illness* 8(4): 325–50.

Bourdieu, Pierre. 1986. "The Forms of Capital." In *Handbook of Theory of Research for the Sociology of Education*, edited by J. Richardson, 241–58. New York: Greenwood Press.

Broom, Dorothy. 2009. "Gender and Health." In *Second Opinion: An Introduction to Health Sociology*, edited by John Germov, 130–55. Melbourne: Oxford University Press.

Broom, Dorothy, and Roslyn Woodward. 1996. "Medicalisation Revisited: Toward a Collaborative Approach to Care." *Sociology of Health and Illness* 18(3): 357–78.

Cameron, E., and I. Bernades. 1998. "Gender and Disadvantage in Health: Men's Health for a Change." *Sociology of Health and Illness* 20(5): 673–93.

Crabtree T., S. Pelletier, T. Gleason, T. Pruett, and R. Sawyer. 1999. "Gender-Dependent Differences in Outcome after the Treatment of Infection in Hospitalised Patients." *JAMA* 282(22): 2143–48.

Curry, Phillip, and Marita O'Brien. 2006. "The Male Heart and the Female Mind: A Study of the Gendering of Antidepressants and Cardiovascular Drugs in Advertisements in Irish Medical Publication." *Social Science and Medicine* 62(8): 1970–77.

Davies, M., and G. Elwyn. 2008. "Advocating Mandatory Patient 'Autonomy' in Healthcare: Adverse Reactions and Side Effects." *Health Care Analysis* 16(4): 315–28.

Delvecchio Good, Mary-Jo, Seth Hannah, and Sarah Willen. 2011. "Shattering Culture: An Introduction." In *Shattering Culture: American Medicine Responds to Cultural Diversity*, edited by Mary-Jo Delvecchio Good, Sarah Willen, Seth Hannah, Ken Vickery, and Lawrence Taeseng Park, 1–30. New York: Russell Sage Foundation.

Dew, Kevin, Anthony Dowell, Maria Stubbe, Elizabeth Plumridge, and Lindsay Macdonald. 2008. "Treating Patients Differently: A Qualitative Study of How Clinical and Social Factors Shape Interactions between Doctors and Patients." *New Zealand Family Practice* 35: 382–86.

Farrimond, Hannah. 2012. "Beyond the Caveman: Rethinking Masculinity in Relation to Men's Health-Seeking." *Health* 16(2): 208–25.

Feyer, A., J. Langley, M. Howard, S. Horsburgh, C. Wright, J. Alsop, and C. Cryer. 2001. "The Work-Related Fatal Injury Study: Numbers, Rates and Trends of Work-Related Fatal Injuries in New Zealand, 1985–1994." *New Zealand Medical Journal* 114(1124): 6–10.

Groopman, Jerome. 2007. "What's the Trouble? How Doctors Think." *New Yorker*, January 29.

Hausken, A. M., S. Skurtveit, E. O. Rosvold, J. G. Bramness, and K. Furu. 2007. "Psychotropic Drug Use among Persons with Mental Distress Symptoms: A Population-Based Study in Norway." *Scandinavian Journal of Public Health* 35(4): 356–64.

Housley, William, and Richard Fitzgerald. 2009. "Membership Categorization: Culture and Norms in Action." *Discourse and Society* 20(3): 345–62.

Institute of Medicine. 2003. *Unequal Treatment: Confronting Racial and Ethnic Disparities in Health Care*. Washington, DC: National Academies Press.

James, T. L., J. Feldman, and S. D. Mehta. 2006. "Physician Variability in History Taking when Evaluating Patients Presenting with Chest Pain in the Emergency Department." *Academic Emergency Medicine* 13(2): 147–52.

Kai, J., J. Beavan, C. Faull, L. Dodson, P. Gill, and A. Beighton. 2007. "Professional Uncertainty and Disempowerment Responding to Ethnic Diversity in Health Care: A Qualitative Study." *PLoS Medicine* 4(11): e323, doi:10.1371/journal.pmed.0040323.

Keskimaki, I., S. Koskinen, M. Salinto, and S. Aro. 1997. "Socioeconomic and Gender Inequities in Access to Coronary Artery Bypass Grafting in Finland." *European Journal of Public Health* 7(4): 392–97.

Lorber, J. 1997. *Gender and the Social Construction of Illness*. Thousand Oaks, CA: Sage.

Lutfey, K. E., K. W. Eva, E. Gerstenberger, C. L. Link, and J. B. McKinlay. 2010. "Physician Cognitive Processing as a Source of Diagnostic and Treatment Disparities in Coronary Heart Disease: Results of a Factorial Priming Experiment." *Journal of Health and Social Behavior* 51(1): 16–29.

Mangione-Smith, R., M. N. Elliott, T. Stivers, L. McDonald, J. Heritage, and E. A. McGlynn. 2004. "Racial/Ethnic Variation in Parent Expectations for Antibiotics: Implications for Public Health Campaigns." *Pediatrics* 113(5): E385–E94.

McKinlay, J., C. Link, K. Freund, L. Marceau, A. O'Donnell, and K. Lutfey. 2007. "Sources of Variation in Physician Adherence with Clinical Guidelines: Results from a Factorial Experiment." *Journal of General Internal Medicine* 22(3): 289–96.

Nazroo, J., A. Edwards, and G. Brown. 1998. "Gender Differences in the Prevalence of Depression: Artefact, Alternative Disorders, Biology or Roles?" *Sociology of Health and Illness* 20(3): 312–30.

Norris, P., S. Horsburgh, K. Lovelock, G. Becket, S. Keown, B. Arroll, J. Cumming, P. Herbison, and P. Crampton. 2011. "Medicalisation or Under-Treatment? Psychotropic Medication Use by Elderly People in New Zealand." *Health Sociology Review* 20(2): 202–18.

Ramani, S., S. Byrne-Logan, K. Freund, A. Ash, W. Yu, and M. Moskowitz. 2000. "Gender Differences in the Treatment of Cerebrovascular Disease." *Journal of the American Geriatrics Society* 48: 741–45.

Robson, Bridget. 2008. "What Is Driving the Disparities?" In *Understanding Health In-equalities in Aotearoa New Zealand*, edited by Kevin Dew and Anna Matheson, 19–31. Dunedin: Otago University Press.

Smedley, Brian, Adrienne Stith, Alan Nelson, and Committee on Understanding and Eliminating Racial and Ethnic Disparities in Health Care. 2003. *Unequal Treatment: Confronting Racial and Ethnic Disparities in Health Care.* Washington, DC: National Academies Press.

Tudor Hart, J. 2000. "Commentary: Three Decades of the Inverse Care Law." *BMJ* 7226: 18–19.

van Ryn, Michelle, and Jane Burke. 2000. "The Effect of Patient Race and Socio-Economic Status on Physician's Perceptions of Patients." *Social Science and Medicine* 50: 813–28.

Vertinsky, P. A. 1994. *The Eternally Wounded Woman: Women, Doctors, and Exercise in the Late Nineteenth Century.* Champaign: University of Illinois Press.

Weisz, Daniel, Michael Gusmano, and Victor Rodwin. 2004. "Gender and the Treat-ment of Heart Disease in Older Persons in the United States, France and England: A Comparative, Population-Based View of a Clinical Phenomena." *Gender and Medicine* 1(1): 29–40.

Williams, David, Kathleen Bennett, and John Feely. 2003. "Evidence for an Age and Gender Bias in the Secondary Prevention of Ischaemic Heart Disease in Primary Care." *British Journal of Clinical Pharmacology* 55(6): 604–8.

Who's the Boss?
Diagnosis and Medical Authority

Tania M. Jenkins

STARTING POINTS

- Society often believes that "doctor knows best," but where did that belief come from?
- Doctors control access to the sick role by making diagnoses.
- Physicians rely on tools, such as technology, to make diagnoses.

The onset was sudden. Laura Hillenbrand, author of the famed book that later became a major motion picture, *Seabiscuit,* was a healthy college student who within weeks became so sick she had to drop out of school. Her symptoms were all over the map: nausea, fever, chills, joint pain, stiffness, sore throat, confusion, disorientation, aphasia, weight loss. Her internist ran test after test but could find nothing wrong with her: "My problem, he said gravely, was not in my body but in my mind; the test results *proved* it. He told me to see a psychiatrist" (Hillenbrand 2003; emphasis added). When she went to see a psychiatrist, he sent her back to her internist. According to him, "I was mentally healthy but suffering from a serious physical illness." Over the course of the next few months, Hillenbrand's condition worsened but she was no closer to a diagnosis. Her peers began to lose patience: "Without my physicians' support, it was almost impossible to find support from others. People told me I was lazy and selfish" (Hillenbrand 2003).

Hillenbrand's experience highlights the power that a diagnosis can carry in legitimizing a **patient**'s suffering, revealing that the process of diagnosis is an act of power, one where the physician traditionally exercises authority over a set of social actors—usually the patient, but also friends, family, and the public at large. This chapter describes how physician authority both manifests in—and gets reinforced by—medical diagnosis. It also examines how recent social changes have affected medical authority, challenging both the legitimacy of and our dependency on the medical profession, with diagnosis at the center of these shifts.

MEDICAL AUTHORITY = LEGITIMACY + DEPENDENCE

To understand how diagnosis and authority interact, we must first establish what we mean by medical authority. In his seminal treatise on the rise (and fall) of the

American physician, Paul Starr (2004) writes that medical authority, "in its classical sense, signifies the possession of some status, quality, or claim that compels trust or obedience" (580). Perhaps this quality is the scientific ability to heal—after all, we do turn to physicians for tried and tested solutions to our medical problems. It is not enough for Starr, however, that physicians lay claim to science for healing purposes, and he points to instances where allopathic (or mainstream) physicians, such as those in Soviet Russia, still used scientific methods but did not rise to the same level of authority as in the West. He goes on to designate two particular dimensions that distinguish Western physicians from other healers; on the one hand, they have legitimacy as a group of professionals, and on the other, there is social dependence on their services. Let us unpack these concepts by seeing how they apply to diagnosis.

A MONOPOLY OVER DEFINING DISEASE

As mentioned above, physicians' monopoly over healing historically came from more than just the improvement in scientific approaches to disease. In fact, the regulation of the medical profession in many countries occurred well before experimentation and the use of statistical tests in assessing clinical effectiveness gained a foothold in medical research (see Hacking 1990; Porter 1995). In the late nineteenth and early twentieth centuries, physicians managed to convince governments that their knowledge was so esoteric (understood by such a small group) that only other physicians could regulate the profession. This control gave doctors government-sanctioned oversight of training, licensing, and ultimately the authority to diagnose (Freidson 1970; Starr 2004). The combination of government support and dominance over other health practitioners gave the medical profession the ultimate authority to name disease, although this power was never an absolute, as "alternative" health practitioners and even laypeople (see chap. 12) have named disease. Nevertheless, medical diagnosis wields power in courts, death certificates, and compensation and insurance claims; allows access to a range of health resources and services; and gives permission to miss work, have special conditions for taking examinations, obtain parking permits, and other special considerations. As a result, diagnosis (or the naming of disease) is inherently a function of the "legitimacy" dimension of physicians' authority.

But Starr and Freidson remind us that having the legitimate right to practice medicine is meaningless without patients' trust in medical professionals. As patients, we trust in and depend on medicine's ability to make use of esoteric knowledge to evaluate and fulfill our health needs (Starr 2004). For medical authority to exist, it must be characterized by both legitimacy and dependence.

The **sick role**, as defined by the well-known American sociologist Talcott Parsons (1951), is a great example of how the two concepts of legitimacy and dependence work together. When a patient receives a diagnosis, she also receives access to the sick role, which is associated with specific rights and obligations. The patient is exempt from the normal duties of everyday life (such as chores and work obligations), and exempt from blame for her inability to fulfill those everyday duties. In exchange for these exemptions (granted by a physician), the patient is required to attempt to get better. That obligation is both defined and facilitated by competent, expert medical help.

The physician in turn has the corresponding obligation to serve the patient's best interests and to do so with professional competence, expertise, altruism, and affective neutrality, the latter being a requirement that all patients should be treated in the same way and that health professionals should not respond in relation to whether they like or dislike a patient (Gehardt 1987). In this way, the sick role is both contingent on physician authority, as it requires the legitimacy of a medical license and expert knowledge, and contributive to that authority, because it establishes that physicians should act in the best interest of their patients, which inspires both trust in—and dependence on—the medical profession. Diagnosis is pivotal for a patient to be a patient, with all of the accompanying social exemptions such as taking time off work, getting light duty, and receiving other special consider-ations. In this way, physicians have the authority to transform social roles through their allocation of the sick role. And while the doctor-patient relationship may no longer conform exactly to the traditional sick role (Parsons 1975; Rier 2010), it remains that the diagnostic encounter, where the sick role is bestowed, is both a manifestation and reinforcement of physician authority.

DIFFERENTIAL DIAGNOSIS

Consider a more concrete example of how diagnosis can be both a cause and consequence of medical authority by looking at the history of psychiatry as a sub-discipline of medicine. Today, physicians pride themselves on espousing rigor-ous scientific principles, such as those contained in **evidence-based medicine** (the **gold standard** of "scientific" medicine), and differential diagnosis, the systematic method of arriving at a diagnosis through a process of elimination. This process of elimination requires adherence to and knowledge of a diagnostic nosology that catalogues various alternative diagnoses for a given symptomatology (see chap. 1, on classification, and chap. 2, on the diagnostic process). This practice of dif-ferential diagnosis lends scientific cred-ibility to the diagnostic process and to the profession as a whole. In some ways, differential diagnosis can be consid-ered a defining characteristic of mod-ern medical practice, distinguishing it from other forms of healing. Without differential diagnosis, the practice of medicine would be considered merely speculative.

The attending interrupts—"What's the differential diagno-sis before we see the CT?" Suggestions get tossed about the room: Could be osteonecrosis? An abscess? Lipoma? "Femoral hernia?," asks one resident. The attending interjects, "Ah, but you'd *feel* it." They decide to look at the CT scan results together. Finally, they stop at a large white spot in the leg and, almost in unison, the doctors nod their heads, murmuring "abscess." The patient will be sent to interventional radiology for treatment. (Author's field notes from ethnographic research at a community hospital)

An example of differential diagnosis.

Making diagnoses on the basis of evidence was not always standard practice for all branches of medicine, however. Until the middle to late twentieth century, psychiatry did not employ differential diagnostic methods, relying instead on psychoanalytic and idiopathic approaches. These approaches viewed each patient as unique and did not attempt to find trends or patterns among symptoms and diseases, thereby making it difficult for psychiatrists to even speak of diagnosis per se, as they did not have the tools to describe commonalities between patients.

This meant that psychiatry also did not have a nosology, or a systematic and hierarchical means of classifying mental disorders. Psychiatry was therefore not as well respected as a subspecialty, and numerous other **professions** in the counseling field encroached upon its authority, a situation that the discipline attempted to remedy with the diagnostic process. Early attempts at a nosology, resulting in the first (1952) and second (1968) editions of the *Diagnostic and Statistical Manual of Mental Disorders* (DSM), were not well organized and thus rarely used. In preparing the third edition, however, psychiatrists wanted to improve their position within the broader profession of medicine and to increase the legitimacy of their work (Young 1997). As a result, they worked within a neo-Kraepelinian framework based on the work of German psychiatrist Emil Kraepelin, who was thought to have come up with the idea of differential diagnosis in mental disorders.

The new framework abandoned the idiopathic approach and advocated careful record keeping in order to uncover the etiologies of mental disorders. The DSM-III, containing 265 disorders, was released in 1980 (up from 106 in DSM-I and 182 in DSM-II) and was considered a major step forward in granting authority to the fledgling discipline. By adopting a nosology with standardized diagnostic criteria, giving psychiatrists the ability to conduct differential diagnosis, psychiatry obtained a monopoly over medically defining mental illness, thereby making it less subjective and more legitimate than other professions, such as psychoanalysis. By improving their legitimacy, psychiatrists also increased patients' dependence on them as the sole arbiters of sanity. In this way, the process of differential diagnosis, made possible by the creation of the DSM-III, both delegated psychiatry authority over mental health vis-à-vis other practitioners and reaffirmed that authority by making patients dependent on psychiatrists for their mental health care.

MEDICALIZATION AND AUTHORITY

Through the creation of new diagnoses, medical subspecialties can enhance their standing within the profession while also extending their authority to new social realms. Stephen Pfohl (1977) has written about pediatric radiologists' "discovery" of "battered child syndrome" (or child abuse) as a diagnostic category in the early 1960s, and about the various circumstances that led to the creation of that diagnosis.

Pfohl describes an American historical tradition that until the first half of the twentieth century legitimized violence toward children, such that parents would only be criminally liable for physically disciplining their children if their actions resulted in permanent injury. In more serious cases, when children were brought to the emergency room after having sustained injuries from their parents, emergency physicians were reluctant to make a diagnosis of abuse because of (1) concerns about doctor-patient confidentiality and fears of litigation; (2) not wanting to get involved in family affairs; (3) disbelief that parents could harm their children in this way; and (4) ignorance that a diagnosis of abuse was even an option, as this diagnosis did not yet exist.

Pediatric radiologists, however, increasingly found that the radiographic evidence did not support the claims that particular injuries were caused by childhood accidents. In 1962, they created the diagnosis of battered child syndrome to rectify this discrepancy. Pfohl (1977) attributes this discovery to three major characteristics that pertain to pediatric radiology: (1) radiologists enjoyed a certain social distance from patients and their parents, such that X-rays "carry little of the horror of bloody assault" (317); (2) at the time, radiologists did not share emergentologists' concerns about violating confidentiality, once again because of this social distance; and, perhaps most relevant to our purposes, (3) the field of pediatric radiology was looking for an opportunity for an intraprofessional advance in prestige and the chance to name and label a disease of its own. Pediatric radiology at the time was marginalized within the profession for not performing risky procedures, not dealing with blood and guts, and having little life-or-death decision-making authority. Of course, professional advancement was not the only motivator for creating the diagnosis of battered child syndrome, but, combined with the undeniable "objective" radiographic evidence before them, the desire to advance the field gave pediatric radiologists the impetus needed to establish a new disease category.

Creating this diagnosis provided pediatric radiologists an opportunity to improve their status within the broader medical profession as they made their entrée into the diagnostic arena: "By linking themselves to the problem of abuse, radiologists became indirectly tied into the crucial clinical task of patient diagnosis" (Pfohl 1977, 318). At the same time, the medical profession as a whole extended its authority into moral and family matters—an area in which government wanted to avoid getting involved. The diagnosis eventually led to the criminalization of child abuse. By capturing this particular action in medical definitional terms (see chap. 8, on **medicalization**), medicine positions itself to make moral judgments, as if it were a "repository of truth, the place where absolute and often final judgments are made by supposedly morally neutral and objective experts" (Zola 2009, 470). The diagnosis of battered child syndrome is a positive intervention, but it also illustrates how medical specialties use diagnosis as a means for overcoming marginalization, and how the profession as a whole works to improve its overall authority within society.

In sum, medical authority is both enshrined in diagnosis and continually reinforced through patients' dependency on physicians for access to resources, achieved through conferring the status of the sick role to patients as well as through the expansion of medicine into new domains. Physicians' authority is not static, however; while there may be several factors that enhance it, as described above, recent changes in the medical system have also challenged physicians' sovereignty. These changes include encroachment by other health practitioners, shifting patient roles, and the divergent effect of technology, which both enhance and undermine physician authority. And yet, despite all of these changes, physicians continue to maintain their authority.

CHALLENGES TO MEDICAL AUTHORITY
The Growing Nonexclusivity of Diagnosis

A number of broad trends during the 1970s and 80s weakened physicians' legitimacy and led to the undoing of medical sovereignty over diagnosis. Poor-quality outcomes, an increasingly specialized yet fractured profession, and, the emergence of antitrust laws prohibiting physicians in the United States from having a monopoly over patient care facilitated the existence of competition (Light 2010; Mendel and Scott 2010; Ritzer and Walczak 1988; Scott 2003). The result is that physicians no longer bear the exclusive right to make diagnoses that allow access to health resources and services; increasingly, other health professionals are permitted to make diagnoses (such as nurse practitioners, optometrists, and even physical therapists), all of which has diluted the exclusivity that physicians traditionally enjoyed.

Nurses who prescribe medicine threaten this exclusivity. In many countries, clinical nurse specialists are joining nurse practitioners to prescribe quasi-independently an ever-growing list of medications. Nurse prescription has selectively shifted responsibility for certain clinical activities from one professional group to another, freeing up physicians to focus their time on more complex medical issues in a system that is already overtaxed (Kemp 2007). By the same token, however, the policy has also shifted part of the authority to diagnose to nurses and away from physicians in a move that can be described as professional encroachment. Similarly, alternative health practitioners are also challenging doctors as diagnosticians by increasingly becoming professionalized and scientized (Goldner 2004; Hirschkorn 2006).

By having lost their monopoly over diagnosis through the encroachment of other health practitioners, physicians have experienced a corresponding decline in authority, which is only exacerbated by the dissemination of medical information to other practitioners and the general public (see below) through channels like the Internet. Yet physicians remain society's primary diagnosticians, and while their authority might be in flux, it is still firmly entrenched. In some jurisdictions, for example, health professionals who can diagnose (such as nurse practitioners and midwives) must still work under the supervision of a physician, suggesting that while there may be a wider variety of diagnosticians in society, physicians still maintain tight control over the process.

[It] is a very specific prescription that actually has *my* signature, *my* name, *my* license number; that's my very own prescription. (Primary care nurse with six years of experience)

Registered nurses in Quebec, Canada, now have the ability to prescribe certain medications after legislation was passed that expanded their clinical responsibilities.

The Empowered Patient

As seen in chapter 4, on the diagnostic relationship, patients are becoming increasingly informed and mobilized as a result of easier access to medical knowledge. Health information has become "e-scaped" through the explosion of web-based resources (Nettleton 2004), providing a leveling effect on the traditionally paternalistic doctor-patient relationship (Bury 2004). Increases in lay knowledge have meant that patients often come to a clinical encounter with a diagnosis in mind, which they put forward and negotiate. Rather than approaching physicians as experts who have unique knowledge (i.e., in a traditional dependence framework set out by the sick role), patients increasingly are consulting doctors for support in making choices—including diagnostic decisions—about their health (in a phenomenon known as "physician compliance"; see Barker 2008). This has meant that physician authority has been countered by rising patient empowerment in the form of medical knowledge and social support, as we are less dependent on physicians than before. About 95% of Americans today (referred to as the "informed-by-Google generation") look for health information on the Internet, where it is available twenty-four hours a day, seven days a week, free of charge (Sanders 2009). Patients are also increasingly turning to the Internet as a source of social support when physicians do not grant them the sick role for medically unexplained symptoms (Barker 2008; Dumit 2006). Disillusioned by physicians' unbridled autonomy, which led to mistakes and quality issues (Light 2010), patients have begun to question medicine's legitimacy and to take matters into their own hands, reducing their dependence on the profession, a position that was less likely only a few decades ago, when information was less accessible.

Despite this growing empowerment, patients' dependence on physicians persists. Recent developments in **health social movements** and health legislation may have improved patients' standing vis-à-vis physicians, but they remain reliant on doctors' social legitimacy (composed, among other things, of specialized knowledge and altruism) in order to access certain resources. Patients might feel like they have more of a say in their health (care) these days, but these choices largely remain within a biomedical framework, where physicians remain at the helm. While patients may have more choices to look elsewhere, those alternatives are largely other medical authorities.

They come to see me, they ask my advice, and then they go tootling off to the Internet to find some website which tells them not to do what I just recommended, and they come back three months later, much worse, and still not willing to follow my advice. What can I do?!

Medical authority is no longer immutable. Access to other forms of information challenges the way doctors practice today.

Social Movements

Patients have become increasingly involved in their health and the health of others, fighting to be heard alongside (or in spite of) dominant medical science. One way they have done this is through health social movements. Brown et al. (2004) have distinguished between three different types of health movements: (1) health access movements that seek to correct inequalities in access to health-care services; (2) constituency-based health movements that seek to redress inequalities in health on the basis of social categories such as race, gender, and sexual preference; and (3) embodied health movements, which are premised on the idea that patients have valuable contributions to debates about disease diagnosis, etiology, and treatment based on their own embodied experience of illness. These movements blur the boundary between experts and laypeople, as individuals driven by their own lived experience of a disease become experts in the science. They therefore also blur the line between what is considered to be "good" and "bad" science, as they often bring to the table more subjective knowledge generated from individual experience, while scientists place priority over so-called rigorous and objective science.

The environmental breast cancer movement is a good example of an embodied social movement, as it centers itself on the body and on the lived experiences of women suffering from the disease. Laypeople draw on their own knowledge production in order to counter common conceptions of etiological processes that lead to disease. Directly challenging the paternalistic model of medicine that reigned during the golden era of the early twentieth century, these movements seek to shift the power dynamic between physicians and laypeople in order to afford individuals a better chance at the diagnostic negotiation table when it comes to determining etiology. They do not, however, seek to overturn physician authority altogether; instead, they often establish citizen-science alliances or "lay-professional collaborations in which citizens and scientists work together on issues identified by lay people" (Brown 2007, 33). In fact, embodied health movements are defined not only by the fact that they challenge current science, but also that they work in collaboration with experts in order to improve treatment, prevention, research, and funding outcomes. In this way, while patients may be growing more empowered, they are still reliant on physician authority to achieve their goals.

A good example of one such citizen-science alliance occurred in Woburn, Massachusetts, in the 1980s. From 1966 to 1986, twenty-eight cases of childhood leukemia developed among Woburn children, a rate four times higher than expected at a national level (Brown and Mikkelsen 1990; Durant et al. 1995). A later study found that six of the children with leukemia lived within close proximity of one another, a staggering seven and a half times the expected number in that geographic location (Cutler et al. 1986). Other health problems were also more common than normal, including adult-onset leukemia and renal cancer (Brown and Mikkelsen 1990). The families of these sick individuals began to suspect that their health problems were linked to drinking water contaminated by dumped industrial waste in the local water source. In 1979, 184 fifty-five-gallon drums were discovered next to the Aberjona River, and water samples from underground wells near the site were found to contain up to forty times the permissible concentrations of known toxic and carcinogenic chemicals (Brown and Mikkelsen 1990; Lagakos et al. 1986).

The discovery of these pollutants and their link to leukemia was largely based on the efforts of the laypeople in Woburn. Families banded together to form the social movement organization For a Cleaner Environment (FACE) to help address the toxic waste problems of the community. This group almost single-handedly detected a cancer cluster, incited the government to clean up the toxic sites, brought two major national corporations to court, pioneered a health study surrounding the effects of toxic chemicals on cancer, and while doing so drew national attention to the broader issue of environmental health (Brown and Mikkelsen 1990). It started in 1979 when two members of the Woburn community (a mother and her pastor) joined forces with a local physician and mapped all the cases of childhood leukemia in the city. This effort eventually led to an alliance with three Harvard scientists and ultimately the design and implementation of the Woburn Harvard/FACE study. The goal of the study was to provide more systematic data on the cancer cluster and its link to contaminated water, and it is now considered a model for citizen-practitioner alliances. A group of 235 volunteers surveyed 57% of Woburn's population, an impressive size given the study's dearth of research funding ($10,000 for a study that would have ordinarily cost between $500,000 and $750,000; Brown and Mikkelsen 1990; Lagakos et al. 1986). Twenty cases of childhood leukemia diagnosed between 1964 and 1983 were further studied alongside a hydrogeological model for the groundwater (Lagakos et al. 1986). Perhaps unsurprisingly, the study found positive significant associations between the toxic water and childhood leukemia, perinatal deaths and certain types of childhood diseases, including congenital abnormalities (Lagakos et al. 1986). These findings were enough to incite eight families to go to trial.

The Woburn case is important because "the children died. Sixteen children died in Woburn. I think it had to do with the fact that the children died of leukemia and some *mothers got very involved*. They tell a very unhappy story and I think people relate to that. It is a human tragedy." (Gretchen Latowsky, community organizer, cited in Brown and Mikkelsen 1990, 47, emphasis added)

Why popular epidemiology came about in Woburn, and why it is such an important case study.

The example above powerfully illustrates the ability of laypeople to piggyback on medical authority by creating links between diagnoses and causes. In other instances, this kind of alliance may be harnessed to recognize and even name diseases. Lyme disease is an important case in point. As Robert Aronowitz (1998) has written, some Connecticut mothers (from the area around the town of Lyme) recognized that a number of children were suffering from similar low-grade fevers, headaches, malaise, and joint pain. Bringing this disease cluster to the attention of the U.S. Centers for Disease Control and Prevention (CDC) with the support of their local doctors was the first step in disease recognition. Had the cases been more geographically dispersed, the sufferers less articulate, or public health officers less receptive to its description as a unified condition, Lyme disease might never have been named.

The fact that the community members, starting with mothers in both of these cases, were able to effectively create new science that in the first case linked toxic chemicals to leukemia, and in the second gave meaning to general systemic symptoms of infectious disease, is evidence of a significant shift in social relations between physicians, scientists, and laypeople. But their efforts were made possible due to the alliances they made with physicians. The people of Woburn encountered initial resistance from the CDC, which would not seriously entertain their requests for water testing, and only agreed after the citizens of Woburn sought a physician's help. While it remains true that social movements sometimes seek to challenge extant social relations between patients and doctors, they also require the authority of physicians to get their message across.

Legal Challenges to Medical Authority

In some cases, it is not social movements that challenge physician authority, but rather social **institutions**, like the law. Patients have become increasingly empowered through the rise of malpractice lawsuits that seek to redress wrongs performed by physicians, especially as a result of not disclosing full information to patients. In part due to health social movements, full disclosure of medical information has become the legal norm, such that patients are expected to want and to be able to handle full disclosure about their diagnosis, prognosis, and treatment. In the United States, the Patient Self-Determination Act of 1991 says that competent individuals have a right to make decisions about their health care, including end-of-life care (Luce and Alpers 2001). This codification of patient autonomy constitutes a major reversal of previous informal practices, where physicians would paternalistically make life-and-death decisions on patients' behalf (Burns et al. 2003; Klawiter 2004; Veatch 2003). Today, patients have increasing control over technical, medical matters that were formerly thought to be too complicated for laypeople to handle (Veatch 2003). Physicians have thus been legally stripped of their exclusive authority to make life-and-death decisions without first consulting their patients.

The result is that patients are now legally included in decision making about their health, which has shifted the way patients are seen by physicians: "The lay person who consults the health care professional is no longer the submissive and compliant 'patient' but an expert *partner* who brings his or her experience of illness to the differentially specialized medical practitioner" (Jutel 2011, 69). But including patients in the decision-making process can lead some physicians to willfully abdicate their responsibility (and perhaps their authority) vis-à-vis patients, as the text box suggests. Consider a patient who enters a doctor's office with a presumptive diagnosis and demands antibiotics for what is clearly (to the physician) a viral respiratory infection: the doctor who complies with this request for fear of being sued or to avoid explaining the pharmacology of antibiotic therapy may in fact be harming her patient. In an attempt to decrease **paternalism** within medicine by including the patient as an active partner, we may

---

When I started residency, I viewed patient autonomy as an absolute good, an ethical imperative that trumped all others . . . Informed consent was supposed to guard against such abuses. But informed consent is practiced very differently from the way ethicists envisioned it. *It was supposed to protect patients from doctors. Instead, it is used to protect doctors from patients, or rather, from the hard decisions that patient care demands.* Doctors nowadays sometimes use informed consent as a crutch to abdicate responsibility. (Jauhar 2008, 231, emphasis added)

Changing attitudes and practices toward patient autonomy.

inadvertently be threatening one of the very cornerstones of sound medical practice and physician authority—discretion.

Professional Challenges to Clinical Authority

This brings us to the issue of how professions can sometimes constrain their own authority. Professional governing bodies establish the standards by which members of their group are held accountable. In the case of medicine, members of the profession must be able to demonstrate how their actions comply with established standards embodied in guidelines, protocols, and practice policies. These are procedural standards that attempt to specify the processes by which diagnoses are made and how treatment plans are determined and implemented (Timmermans and Berg 2003). Practitioners are also regularly assessed by quality assurance and quality improvement processes. Deviations from such standards must be justified by a warrant for their nonconformity. The individual clinician's authority is thus challenged in relation to professional standards, which attempt to standardize medicine and in so doing define medical practice as the logical and sequential application of science.

Standardization is a way of dealing with huge variations in medical practice with widely varying outcomes, but one of its consequences is limiting clinical autonomy and patient choice. It cannot be assumed that attempts to standardize medical practices through such means as requiring the use of protocols will have the intended outcome. As demonstrated by detailed analysis of interactions between patients and clinicians, there are many means by which clinicians can ignore, undermine, or utilize protocols and standardized procedures (Dew et al. 2005; 2010)

As Freidson (1970) writes, "In order to provide a truly human service, practitioners must have a significant degree of autonomy within reasonable limits dictated by patients' rights, official standards, and accountability" lest we "reduc[e] practitioners to passive cogs in a rationalized system" (391). Despite these warnings, however, it appears that enshrining patient autonomy in the law and clinical accountability in protocols has not gone so far as to completely eradicate physician authority in the context of medical decision making. Patient autonomy laws and attempts to standardize clinical practice might challenge this authority, but it is a long way from being undermined altogether.

Technology as a Double-Edged Sword

As discussed in chapter 10, on diagnostic technology, while most doctors can interpret some diagnostic tests (complete blood count, for example), specialist medical interpretation may be required for others, such as magnetic resonance imaging (MRI) and other technical imaging procedures. The need for specialization adds to the dependence dimension of their authority; we are dependent on physicians for access to certain resources, including technology. But this monopoly can also (paradoxically perhaps) threaten clinical legitimacy. Having control over diagnostic technologies may enhance physicians' ability to diagnose, but overreliance on technology can also lead to mistrust and devaluation of clinical acumen: "the development of newer and better technologies—the mammogram, ultrasound and most recently the MRI—has caused doctors to doubt the value of what their hands can tell them" (Sanders 2009, 52). Some fear that advances in technology are leading to the demise of the physical exam, which used to be at the center of diagnosis but is now only performed perfunctorily. Some physicians view it as a waste of time, and while most agree that the physical exam is important, it is often subtly dismissed as unreliable compared to the results of diagnostic technology.

Seeing the physical exam as being potentially unreliable can have important implications for physician authority as it affects the sick role; according to Parsons (1951), physicians ought to have unimpeded access to the body in order to reach a diagnosis. As physician Lisa Sanders (2009) writes, "the act of placing your hand upon another's body is, in many ways, the hallmark of the physician" (47). Given that the increasing use of technology detracts from the importance of the "laying of hands" upon patients' bodies and that these technologies can make physicians doubt their own clinical acumen, does this start to undermine patient dependence on the physician? The fine line between the authority of having control over access to diagnostic technologies and the reduced importance of the actual clinical skills of the physician will become increasingly tricky to navigate in the future, as diagnostic technologies proliferate even further.

DIAGNOSIS: A PRODUCT AND ENGINE OF MEDICAL AUTHORITY

Diagnosis is both a manifestation and reinforcement of physician authority. But that authority is also contingent upon broader social changes, such as the rising professionalization of other health practitioners and shifts in power between doctors and patients. As a clinician, it is important to be aware of how diagnosis is embedded not only in scientific knowledge but myriad social relations that variously affect our dependency on the medical profession and its legitimacy.

This brings us full circle to Laura Hillenbrand's ordeal. Nearly a year after the initial onset of her symptoms, Hillenbrand was diagnosed with chronic fatigue syndrome, a poorly understood, incapacitating illness. By getting that label from a physician, she was able to receive the support and recognition she needed from her peers. She—just like all of us—was dependent on the authority vested in her physician to pronounce a diagnosis, which granted her access to the resources necessary to get help. In this way, her diagnosis was both a product and an engine of medical authority.

TAKEAWAY POINTS

- Diagnosis is an act of power.
- Medical authority is manifested and reinforced by diagnosis.

- Diagnosis can also challenge medical authority, especially when other actors (including patients and other professionals) compete for access to the diagnostic process.
- Diagnosis is embedded in scientific knowledge as well as the social relations that variously affect our dependency on the medical profession.

DISCUSSION QUESTIONS

1. Reflect on a recent diagnostic encounter where you were either patient or clinician. In what ways was authority present in this encounter? Are there ways in which your clinician (if you were the patient) or you (if you were the clinician) can become more aware it?
2. How do you feel about challenges to physicians' authority? Do you think there ought to be more checks and balances to keep physicians from having too much power, or should they be given even more authority to exercise full clinical discretion?
3. Can you think of any diagnoses in your field that may have been linked to a power struggle by the profession?

REFERENCES

Aronowitz, R. 1998. *Making Sense of Illness: Science, Society and Disease.* Cambridge: Cambridge University Press.

Barker, K. 2008. "Electronic Support Groups, Patient-Consumers, and Medicalization: The Case of Contested Illness." *Journal of Health and Social Behavior* 49(1): 20–36.

Brown, Phil. 2007. *Toxic Exposures: Contested Illnesses and the Environmental Health Movement.* New York: Columbia University Press.

Brown, Phil, and Edwin J. Mikkelsen. 1990. *No Safe Place: Toxic Waste, Leukemia and Community Action.* Berkeley: University of California Press.

Brown, Phil, Stephen Zavestoski, Sabrina McCormick, Brian Mayer, Rachel Morello-Frosch, and Rebecca Gasior Altman. 2004. "Embodied Health Movements: New Approaches to Social Movements in Health." *Sociology of Health and Illness* 26(1): 50–80.

Burns, J. P., J. Edwards, J. Johnson, N. H. Cassem, and R. D. Truog. 2003. "Do-Not-Resuscitate Order after 25 Years." *Critical Care Medicine* 31(5): 1543–50.

Bury, M. 2004. "Researching Patient-Professional Interactions," supplement, *Journal of Health Services Research and Policy* 9(1): 48–54.

Cutler, J. J., G. S. Parker, S. Rosen, B. Prenney, R. Healey, and G. G. Caldwell. 1986. "Childhood Leukemia in Woburn, Massachusetts." *Public Health Reports* 101(2): 201–5.

Dew, K., J. Cumming, D. McLeod, S. Morgan, E. McKinlay, A. Dowell, and T. Love. 2005. "Explicit Rationing of Elective Services: Implementing the New Zealand Reforms." *Health Policy* 74(1): 1–12.

Dew, K., Maria Stubbe, Lindsay Macdonald, Anthony Dowell, and Elizabeth Plumridge. 2010. "The (Non) Use of Prioritisation Protocols by Surgeons." *Sociology of Health and Illness* 32(4): 545–62.

Dumit, J. 2006. "Illnesses You Have to Fight to Get: Facts as Forces in Uncertain, Emergent Illnesses." *Social Science and Medicine* 62(3): 577–90.

Durant, J. L., J. Chen, H. F. Hemond, and W. G. Thilly. 1995. "Elevated Incidence of Childhood Leukemia in Woburn, Massachusetts: Niehs Superfund Basic Research-Program Searches for Causes," supplement, *Environmental Health Perspectives* 103(6): 93–98.

Freidson, Eliot. 1970. *Profession of Medicine: A Study of the Sociology of Applied Knowledge.* Chicago: Chicago University Press.

Gerhardt, U. 1987. "Parsons, Role Theory, and Health Interaction." In *Sociological Theory and Medical Sociology*, edited by G. Scambler, 110–33. London: Tavistock.

Goldner, M. 2004. "The Dynamic Interplay between Western Medicine and the Complementary and Alternative Medicine Movement: How Activists Perceive a Range of Responses from Physicians and Hospitals." *Sociology of Health and Illness* 26(6): 710–36.

Hacking, Ian. 1990. *The Taming of Chance.* Cambridge: Cambridge University Press.

Hillenbrand, Laura. 2003. "A Sudden Illness." *New Yorker*, July 7, 56–65.

Hirschkorn, K. A. 2006. "Exclusive versus Everyday Forms of Professional Knowledge: Legitimacy Claims in Conventional and Alternative Medicine." *Sociology of Health and Illness* 28(5): 533–57.

Jauhar, Sandeep. 2008. *Intern: A Doctor's Initiation.* New York: Farrar, Strauss and Giroux.

Jutel, Annemarie Goldstein. 2011. *Putting a Name to It: Diagnosis in Contemporary Society.* Baltimore: Johns Hopkins University Press.

Kemp, K. A. 2007. "The Use of Interdisciplinary Medical Teams to Improve Quality and Access to Care." *Journal of Interprofessional Care* 21(5): 557–59.

Klawiter, M. 2004. "Breast Cancer in Two Regimes: The Impact of Social Movements on Illness Experience." *Sociology of Health and Illness* 26(6): 845–74.

Lagakos, S. W., B. J. Wessen, and M. Zelen. 1986. "An Analysis of Contaminated Well Water and Health Effects in Woburn, Massachusetts." *Journal of the American Statistical Association* 81(395): 583–96.

Light, Donald W. 2010. "Health-Care Professions, Markets, and Countervailing Powers." In *Handbook of Medical Sociology*, edited by Chloe E. Bird, Peter Conrad, Allen M. Fremont, and Stefan Timmermans, 270–89. Nashville, TN: Vanderbilt University Press.

Luce, J. M., and A. Alpers. 2001. "End-of-Life Care: What Do the American Courts Say?" *Critical Care Medicine* 29(2): N40–N45.

Mendel, Peter, and W. Richard Scott. 2010. "Institutional Change and the Organization of Health Care: The Dynamics of 'Muddling Through.'" In *Handbook of Medical Sociology*, edited by Chloe E. Bird, Peter Conrad, Allen M. Fremont, and Stefan Timmermans, 249–69. Nashville, TN: Vanderbilt University Press.

Nettleton, Sarah. 2004. "The Emergence of E-Scaped Medicine." *Sociology* 38(4): 661–79.

Parsons, Talcott. 1951. "Social Structure and Dynamic Process: The Case of Modern Medical Practice." In *The Social System*, 436–39. New York: Free Press.

———. 1975. "The Sick Role and the Role of the Physician Reconsidered." *Milbank Memorial Fund Quarterly: Health and Society* 53(3): 257–78.

Pfohl, Stephen J. 1977. "The 'Discovery' of Child Abuse." *Social Problems* 24(3): 310–23.

Porter, Theodore. 1995. *Trust in Numbers: The Pursuit of Objectivity in Science and Public Life.* Princeton, NJ: Princeton University Press.

Rier, David A. 2010. "The Patient's Experience of Illness." In *Handbook of Medical Sociology*, edited by Chloe E. Bird, Peter Conrad, Allen M. Fremont, and Stefan Timmermans, 163–78. Nashville, TN: Vanderbilt University Press.

Ritzer, G., and D. Walczak. 1988. "Rationalization and the Deprofessionalization of Physicians." *Social Forces* 67(1): 1–22.

Sanders, Lisa. 2009. *Every Patient Tells a Story*. New York: Broadway.

Scott, W. Richard. 2003. "The Old Order Changeth: The Evolving World of Health Care Organizations." In *Advances in Health Care Organization Theory*, edited by Stephen S. Mick and Mindy E. Wyttenbach, 23–43. San Francisco: Jossey-Bass.

Starr, Paul. 2004. "Précis of Paul Starr's the Social Transformation of American Medicine." *Journal of Health Politics, Policy and Law* 29(45): 575–620.

Timmermans, Stefan, and Marc Berg. 2003. *The Gold Standard: The Challenge of Evidence-Based Medicine and Standardization in Health Care*. Philadelphia: Temple University Press.

Veatch, R. M. 2003. "Do Not Resuscitate: Ordering Nonassault and Charting Patients' Decisions to Forgo Cardiopulmonary Resuscitation." *Critical Care Medicine* 31(5): 1593–95.

Young, Allan. 1997. *The Harmony of Illusions: Inventing Post-Traumatic Stress Disorder*. Princeton, NJ: Princeton University Press.

Zola, Irving Kenneth. 2009. "Medicine as an Institution of Social Control." In *Sociology of Health and Illness*, 9th ed., edited by Peter Conrad, 470–80. New York: Worth.

Is This Really a Disease?
Medicalization and Diagnosis

Annemarie Goldstein Jutel, Andrew Greenberg, and Barbara Katz Rothman

STARTING POINTS

- The term "medicalization" emerged in the 1970s and was initially used by Ivan Illich (1976) and other critical commentators to suggest medical imperialism.
- Medicalization is the placing under medical authority life events or dysfunctions that are arguably not medical in nature.

How have medicine and medical professionals come to exert such influence in so many areas of our lives? In such diverse areas as birth, exercise, child rearing, death, diet, education, sexuality, sadness, criminal interrogation, and war, medicine wields influence, control, and expertise. You probably have heard and maybe used the term **medicalization**. It is a sociological term that worked its way into the vernacular, and captures this picture of medicine's influence over daily life.

To see an entity is already to foresee an action. (Canguilhem 1991)

Common usage of "medicalization" infers that everything is now a disease or symptom and possibly that there is some medical intent or conscious manipulation to bring additional events and conditions under the control of medicine. But a sociological understanding differs in two important aspects. First, from the sociological perspective, the question is not only if something is medicalized, but also which social forces pushed it to be medicalized and what interests are served by particular phenomena being considered medical in nature. For example, the process by which **direct-to-consumer** advertising of Paxil promoted the diagnoses of both social anxiety disorder and generalized anxiety disorder is quite different from the social movement–oriented demand of veterans following the Vietnam War to have posttraumatic stress disorder (PTSD) recognized and covered by veteran's benefits (Scott 1990). The sociological understanding of medicalization includes, but is not limited to, the emphasis on overmedicalization.

A second difference between the sociological idea of medicalization and the lay understanding of the term is that in sociology, medicalization is not an isolated concept; rather, it is related to social theories. Early theorists on medicalization such as Zola (1972, 1983) and Freidson (1972) were interested in the concept of social control and professional dominance. Here the question of medicalization is part of a larger question, namely, how a society controls its members. In a somewhat cartoonish history we can demonstrate how the responsibility of control has moved from religious **institutions** such as the church to secular institutions such as medicine.

While we are tempted to quickly add meaning to this transition, our real jumping-off point must be an interest in the details of how it happened. It may be uncomfortable when key concepts we use to make sense of our world—like disease—are threatened. It is easy to feel smug when we discuss the medicalization of masturbation at the turn of the nineteenth century, as if we now have facts and criteria that should separate all these social questions from real medicine. However, the "realness" of a disease is often unimportant insofar as diseases become social actors with real effects. To be labeled a witch in the seventeenth century, a homosexual in the nineteenth, a neurotic in the twentieth, or clinically obese in the twenty-first is to suffer a significant impact. All of these labels are real for those with the labels and those who do the labeling. In this chapter we don't question whether the conditions being medicalized should be part of the medical understanding of life, simply that they are. We then consider the consequences of this conceptualization.

Here we review what medicalization is and how the concept has changed and evolved, and we discuss various medicalized conditions from both historical and contemporary medical practice. Mainly we reflect upon how medicalization is both enabled by and enables diagnosis, providing yet another interesting, albeit challenging, social factor to the clinical work of the diagnostician.

WHAT IS MEDICALIZATION?

The term "medicalization" surfaced in critical writing in the late 1960s buttressed by the widely read and controversial works of authors such as Ivan Illich (1976), Thomas Szasz (1970), R. D. Laing (1967), and Michel Foucault (1963), who sought to understand the origin of myriad social ills. They focused on how technical knowledge was being used to marginalize and label youth culture, draft resisters, and other countercultures (Nye 2003). Their work emerged at a transformative moment in the social landscape, when doctors and other social authorities were demonized by some as tools of the establishment. The medicalization of the 1960s and early 1970s was a phenomenon characterized as medical imperialism, with a profession intent upon grasping power and exerting control, much of it through diagnostic machinations. Illich (1976) saw the focus on disease as disempowering. It "always intensifies stress, defines incapacity, imposes inactivity, and focuses apprehension on non-recovery, on uncertainty, and on one's dependence upon future medical findings" (104). He described "therapeutic culture" as a means by which the healthy individual could be classed as deviant for radical or independent thinking. In this way, diagnosis was used as a tool for political oppression.

Dissent, for example, has been treated as mental illness. Robin Munro (2002) writes of a Chinese diagnosis of "political mania," a form of paranoid psychosis. Lest one rule this diagnosis irrelevant and a non-Western seepage of the political into the psychiatric, consider the UK Department of Health's definition of dangerous and severe personality disorder: individuals over the age of eighteen "who have an identifiable personality disorder to a severe degree, who pose a high risk to other people because of serious antisocial behaviour resulting from their disorder . . . [the] overwhelming majority are people who have committed serious offences . . . a small minority who have not committed any serious offence remain at large in the community" (Corbett and Westwood 2005). As Corbett and Westwood point out, this definition focuses on the social, as opposed to the psychiatric, and could clearly be used in the practice of social control.

Irving Zola jumped into the debate on medicalization in the early 1970s, concerned by the great public popularity of antiestablishment writers such as Thomas Szasz, whom Zola believed had undertaken inadequate reflection about the structure of medicine as a social institution. In his "Medicine as an Institution of Social Control," Zola (1972) described the theoretical and historical cornerstones of contemporary medicalization.

Zola (1972) defined medicalization as the process by which medicine has taken within its jurisdiction aspects of everyday life that previously were not under its control. His definition does not suggest that medicine itself has appropriated a particular aspect of everyday life, nor does it imply that specific social institutions assign this appropriation. Notably, he wrote that medicalization was not the result of medical imperialism or of "misguided human efforts or motives" (487). Instead, medicalization was strongly grounded in social reliance upon the expert.

He explained that there are four ways in which medicine was awarded jurisdiction over ever-expanding realms of human existence. First, there is an expansion of what is deemed relevant to the good practice of medicine. If **patient** behavior (lifestyle, exercise, diet) contributes to particular chronic illnesses, for example, then the physician is justified in making these behaviors part of her business. Second, the retention of control over certain technical procedures reinforces medical control over death, birth, and other life events. In this case, one might consider access to pain medication as an example. Narcotic substances might be useful in death as in birth, but to access in either circumstance, one must call upon the physician. Third, Zola (1972) writes that retention of near-absolute access to certain taboo areas (aging, drug addiction, pregnancy) further extends the medical jurisdiction. Finally, expansion of how the rhetoric of medicine is used to advance any cause reinforces the importance of medicine in realms not necessarily previously considered its own. Didier Fassin (2009) reinforces this point when he describes how diagnoses bear witness to the world in authoritative ways. The suffering of survivors of natural disaster, war, or a combination of both, when expressed as cases of PTSD, brings an accounting of misery with credible substance. The diagnosis substitutes the words of the expert for the voice of the sufferer.

Conrad (1992) builds on Zola's work, writing about how medicalization suggests a particular framing of the problem in question. The problem becomes redefined: it may get a new name (a diagnosis), and its remedy is thought to be in medicine as opposed to somewhere else. While medicalization is frequently thought to refer to problems where alternative (and possibly more appropriate) frames to medicine could or should be applied, for Conrad, it is a neutral term referring to any problem that is newly defined in medical terms.

Conrad describes medicalization on three levels: (1) a conceptual approach defining the problem in medical terms, (2) an institutional level where a medical approach is adopted to treat the problem, and (3) and interactional level where the patient sees a doctor for medicalized condition and receives diagnosis, treatment, prognosis, and so forth. What is important in Conrad's understanding of medicalization is that he is not concerned with whether a particular phenomenon is really a disease; rather, he wants to know how the problem has come to be considered in medical terms at all. What are the social circumstances that make a problem recognizable by medicine, to be described in the idiom of disease? That we should consider social problems in diagnostic language is both to punctuate the extent to which diagnosis helps us to make sense of the world, and to underline the way in which medicalization limits the range of possible understandings of our problems and challenges.

The discussion of medicalization is not solely one of adjudication, although it often is. As discussed in chapter 11, medicalization is one site of contention in the arena of the contested diagnosis. But medicalization is intimately involved with the problems of meaning and power. The question of who governs our understanding of a particular problem (in the case of medicalization, it is clearly medicine) has an important effect on the range of meanings permitted for a particular situation. Medical historian Charles Rosenberg (2002) writes that diagnosis "constitutes an indispensable point of articulation between the general and the particular, between agreed upon knowledge and its application. It is a ritual that has always linked doctor and patient, the emotive and cognitive, and in doing so, has legitimized physicians and the medical system's authority while facilitating particular clinical decisions and promoting cultural agreed upon meaning for individual experience" (240). When medicalization and diagnosis become everyday phenomena, when bodily sensations transform into symptoms, and when every aspect of our lives becomes useful for the doctor to diagnose our condition, even if our condition might be considered normal when viewed from a different angle, then what is at stake is precisely how we attach meaning to individual experience.

If we follow this idea to its conclusion, then diagnosis becomes a complicated idea. On the one hand, it is a ritual and set of tools for understanding and treating a patient; on the other, insofar as the diagnosis creates meaning for the patient and defines the situation, diagnosis is not only a way of understanding the world, it is also a way of creating a world.

EXAMPLES OF MEDICALIZATION

History gives us a kind of distance from which we can see how particular conditions have previously been medicalized. To think of slave insubordination in medical terms, as did Cartwright (1981) when he referred to "dysaethesia aethiopica" as a "disease of negroes" causing rascality, is clearly an example of how social expectations of the Africans brought to North America were based on a social order we refute absolutely today. Similarly, that homosexuality was actually contained in the *Diagnostic and Statistical Manual of Mental Disorders* (DSM) as a mental disorder, rather than a variant within the range of possible human sexualities, speaks to heteronormativity in the Western world. However simple it would seem to attribute these examples to historic idiosyncrasy, or even to the ever-progressing advancement of human knowledge, it would be a mistake. There are many examples of medicalization present in contemporary society. Among these examples are many that are neither knowledge based nor idiosyncratic (although some examples are both). In the following paragraphs we provide a few examples of medicalization through diagnosis and identify the groups, values, and pressures that may explain how these particular conditions happen to be defined in medical terms.

Female Hypoactive Sexual Desire Disorder

In the early part of this century, renewed interest in a condition found in the DSM-III-R, called hypoactive sexual desire disorder (HSDD), surfaced in both medical and lay circles (Jutel 2010). The condition was described as "Persistently or recurrently deficient or absent sexual fantasies and desire for sexual activity. The judgment of deficiency or absence is made by the clinician, taking into account factors that affect sexual functioning, such as age, sex, and the context of the person's life" (American Psychiatric Association Work Group to Revise DSM-III 1987, 293). HSDD was consciously promoted as a prevalent problem among Western women. Commercial forces played an important role in putting HSDD in the public and professional light. After the overwhelming success of Viagra as a response to male erection problems, the pursuit of an equivalent magic pill for woman (dubbed the "pink Viagra") was high on the minds of pharmaceutical industry executives. When a compound being tested for its antidepressive effects was fortuitously identified as potentially having female erotogenic properties, the pharmaceutical industry took a number of steps to capitalize on the findings.

Female sexual dysfunction is a multicausal and multidimensional problem combining biological, psychological, and interpersonal determinants. It is age related, progressive and highly prevalent, affecting 20% to 50% of women. Based on epidemiological data from the National Health and Social Life Survey a third of women lack sexual interest and nearly a fourth do not experience orgasm. (Basson et al. 2000)

Specialists friendly with the pharmaceutical industry easily typify problematic sexual function as a serious medical problem.

First, a meeting of industry-friendly doctors was convened to produce a consensus statement lamenting the absence of research on female sexuality and to highlight the supposed prevalence of sexual dysfunction in women. Second, extensive funding was provided for research to develop screening tools and diagnostic frameworks for this putative condition. Third, the idea of hypoactive sexual desire disorder was vigorously promoted in public awareness campaigns, using high-profile actresses to discuss the relief they felt at finally realizing that their lack of lust was a disease, not "in their heads." Of course, this all took place against the backdrop of the commodity culture, where female hypersexuality is constantly marketed as the norm, and treatment for its absence is presented as an imperative (Spurgas 2012). Finally, numerous pharmaceutical companies (notably Boehringer Ingelheim, or BI) went to work trialing various compounds and delivery methods to find the magic bullet that would transform the lustless heterosexual woman into a willing sexual partner.

Many social theorists would argue, as did Naomi McCormick (in Rothblum and Brehony 1993), that "the absence of genital juxtaposition hardly drains a relationship of passion or importance" and that the demand of sexual pleasure as proxy for partnership is a reflection of an androcentric approach to sexuality. This particular example of the medicalization of women's sexuality is one that was resisted, and ultimately may lead to the shelving of HSDD. The U.S. Food and Drug Administration did not give authorization for the compound identified by BI. Strong protest and advocacy from a number of antimedicalization groups, as well as poor performance of the medication in the trials, resulted in BI changing tack, abandoning the actual product development, but perhaps leaving in the minds of those who had read the advertising copy and media promotion a persistent sense of low sexual drive as disease.

Depression

Major depressive disorder, or MDD, has become the most commonly treated mental disorder in the Western world (Horwitz and Wakefield 2007). The increasing prominence of the disorder could represent an unprecedented increase in mental suffering, or it could signal the medicalization of the type of everyday sadness resulting from exposure to trying life events. The latter is widely supported by a range of social scientists, and could be explained by the DSM's redefinition of MDD born of interprofessional politics, the promotion of (and disease **branding** for) commercial products designed to alleviate MDD, and advocacy groups (Horwitz 2011). In the following paragraphs, we discuss what Mayes and Horwitz (2005) have referred to as "the loss of sadness," or the mechanisms by which medicine has expanded its jurisdiction to include sorrow.

As Mayes and Horwitz (2005) discussed at length, the DSM underwent significant transformation in its third revision. The first revision of the DSM took place in 1968 and represented a minor exercise in categorical alignment rather than the controversial conceptual and political modification that the DSM revisions were to become. The changes to the DSM-III, however, were motivated by subspecialty politics. Psychiatry had been marginalized within the medical community, its therapeutic roles subsumed by nonmedical professionals and its scope of practice restricted by those who funded care. Tensions within the field and a bourgeoning antipsychiatry movement led the psychiatric discipline to reconstruct psychiatric classification around symptom-based categorical diseases rather than etiologically defined entities. According to Mayes and Horwitz (2005), the new manual "transformed the little-used mental health manual into a biblical textbook specifically designed for scientific research, reimbursement compatibility, and by default, psychopharmacology" (263).

The symptom-based approach led to the adoption of a set of criteria for MDD that could be precisely identified and measured. These criteria included either a dysphoric mood or a loss of interest or pleasure in usual activities, accompanied by the daily presence of at least four other common symptoms (appetite, weight change, sleep, libido, fatigue, feelings of worthlessness or guilt, lack of focus, or suicidal ideation) for at least two weeks' duration. Exclusion is made of the presence of this symptom cluster when it appears after spousal bereavement (Horwitz 2011).

What Horwitz (2011) and others have made clear is the extent to which these symptoms are common in the presence of the normal reactions to sorrow and stress. Two weeks is a short time frame for concluding that a major depressive illness is present, as opposed to the expected reaction in the face of situational depression. Writes Horwitz (2011), "MDD in the DSM-III encompasses both symptoms that typify very severe and enduring symptoms as well as those that are short-lived signs of distress" (48).

In the most recent revision of the DSM, exclusion criteria have been removed, further widening who may be considered depressed. Where a bereaved person previously would have to have either self-destructive symptoms or to have been bereaved for more than two months before receiving a diagnosis depression, in the DSM-5, the exclusion has been removed, and depression may be diagnosed as soon as two weeks after a death.

Here again, the pharmaceutical industry has been quick to jump on a bandwagon that considers sorrow as disease. With this position strongly anchored, antidepressants solidify their position in the therapeutic armory. Not only do the industry players attempt to increase physician awareness of depression and their related pharmaceutical therapies, antidepression campaigns are funded by the industry even while many question the value of the drug treatment of unhappiness in primary care (Moncrieff et al. 2005).

Infertility

Infertility provides an example of how medicalization works in the realm of the tangible and the physiological, rather than in the less measurable world of the psychological, where, as discussed above, the signs and symptoms are subjective assessments. Infertility is a material failure to conceive. Medicine offers therapeutic means to remedy what ails the infertility patient. As Becker and Nachtigall (1992) have pointed out, however, infertility could be just as easily considered in the social frame of unwanted childlessness, and understood as a condition related to the social imperative to have a genetic heir.

In diagnostic language, not being able to have a child becomes either female or male infertility in the pages of the *International Classification of Diseases* (ICD). It may be of tubal or of uterine origin, associated with anovulation, azoospermia, or extraefferent duct obstruction or of unspecified origin. The diagnosis of infertility embodies a shift from a previously unmedicalized consideration of involuntary childlessness—the solution to which might be found in adoption, fostering, or child-related occupations—to the biomedical realm. As Becker and Nachtigall (1992) write:

> While medical diagnosis may provide an explanation for the inability to conceive and may even provide temporary relief from feelings of failure, individuals' feelings of abnormality may intensify if expectations that medical treatment will quickly cure the problem are not realised. Although individuals seek to solve the problem of childlessness by seeking medical treatment, treatment reflects the same dilemma they experience in daily life: cultural norms are reflected in medical treatment, and childlessness is consequently viewed as abnormal. (460)

The shift offers, of course, a different range of options for palliation of the social problem of not having a child. And it perhaps uniquely offers the solution of the child who is genetically related to the parents. These options are some to which patient activists are eager to ensure access. In vitro fertilization (IVF) and other reproductive technological procedures are clearly linked to diagnostic recognition of infertility. In the United States, without a diagnosis, insurance plans will not cover the cost of treatment. At the writing of this chapter, a few states, including Illinois and New Jersey, have passed legislation mandating that infertility is a disease, and every person who seeks treatment for infertility has a right to access it. In New Jersey, insurers must cover the expenses of two rounds of IVF.

But a medical approach is not without its limitations. Casting the inability to produce genetic offspring as a disease reinforces a particular norm, framing childless individuals as deviant. Fertility treatment itself can be stressful, divisive, unsuccessful, and stigmatizing. It can result in multiple births, which in some countries can lead to selective termination of multiple fetuses. Nor is the promise embodied by the diagnostic status of infertility complete. Some forms are, as the ICD recognizes, "unspecified" and unresponsive to medical treatment.

In medicine, where certainty reigns, the frequent inability to identify and remedy infertility is troublesome. A social frame might be more helpful, yet is frequently seen as a second-rate solution as a result of its normative co-construction as a medical problem.

WHAT DRIVES MEDICALIZATION AND DIAGNOSIS?

Another way of understanding medicalization is to ask what social forces propel it. Why are some conditions like baldness and erectile dysfunction medicalized, and others not? We have alluded to many of these forces above; Conrad (2005) has nicely summarized them as "engines of medicalization." These engines, or drivers, include: biotechnology, consumption, and, in the United States, managed care.

The female HSDD example described above typifies the pharmaceutical industry's involvement in the medicalization of particular disorders. But it is not restricted to this or any one disorder. From HSDD to depression, bipolar disorder, obesity, social phobia, social anxiety disorder, avoidant personality disorder, and so on, industry players often identify and promote the expansion of diagnostic categories in order to sell the concomitant treatment. While not wishing to minimize the role of the pharmaceutical industry, which cannot be underestimated, it is not alone with commercial interests in the promotion of disease awareness.

As Mary Ebeling writes in chapter 9, other forms of technology, including screening practices and self-diagnostic tools, are prevalent and powerful in the promotion of diagnosis or disease risk. Conrad (2005) sees potential areas for growth around medicalization in the area of genetic screening and medical intervention for enhancement. While this scenario may seem far-fetched, there is precedent. The availability of synthetic human growth hormone (HGH) has led to its use in short-statured children. The administration of HGH constitutes the kind of "technical procedure" that Zola (1972) refers to as reinforcing medical control. (It also reinforces short stature as problematic, rather than as one range of heights on the continuum of heights that an adult might achieve.) A range of "lifestyle drugs" are openly marketed to treat problems that fall somewhere between the medical and social definitions of health (Lexchin 2001). One perverse example was the practice of giving girls estrogen to restrict their growth and to prevent them from becoming too tall (Alcock 2010).

Adele Clarke et al. (2003) suggest the term "biomedicalization" to describe this phenomenon. They write: "Medicalization practices typically emphasize the exercising *control over* medical phenomena—diseases, illnesses, injuries, bodily malfunctions. In contrast, biomedicalization practices emphasize *transformations of* such medical phenomena and of bodies, largely through sooner-rather-than-later technoscientific interventions not only for treatment but also increasingly for enhancement" (2).

Yet medicalization is also driven from outside the technical realm. As the examples above illustrate, the patient as consumer takes a driving seat in ways that were historically less prevalent. The example of infertility highlights how lay activism plays an important role in promoting medicalization. It is not alone in its genre. From PTSD to Lyme disease, Alzheimer disease, prostate cancer, and many other conditions, the interests of particular groups of laypeople may be instrumental in highlighting how a particular condition can be defined in medical terms. **Health social movements** provide an important political force to address access to or provision of health services; the experiences of disease, illness, and disability, particularly contested illness; and health inequality and inequalities related to ethnicity, race, gender, class, and sexuality (Brown et al. 2004). Health social movements engage with medical science and public health to encourage favorable research, utilize resources, and produce their own knowledge.

Patient advocacy groups and individual patients may be buttressed or even wholly created and financed by industry. Their information may come from industry-sponsored patient education documents, and companies who stand to benefit in various ways from the increasing recognition of the condition in question may sponsor their activities, support groups, and information sites. This is not to say that patients are dopes, nor does it mean that their suffering isn't real. It is simply to acknowledge medicalization as process, and why and how groups seek to give medical meaning to particular forms of suffering.

One important such group was the Alzheimer's Disease and Related Disorders Association (ADRDA), which took the then–reasonably obscure condition of Alzheimer disease out of the shadows to become the prominent and well-recognized condition we know today (Fox 1989). Forging alliances with the ADRDA, an organization established to support the caregivers of people with Alzheimer disease, the National Institute on Aging raised public awareness, funds, research, and recognition of this specific disorder. This "unifying construct" (59) of scientists, lay organizations, and government agencies was responsible for identifying and addressing early onset senility as a disease, and for recasting it as one of the most common causes of death in the United States.

BEYOND DIAGNOSIS

Diagnosis is not the only vehicle by which medicalization occurs, although it is a prominent one. Birth provides an excellent example of another means of medicalization. The vocabulary of illness colors discussions of pregnancy in medical and in lay publications alike. The determination of pregnancy itself, for example, is still referred to as a "diagnosis," and the changes of normal pregnancy are its "symptoms." The medicalization of birth happens through its language, but also on a trifecta focus on preparation, pain, and risk.

The management of pregnancy as practiced in North America focuses on preparation for birth. "Natural childbirth" may be proposed as an option, on the surface, suggesting a demedicalized approach. But natural childbirth is a slippery concept; one would be hard put to claim that anything people do is "natural." In the world of birth, "natural" is used for anything from a vaginal (as contrasted to a cesarean) birth, and whether the woman was conscious, to a completely "nonmedicated" birth. "Prepared childbirth" is a more useful concept for viewing hospital births; it has come to mean the use of breathing or relaxation techniques, and particularly taking childbirth preparation courses to learn about birth or the medical management of the childbirth process: Most of the preparation courses, many offered by the hospitals themselves, are designed to prepare the woman for the hospital experience she is expected to have.

> The diagnosis of pregnancy requires a multifaceted approach using 3 main diagnostic tools. These are history and physical examination, laboratory evaluation, and ultrasonography. Currently, physicians may use all of these tools to diagnose pregnancy at early gestation and to help rule out other pathologies. (Shields 2012)
>
> *Using medical language to describe pregnancy colors its discussions and places it under medicine's jurisdiction.*

And what is that experience? Largely it is understood in terms of pain: pain experienced and pain avoided. There are a number of reasons why pain is a central issue in hospitalized births. First, birth in hospitals is almost certainly experienced as more painful than birth outside of hospitals. Before the pressures of the prepared-childbirth movement brought husbands or other companions into the labor room, laboring women were routinely left alone or with another laboring woman on the other side of a curtain, or a nurse who would stop in now and again (Simonds et al. 2006).

Second, the physical management of birth may make it more painful. Confinement to bed prolongs labor, and the comparatively inefficient contractions in the horizontal position may also make it more painful. When a woman is upright, each contraction presses the baby down against her cervix, opening up the birth passage. When she is lying down, the weight of the baby presses on her spine, increasing her discomfort (Simonds et al. 2006).

Third, the medical management of labor produced and reproduced birth as necessarily medical. The lithotomy position, flat on the back with legs in stirrups, was invariably used since the 1930s and even today for medical convenience. Doctors felt that this position gave them the most control, with total access to the woman's exposed genitals (Simonds et al. 2006). But doctors' control came at the expense of mothers. In this position, the baby had to be moved (pushed or pulled) upward because of the curve of the birth canal. It also prevented the woman from being able to help herself, with her limbs immobilized. Conceptualizing the woman's experience as work would have moved control to the woman and would have enabled her to seek a range of potential positions, some for their effectiveness, others for their comfort.

The infiltration of medicalization in childbirth is also evident in the concept of risk. Medicine can claim jurisdiction not only over illness, as described above, but also over the possibility of illness. What David Armstrong (1995) refers to as "surveillance medicine" and what serves as another cornerstone of the medicalization of birth is the idea that every health event or individual is always teetering precariously between health and disease, and that the potential for disease—or, in the case of childbirth, complications—to strike without warning rationalizes the importance of continual medical surveillance, all in the interest of health of course, but paradoxically at its expense, too.

Continual fetal monitoring, in which external electrodes measure the heart rate of the fetus throughout the birthing process, is one of many examples of medical surveillance of the normal birth. While it may intuitively seem a good way to prevent the risk of harm to the fetus, the benefits of its use are questionable. It has only been shown to have a small potential clinical benefit in the prevention of neonatal seizures, while contributing to an increase in caesarean and operative vaginal delivery with their own concomitant complications (Thacker et al. 2001).

MEDICALIZATION: OPENING AND CLOSING

Diagnosis plays an important enabling role in medicalization. It sanctions anxiety about particular conditions in a medical idiom, transferring jurisdiction in an immediately recognizable form. As our opening box underlines, once something becomes named a "thing," differentiable from other things by its very naming, it becomes a point of action. Once a condition becomes a medical thing, accordingly named, filed in medicine's taxonomies, and thus highlighted as medicine's responsibility, it becomes difficult to consider other avenues for action.

We can see that putting conditions under medicine's jurisdiction has distinct benefits. It decriminalizes psychosis, for example, and provides a scientific, rather than a commercial, source for problem solving. It provides mechanisms for alleviating suffering, and for focusing funds and interests on cures, or at least on palliation of troubling problems.

As described above, however, it is not without problematic consequences, and that fact should be taken into consideration by all who use medical labels, be they professionals, laypeople, or other agents. Considering a problem from all angles may also provide avenues for alleviating suffering, as well as robust solutions to tenacious problems. Finally, by medicalizing particular conditions (the above examples of sadness and short stature are salient), we also narrow the range of what is considered to be normal. Medicalization restricts what we are able to see, and how we judge things to be. It reduces, rather than enlarges, our possibilities.

TAKEAWAY POINTS

- Medicalization is a reflection of the importance and influence afforded to medical authority.
- Medicalization can be detrimental to health outcomes.
- Numerous industries and institutions promote medicalization by referring to medical authority to enhance their own interests.
- By seeing some conditions as medical in nature, other potential avenues for reducing individual suffering may not be explored.

DISCUSSION QUESTIONS

1. In mystery novels, the police often send for the doctor to attend to the murder victim's bereaved widow. Why is the doctor identified in literature as the typical support person in this situation of intense grief? Is this the doctor's proper role? Why or why not? What are the limitations of medical education for assuming this role?
2. A mother comes to see you, stating that the school nurse has recommended her child take medication for attention deficit disorder. She gives you a list of symptoms that the school nurse said confirm her child's disease. Your assessment is that the child is highly active and a "handful," but does not have a disease. How do you manage this situation?
3. There is increasing interest in medical and popular literature about "compassion fatigue" as a disease state experienced by doctors, nurses, and other health professionals in high-intensity settings. Provide an alternative nonmedicalized

framework for the problematic state of being. What are the advantages and disadvantages of the respective frameworks for assisting the distressed individuals?

4. List five potentially negative outcomes of diagnosing sadness as depression. Explain your answers.

REFERENCES

Alcock, Katie. 2010. "Can You Be Too Tall?" *BBC*, http://www.bbc.co.uk/news/health -11261760.

American Psychiatric Association Work Group to Revise DSM-III. 1987. *Diagnostic and Statistical Manual of Mental Disorders: DSM-III-R*. Washington, DC: American Psychiatric Association.

Armstrong, D. 1995. "The Rise of Surveillance Medicine." *Sociology of Health and Illness* 17(3): 393–404.

Basson, R., J. Berman, A. Burnett, L. Derogatis, D. Ferguson, J. Fourcroy, I. Goldstein, A. Graziottin, J. Heiman, E. Laan, S. Leiblum, H. Padma-Nathan, R. Rosen, K. Segraves, R.T. Segraves, R. Shabsigh, M. Sipski, G. Wagner, and B. Whipple. 2000. "Report of the International Consensus Development Conference on Female Sexual Dysfunction: Definitions and classifIcations." *Journal of Urology* 163(3): 888–93.

Becker, G., and R. D. Nachtigall. 1992. "Eager for Medicalisation: The Social Production of Infertility as a Disease." *Sociology of Health and Illness* 14(4): 456–71.

Brown, P., S. Zavestoski, S. McCormick, B. Mayer, R. Morello-Frosch, and R. G. Altman. 2004. "Embodied Health Movements: New Approaches to Social Movements in Health." *Sociology of Health and Illness* 26(1): 50–80.

Canguilhem, G. 1991. *The Normal and the Pathological*. New York: Zone Books.

Cartwright, S. 1981. "Report of the Diseases and Physical Peculiarities of the Negro Race." In *Concepts of Health and Disease*, edited by A. Caplan, H. T. Englehardt, and J. McCartney, 305–26. Reading, MA: Addison-Wesley.

Clarke, A. E., J. K. Shim, L. Mamo, J. R. Fosket, and J. R. Fishman. 2003. "Biomedicalization: Technoscientific Transformations of Health, Illness, and U.S. Biomedicine." *American Sociological Review* 68(2): 161–94.

Conrad, P. 1992. "Medicalization and Social Control." *Annual Review of Sociology* 18: 209–32.

———. 2005. "The Shifting Engines of Medicalization." *Journal of Health and Social Behavior* 46(1): 3–14.

Corbett, K., and T. Westwood. 2005. "'Dangerous and Severe Personality Disorder': A Psychiatric Manifestation of the Risk Society." *Critical Public Health* 15(2): 121–33.

Fassin, D. 2009. "Global Public Health." Paper presented at the Medical Anthropology at the Intersections: Celebrating 50 Years of Interdisciplinarity meeting, Yale University, New Haven, CT.

Foucault, M. 1963. *Naissance de la clinique*. Paris: Presses Universitaires de France.

Fox, P. 1989. "From Senility to Alzheimer's Disease: The Rise of the Alzheimer's Disease Movement." *Milbank Quarterly* 67(1): 58–102.

Freidson, E. 1972. *Profession of Medicine: A Study of the Sociology of Applied Knowledge*. 4th ed. New York: Dodd, Mead.

Horwitz, A. V. 2011. "Creating an Age of Depression: The Social Construction and Consequences of the Major Depression Diagnosis." *Society and Mental Health* 1(1): 41–54.

Horwitz, A., V., and J. C. Wakefield. 2007. *The Loss of Sadness: How Psychiatry Transformed Normal Sorrow into Depressive Disorder.* New York: Oxford University Press.

Illich, I. 1976. *Limits to Medicine—Medical Nemesis: The Expropriation of Health.* Middlesex: Penguin.

Jutel, A. 2010. "Framing Disease: The Example of Female Hypoactive Sexual Desire Disorder." *Social Science and Medicine* 70: 1084–90.

Laing, R. D. 1967. *The Politics of Experience and the Bird of Paradise.* Harmondsworth: Penguin.

Lexchin, J. 2001. "Lifestyle Drugs: Issues for Debate." *Canadian Medical Association Journal* 164(10): 1449–51.

Mayes, R., and A. V. Horwitz. 2005. "DSM-III and the Revolution in the Classification of Mental Illness." *Journal of the History of the Behavioral Sciences* 41(3): 249–67.

Moncrieff, J., S. Hopker, and P. Thomas. 2005. "Psychiatry and the Pharmaceutical Industry: Who Pays the Piper?" *Psychiatric Bulletin* 29: 84–85.

Munro, R. J. 2002. "Political Psychiatry in post-Mao China and Its Origins in the Cultural Revolution." *Journal of the American Academy of Psychiatry and the Law* 30(1): 97–106.

Nye, R. A. 2003. "The Evolution of the Concept of Medicalization in the Late Twentieth Century." *Journal of the History of the Behavior Sciences* 39(2): 115–29.

Rosenberg, C. E. 2002. "The Tyranny of Diagnosis: Specific Entities and Individual Experience." *Milbank Quarterly* 80(2): 237–60.

Rothblum, E. D., and K. A. Brehony. 1993. *Boston Marriages: Romantic but Asexual Relationships among Contemporary Lesbians.* Amherst, MA: University of Massachusetts Press.

Scott, W. J. 1990. "PTSD in DSM-III: A Case in the Politics of Diagnosis and Disease." *Social Problems* 37(3): 294–310.

Shields, Andrea D. 2012. "Pregnancy Diagnosis." *Medscape Reference*, http://emedicine.medscape.com/article/262591-overview.

Simonds, W., B. Katz Rothman, and B. M. Norman. 2006. *Laboring On: Birth in Transition in the United States.* New York: Routledge.

Spurgas, A. 2012. "Where Is My Subjectivity? Techno-Imagery, Femininity and Desire." *Social Text,* http://www.socialtextjournal.org/periscope/2012/04/where-is-my-subjectivity-techno-imagery-femininity-desire.php.

Szasz, T. S. 1970. *The Manufacture of Madness: A Comparative Study of the Inquisition and the Mental Health Movement.* New York: Harper Colophon.

Thacker, S. B., D. Stroup, and M. Chang. 2001. "Continuous Electronic Heart Rate Monitoring for Fetal Assessment during Labor." *Cochrane Database of Systematic Reviews* 2: CD000063.

Zola, I. K. 1972. "Medicine as an Institution of Social Control." *Sociological Review* 20: 487–504.

———. 1983. *Socio-Medical Inquiries: Recollections, Reflections, and Reconsiderations.* Philadelphia: Temple University Press.

The Promotion of Marketing-Mediated Diagnosis
Turning Patients into Consumers

Mary Ebeling

STARTING POINTS

- Medical marketing can influence clinical decision making.
- The pharmaceutical industry makes contact with doctors and medical students through visits, promotional events, and sponsorship of research and education.
- Insurance and publicly funded health systems shape diagnostic outcomes.

MARKETING AND DIAGNOSIS

As a student or practitioner in the medical and health-care fields, you have no doubt encountered the pervasive marketing and promotional efforts from pharmaceutical and medical device companies. If you are a medical student, depending on where you are studying, from the moment you enter the field to pursue a career in medicine, you receive visits from sales representatives who offer a range of free samples, symptom checklists, desk displays, all-expenses-paid "educational" seminars promoting a new drug or device, and script pads and pens emblazoned with a drug company's brand. A 2005 study focused on American medical students' exposure to and attitudes about drug companies on campus and found that students receive a gift or attend a sponsored event once a week on average while earning a medical degree (Sierles et al. 2005). Advertisements for a branded drug with a newly innovated formula or an implantable medical device are also common in medical and trade journals. It is possible that one of the articles you've read recently by a clinical researcher or medical practitioner was actually ghostwritten by a drug maker's public relations specialist. You may already be a well-seasoned and perhaps highly skeptical spectator of the endless parade of medical advertisements and marketing gimmicks.

As a student on the path to become a medical practitioner, you may have idealized the process of diagnosis as a relationship between a doctor and her **patient**, a social situation where your years of study, knowledge, and training come to bear on the symptoms and signs displayed in the patient. Yet you and your patient are not alone in the examination room. There are several other unseen stakeholders who have a keen interest in influencing the outcome of that **diagnostic moment**. You are not only training to become a doctor or health-care provider, you are being socialized into a thoroughly commercialized medical industry that affects and provides the context for diagnosis. Diagnosis is ensnared in a web of contending interests from all corners of the health industry. Doctors and medical researchers increasingly have financial interests and commercial ties to any number of companies in the life sciences or in pharmaceuticals and medical devices, and these interests shape diagnosis. Directors of large hospital systems as well as managers of small clinics and private practices, concerned with the balance between what is best for their patients' health and their businesses, all strain against the demands of health insurers or nationalized health systems to cut costs or to limit resources through the diagnostic process. Patients and patient advocates increasingly have become activists around any number of diagnostic categories, from autism spectrum disorders to fibromyalgia, who collaborate with doctors and researchers to define and shape diagnosis. All of these pressures, constraints, and interests have a significant influence on how diagnostic categories are built, how diagnosis is practiced, and the medical understanding of disease and wellness more generally.

The imperatives of medical marketing increasingly have a strong sway on diagnoses. This chapter describes how medical marketing can shape, influence, construct, or disrupt diagnostic categories and relationships. It provides two cases from a selection of health and medical industrial sectors to illustrate how diagnosis is shaped and influenced by the forces of marketing. First is the construction and promotion of new diagnostic categories by pharmaceutical companies that align with a drug's approved indications and **direct-to-consumer** marketing of drugs as well as diseases. The second case examines the marketing advancement of self-diagnosis through genetic diagnostic tests that create "patients-in-waiting" and that shape a patient's disease narratives to fit particular diagnostic categories. Specifically, by looking at these two instances, we examine in detail how medical marketing and advertising affect the diagnostic category and process.

You have already read throughout this book about how social scientists understand diagnosis as a socially mediated phenomenon that at times can be contested and controversial. Often these diagnostic controversies can include power struggles about nosology, or how a disease is defined and categorized; controversies over the very recognition of certain diagnoses, such as fibromyalgia; tensions over how much control patients should have over the diagnostic process; and the potential harmful and stigmatizing effects that certain diagnoses can have on a patient's social and working life, to name a few (see chaps. 7, 11, and 12). The aim here is to understand how powerful commercial interests shape and even dominate diagnosis, especially in the United States. Let's begin with a personal story that demonstrates how commercial forces can influence the diagnostic process.

Not long ago I was going through a period of mourning after experiencing several losses and problems with my health. At the time, I sought the support and guidance of a therapist to help me through this period of sadness. I knew that the blues I was experiencing were part of a normal and healthy response to what life had thrown at me, and that it would pass eventually, but at that moment I needed a little extra help in working through my sadness. Fortunately, I had health insurance and my plan covered six months of therapy. Because I live in the United States, my health insurer required that I be given a diagnosis, or they would not pay for treatment. As we were completing paperwork during the first session, my therapist pulled out the *Diagnostic and Statistical Manual of Mental Disorders* (DSM) and turned to the category "Depressive Disorders Not Otherwise Specified." While acknowledging that this was simply a way for us to find a diagnosis to satisfy my insurer, she explained that though it was a rather perfunctory exercise, we nonetheless had to find a diagnosis that would be convincing. She read out several disorders and asked me to choose the one I thought best described my present state. We settled on adjustment disorder with depressive mood.

This classification system my therapist was using, the DSM, was going through its fifth revision at the time, and this revision has received much criticism. The widely used diagnostic manual had come under fire when it was revealed that 70% of the panel members tasked with its revision had significant financial ties with pharmaceutical companies (Bursztajn et al. 2009). Such ties, many feared, bound these clinicians to their corporate paymasters, influencing them to define diseases not on the basis of medical and clinical evidence but by the marketing priorities of pharmaceutical companies or "marketing-based" medicine (Spielmans and Parry 2010). These priorities included expanding diagnoses of disorders and diseases in people experiencing what had previously been considered normal mood fluctuations that go with life, such as sadness during a period of loss, just as I was experiencing. This concern was so great that one member of the working group stepped down in protest, fearing that expanded categories would create "false epidemics" that could lead to the "medicalization of everyday behavior" (Urbina 2012).

I left our first appointment with mixed feelings. On the one hand, it was my first experience as a patient whose doctor collaborated so explicitly in determining what was "wrong with me." On the other, I colluded with my doctor in labeling myself as "maladjusted," and having "something wrong" with me when all I wanted was someone to talk to. Together my doctor and I rendered what we both thought was a normal response to loss experienced in life as something "unhealthy" and abnormal in order to satisfy the demands of my insurer, the DSM, and the pharmaceutical companies that had a large role in rewriting the diagnostic categories of the manual. This diagnostic moment has come to symbolize for me how the marketing and commercial interests in medicine exert influence on diagnosis. When I chose to seek out support from a health professional, my experience became medicalized because of a range of commercial interests. The health insurance industry, the DSM, antidepressant manufacturers, and even my therapist's need to retain patients all required that I be given a diagnosis.

COMMERCIALIZING DIAGNOSIS AND MEDICINE

While many Western economies have commercialized medical systems to varying degrees, combining some amount of privatized and public health care, most countries, regardless of the tight regulations that may be in place on consumer marketing, allow for extensive and often hidden medical marketing to medical professionals. Since the focus of this chapter is how the highly consumerist and hotly contested context of the American health-care system shapes the process of diagnosis, it is important to compare the financial burden many Americans face when it comes to health costs as compared with other countries. The complex, global medical marketing regulatory field is always shifting, and since the American medical market is the largest in the world, for these reasons we focus on marketing's impact on diagnosis within the United States. In order to better understand the impact of marketing, especially direct-to-consumer (DTC) marketing, of medical goods and services on the process of diagnosis, we examine some of the history of American pharmaceutical advertising.

Americans spend more on health care than any other Organisation for Economic Co-operation and Development (OECD) country: in 2010, Americans spent on average $8,233, compared with the average for all OECD countries, $3,265 (OECD 2012). Even though many Americans have some kind of health insurance coverage or access to varying levels of health care, there are still more than forty-nine million who are uninsured, and most who have coverage overwhelmingly depend upon employer-provided private health insurance. This places the burden of financing health care squarely on the shoulders of employers and patients, with the rise in insurance premiums outpacing the average increase in earnings by roughly four times (Ginsburg 2008; Kaiser Family Foundation 2011).

The typical insured family pays more than a sixth of its annual income toward health care, yet many Americans do not experience improved health outcomes when compared with residents of other OECD countries (Sered and Fernandopulle 2005). These health-care costs are due to many factors, including private and for-profit health care and health insurance, the rise in chronic diseases as more Americans live longer, and the highly complex health system, but the high costs of medical technologies and prescription drugs cannot be minimized. Out of the total that American patients spend on health care, $792 is spent per capita on prescription drugs (almost twice the average $401 spent per capita in other OECD countries), with the United States accounting for 45% of total global drug sales, making America the world's largest pharmaceutical market (Ebeling 2011; OECD 2008). Some have argued that the cause behind the high costs of prescription medicines is largely the expenses associated with marketing and promotion. Indeed, more financial resources are dedicated to marketing than to the research and development of new drugs (Gagnon and Lexchin 2008), and patients pay for this marketing in the high price of medicines and medical technologies that they use and consume.

The United States and New Zealand are the only countries whose regulatory bodies allow for DTC marketing of branded pharmaceuticals and medical devices. Most other countries and regions, such as the European Union, have outright bans on DTC marketing and advertising. Despite these bans, intense drug and device marketing targeting doctors and medical professionals is typical.

Marketing strategies such as "detailing" (a practice involving personal visits by pharmaceutical sales representatives to individual doctors, often accompanied by small gifts as simple as a penlight with the company's logo, trips, larger gifts and meals), promotional educational events at resorts, free samples, and institutional advertising account for the bulk of promotional budgets (Gagnon and Lexchin 2008; Greene 2005). In fact, in 2011, estimates of promotional spending by the industry globally range around $92.2 billion, of which $30.6 billion was spent in North America on total drug promotion activities. Only a fraction of that figure, $4.3 billion, was spent on DTC marketing in the United States (Arnold 2012; Mack 2012; SK&A 2012). Official estimates of spending like the ones above are notoriously underestimated, and, as Marc-André Gagnon and Joel Lexchin note, most official estimates are misleading and likely less than half of what the industry actually spends on promotional activities (Gagnon and Lexchin 2008).

The high visibility of DTC drug marketing, however, tends to attract enormous attention and concern over whether the marketing of pharmaceuticals and diseases is helping us or harming us. Still, the pharmaceutical industry deploys "hidden" marketing tactics to promote their brands. Most pharmaceutical marketing efforts aim to reach the medical practitioners who make diagnoses and write scripts: doctors and, increasingly, nurses. And there is evidence that this has an impact on how doctors diagnose.

The power of advertising to doctors in promoting simplistic *stereotypes* or misleading information about a disease, for example, can have an influence on how doctors diagnose. While there is ample clinical research demonstrating that men suffer from rates of depression on par with women, a study examining the gendering of disease in marketing showed that drug advertising that targeted doctors tended to depict depression as a disease typically afflicting women and affected the likelihood of a depression diagnosis being made for a male patient (Curry and O'Brien 2006).

All of these marketing efforts can have profound impacts on how we understand diagnosis and on the outcomes of a patient's health and treatment options. And that is the purpose of such marketing—to shape, influence, and be central to the diagnostic process. Physician and historian of medicine Jeremy Greene has noted that the diagnosis of disease "has become simultaneously an epidemiological event and a marketing event" (Greene 2007, ix). In what follows, we seek to understand how the diagnosis has become a marketing opportunity for the medical industries.

MEDICAL MARKETING IN THE UNITED STATES

American culture is a consumer culture that is often expressed through advertising. Marketing messages are so common that many times we are barely aware of them: the average city dweller in the United States sees more than five thousand advertisements every day (Story 2007). Compared to thirty years ago, when during a typical day an American could see as few as five hundred promotional messages, it is fair to say that marketing, **branding**, and advertising is the white noise in our daily lives. And this almost-inescapable marketing environment extends to the health-care and medical industries. Patients and medical professionals are all subjected to intense marketing. A patient may see a commercial that is tailored (and regulated) specifically for her, and her doctor might receive a visit from a sales rep. While the messages may be tweaked for each group, they are nonetheless ubiquitous and expand across virtually all media. There are advertisements for educational toys printed on the paper liners of pediatricians' examination tables; the brand names of drugs decorate the pens and charts in doctors' offices; and mobile phone applications "help" patients determine if a set of symptoms can be a sign of a disease. These messages are undoubtedly intended to shape how both patients and physicians understand health and wellness, the meaning of symptoms and diagnoses.

America's highly commercialized media environment started to take shape when the emergence of industrialized, large-scale consumer goods production in the middle to late nineteenth century created a need for manufacturers to promote these products to the new consumer classes, giving rise to mass advertising and marketing. Advertising, then as well as now, functioned to distinguish manufactured goods that often were hardly different from one another. These early advertisers paved the way for marketing messages that are now all too familiar. Advertisements, especially those for what were called "patent" medicines, often did not pitch an appeal on the discernible qualities of the product but rather strategically played on a consumer's fears of ill health; insecurities about gender roles, class status, aspirations, and, above all, the crushing guilt of not taking action. What is more, most Americans had little or no access to physicians, or did not trust some of the dangerous treatments that were commonly practiced at the time, such as leeching, purging, or blistering. Access to what was called "ethical" medication, the drugs formulated by pharmacists, was even lower, and forced many to turn to self-help, self-diagnosis, and self-medication (Conrad and Leiter 2008, 826).

In an effort to distinguish their compounds from those patent medicines that were considered more nefarious and overly commercialized, several North American drug manufacturers marketed their therapeutics as "ethical" medicine, or standardized formulas that were made in accordance with the *United States Pharmacopeia* and marketed under the American Medical Association's *Code of Ethics* (Greene and Herzberg 2010, 794). Though voluntary and not required by any regulatory body, the manufacturers of ethical drugs chose not to advertise widely or directly to consumers, but rather focused on institutional advertising and marketing efforts targeted solely to medical professionals as a way to further distinguish the industry from the unsavory marketing tactics of patent medicines.

Despite their name, patent medicines were neither under patent nor had their formulas been tested for safety and efficacy; the label simply meant they were trademarked. They were the nostrums, elixirs, and potions largely associated in the public's mind with itinerant "snake oil" salesmen peddling hokum. Patent medicines were secretly formulated with either ineffective or potentially dangerous ingredients (Fox 1997, 16). Often these nostrums were labeled and promoted with misleading, wildly exaggerated, and patently false claims in regard to the symptoms treated and to the medicine's effectiveness.

This early instance of medical advertising had profound effects on the bottom lines of producers. As advertising historian Stephen Fox notes, sales of one of the

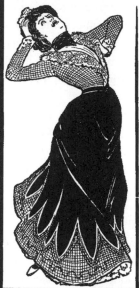

Sudden Death

If you have heart disease you are in grave danger.

You may die any minute—anywhere. Heart troubles, dangerous as they are, can be instantly recognized by all. No doctor can tell better than you if your heart is out of order. If you have any of the following symptoms, don't waste any time. Get my Heart Tablets at once.

Fluttering, palpitation, or skipping beats (always due to weak or diseased heart); shortness of breath from going upstairs, walking, etc.; tenderness, numbness or pain in left side, arm or under shoulder blade; fainting spells, dizziness, hungry or weak spells; spots before the eyes; sudden starting in sleep, dreaming, nightmare;

Heart Disease

choking sensation in throat; oppressed feeling in chest; cold hands and feet; painful to lie on left side; dropsy; swelling of the feet or ankles (one of the surest signs); neuralgia around the heart; sudden deaths rarely result from other causes.

They will restore you to health and strength as they have hundreds of other men and women.

FREE To prove how absolutely I believe in them, to prove that they will do exactly what I say, I will send a box free to any name and address sent me. One trial will do more to convince you than any amount of talk. It will cost you nothing, and may save your life. Send for a trial box and enclose stamp for postage.

DR. F. G. KINSMAN, Box 954 AUGUSTA, MAINE.

Figure 9-1. This patent medicine advertisement, which appeared in an unidentified American magazine from the 1910s, employs scare and guilt tactics to persuade potential consumers to buy the product. While today there is much legislation in place to protect patients from such blatant manipulation, many drug advertisements still use similar techniques to promote sales. *Source: MagazineArt.org, reprinted with permission*

era's most popular preparations, Lydia Pinkham's Vegetable Compound, a formulation purported by its makers to address all female ailments and "complaints," increased by 2500% over ten years after the company began advertising (Fox 1997, 19). At the time, the patent medicines were the first products to be advertised widely and nationally, so much so that in the public's mind the two were inextricably connected (16–19). In fact, the push to nationally advertise patent medicines helped to create not only the first advertising agencies, where more than half of agencies' revenues came from the patent medicine industry, but also helped to prompt a massive increase in magazine publishing (Goodrum and Dalrymple 1990, 29–30). By the late nineteenth century, several magazines were founded to serve solely as vehicles for advertising, and magazines quickly subverted the traditional model of advertising: they went from selling products to potential consumers to becoming instruments that collected and sold consumers to advertisers, much like what most contemporary media now do.

But it was a magazine, *Ladies' Home Journal*, that helped to blow the lid off of the unethical marketing tactics of the proprietary drug makers. In 1892, it refused to accept any more patent medicine advertising and conducted a series of investigative articles on the safety of patent medicines.

The articles in *Ladies' Home Journal* as well as similar investigative pieces that appeared in *Collier's Weekly* led directly to the passing of the 1906 Pure Food and Drug Act, legislation that instituted the U.S. Food and Drug Administration (FDA; Bok 1921). Before 1906, false and misleading labeling of patent drugs was widespread. With the passing of the act, the accurate labeling of drugs was mandated. The regulation of drug advertising, however, especially consumer advertising, would not be regulated until 1938, when the Food, Drug and Cosmetic Act (also known as the Wheeler Lea Act) granted regulatory jurisdiction over pharmaceutical advertising to the U.S. Federal Trade Commission (Palumbo and Mullins 2002).

Soliciting highly personal letters from women as a marketing method was common for patent medicines, especially those marketed to women. A 1911 collection of "nostrums and quackery" advertisements collected by the American Medical Association includes evidence from the Mrs. Cora B. Miller Company, owned and operated by Mr. Frank D. Miller, that had their "young women clerks and stenographers" compounding the toxic formula for "female weakness" and responding to letters from unsuspecting "marks," or women seeking relief through these mail-order treatments (American Medical Association 1911, 194–201).

In an effort to eliminate the duplication of efforts as well as to tighten rules on drug marketing, the FDA took over the regulation of drug advertising in 1962 as legislated by Congress through amendments to the earlier acts. Included in these changes were the Kefauver-Harris drug amendments, which stipulated that all drugs must be proven safe and effective before being marketed to the public. During the mid-twentieth century, most pharmaceutical companies did not pursue DTC marketing and instead focused efforts on advertising directed toward medical professionals. Doctors and practitioners were reached primarily through office visits by drug company sales representatives, in trade and medical journals, and in corporately sponsored research journals—journals often published by the public relations departments of drug manufacturers. By the close of the decade, the FDA issued guidelines for pharmaceutical advertising, which required that the information in advertisements be truthful and not misleading, as well as be "material" to the approved indications for the drug; provide a "fair balance" of information on both the benefits and risks associated with a drug; and, most importantly, offer a "brief summary" on all known risks (Ventola 2011).

It wasn't until the early 1980s, when drug makers began to advertise directly and more heavily to consumers, that the FDA implemented a brief moratorium on the consumer marketing of pharmaceuticals (Palumbo and Mullins 2002). After the moratorium was lifted in 1985, the regulatory body announced that the instated regulations were sufficient, but ostensibly only allowed advertisers to directly promote their products to consumers in print, because the requirements to provide "brief summaries" on the risks, side ef-

There are generally three categories of drug advertisements that are recognized by the FDA: (1) reminder ads, which are those that name a drug, and the form it takes, but not its uses; (2) help-seeking ads that don't mention a brand-named drug but focus on a disease state or categorizes symptoms, which are often called "disease-awareness" ad campaigns and often say "see your doctor if you have these symptoms"; and (3) product claim ads, which state the brand name and mention indications, efficacy, and risk information (Palumbo and Mullins 2002; Ventola 2011).

fects, and contraindications of a drug were too cumbersome for a thirty-second broadcast spot. By 1997, however, after a series of public hearings, the FDA loosened DTC restrictions for broadcast advertising under draft guidance, which was finalized in 1999 (Palumbo and Mullins 2002, 430). In the intervening years since DTC took off in the United States, the FDA has extended DTC advertising and marketing regulations to include medical devices.

Direct-to-Consumer Drug Marketing, Disease Awareness, and Self-Diagnosis

What has been the impact of such marketing on diagnosis? To answer this question, we look at two types of marketing: disease awareness marketing and DTC pharmaceutical marketing. These two instances provide clear examples of how marketing shapes the definition of disease by influencing the construction of categories and what symptoms mean in regard to health and illness. One of the implicit aims of marketing is to encourage patients to self-diagnose, which on the face seems empowering to the patient and disruptive of traditional power relationships in medicine. But it is really a marketing strategy not unlike that seen in nineteenth-century patent medicine—to spur the sales of drugs, disease screenings, and diagnoses of diseases that are marketed by the pharmaceutical makers. These new approaches to marketing pose a new challenge in the lay-professional relationship discussed throughout this book (see chaps. 4, 7, 11, and 12).

In a little over fifteen years, the DTC marketing of medicine, pharmaceuticals, and devices has grown exponentially in the United States. Those opposed to drug advertising point to harmful health effects such as overprescribing, overdiagnosing, or increased misdiagnoses, which are all attributable to such marketing. Those in favor believe that DTC marketing provides necessary and empowering health information to patients.

Remember the television commercials for GlaxoSmithKline's (GSK) branded drug Requip (ropinirole), marketed as a treatment for restless leg syndrome (or RLS, also known as Willis-Ekbom disease), a condition rebranded by the drug manufacturer when it sought FDA premarket approval for its drug? The commercials and print ads were ubiquitous in the mid-2000s across the United States, so much so that RLS became the butt of many comedians' jokes. A neurologist at the Center for Restless Legs Syndrome at Johns Hopkins University, Dr. Christopher Jenkins, noted at the time that the condition had gained "out-of-the-blue disease" status and that RLS advertising was creating an increased consumer demand for the diagnosis, a condition with a low prevalence in the general population (Aleccia 2008). While seen as a transparent attempt on GSK's part to flog drugs by creating a disease where one didn't exist (or at least not as it was branded or at the rate suggested), the campaign quickly became symbolic of all that is harmful with consumer drug advertising.

GlaxoSmithKline's RLS campaign is an example of what is termed **disease awareness marketing**. A significant portion of industry marketing efforts across both DTC and marketing to health-care providers involves the promotion of certain diagnoses and diseases to the public as well as to the medical profession. There are a number of features that distinguish disease awareness campaigns from other forms of health marketing. These campaigns do not explicitly promote a product; they tend to be "unbranded," which means they do not mention the name of the drug maker sponsoring the advertisement, and they can appear to be sponsored by a research foundation or patient advocacy group organized to fight for recognition or a cure for the disease.

Pharmaceutical companies expend huge financial resources to ensure that identified symptoms converge with the approved indications of the drugs that they brand and market. These disease marketing campaigns often begin years ahead of regulatory approval for a company's drug. Most promotional planning begins in the preclinical development of compounds in the laboratory, years before regulatory approval and legal marketing begins (Fugh-Berman and Dodgson 2008). American pharmacological marketing textbooks published as early as the 1950s noted that product marketing and clinical research are essentially interwoven processes, where the development of compounds and how those drugs are marketed to treat disease or symptoms are inextricably linked (Greene 2005).

In the early 1980s, in a rather blatant attempt to invent a disease to protect market interests, during FDA hearings on the safety and reclassification of silicone breast implants as Class III medical devices, the American Society of Plastic Surgeons (ASPS) created a diagnosis of "micromastia," or "small breasts," a deformity the ASPS claimed at the time had detrimental effects on women suffering from the "disease" and whose only remedy was augmentation surgery (Cohen 1994, 169). The ASPS used its power as a lobbying organization to create a definition of disease in order to protect its market interests.

In another widely discussed case, Eli Lilly's exerted strong influence on the work group responsible for the definition of premenstrual dysmorphic disorder (PMDD) in the revision of the DSM-IV. By placing clinical psychiatrists under the pay of Eli Lilly into positions of responsibility with regard to the disease categorization for the revised DSM, the pharmaceutical maker was assured that the associated symptoms of the controversial disorder neatly fit the reapproved indications of Prozac, which was rebranded as Sarafem, a treatment for PMDD (Ebeling 2011).

Conditions, diseases, and diagnoses that are now widely recognized and rarely disputed, at least publicly, are promoted in order to sell the given diseases or diagnoses to physicians, to the larger health industry (including insurers and regulators), and to the public. Commonly recognized health problems such as hypercholesterolemia or hypertension were linked to heart disease in part through the tireless marketing efforts of drug maker Merck during the middle to late twentieth century (Greene 2007). Through Merck's pursuit to build a market for its compounds, company marketers and product developers collaborated with chemical engineers and clinicians to construct a relationship between diagnostic categories, chronic diseases, and the drugs under development in order to promote both conditions as seriously underdiagnosed problems afflicting millions. Through the aggressive marketing of three drugs in particular—Diuril, a diuretic; Orinase, an antidiabetic taken orally; and Mevacor, the first statin on the American market—diagnostic screenings were extended to apparently healthy and asymptomatic patients and assured that the pharmaceutical industry, through a universe of chronic disease that could expand ad infinitum, would realize an equally expandable and profitable market (Ebeling 2011; Greene 2007).

Routine scanning even in the absence of symptoms has become part of a dominant public health discourse, at least in the highly marketing-mediated health environment of the United States. Once an individual reaches a milestone age, the American Cancer Society (and other similar organizations) promote annual screenings in otherwise healthy patients, such as mammograms for women beginning at age forty, or prostate-specific antigen tests to screen for prostate cancer in men at age fifty onward (Cassels 2012). The fact that much of this testing can lead to false positives or unnecessarily alarmist diagnoses that have profound, cascading health implications is of course not part of any of the promotional marketing of these tests or public health messages (Cassels 2012; Welch et al. 2011).

The mainstay of these campaigns, however, is to promote awareness of particular symptom clusters. These campaigns then project a specific diagnosis to these symptom clusters, one for which the drug company's branded drug is an approved treatment. This enables the pharmaceutical company to assist individuals to speak of their own symptom clusters in ways that align with the approved indications for their drugs. Patients then bring this language of marketing to discuss with their doctors. This way, a drug maker can stake a claim for a particular disease, predicate its treatment, and inextricably link the illness and the cure together in the public's mind, much like Eli Lilly did with depression and Prozac. Through marketing, Prozac defined depression.

Advancements made in diagnostic technologies, particularly "at-home" tests and diagnostic assessments administered by patients themselves, when coupled with DTC marketing of diagnoses and disease states, likewise make it easier for patients to see themselves as diseased and in need of medical or pharmaceutical intervention. More testing, and more marketing of testing, leads to more intervention, necessary or otherwise. While self-diagnosis of some illnesses may not necessarily be negative, and can be the first step for a patient to seek out support and guidance from her physician (public health disease awareness campaigns may use the same tools as commercial enterprises), the promotion of self-diagnosis by medical marketing is not designed to benefit the patient. Its purpose is to sell drugs, tests, and services that may not all benefit the patient.

Many critics argue that little has changed since the days of patent medicines and hokum, at least in regard to some of the tactics used in DTC drug advertising and disease awareness marketing. As with patent medicines of one hundred years ago, contemporary pharmaceutical marketing campaigns attempt to persuade patients to recognize symptoms or even asymptomatic conditions as disease, as well as to diagnose themselves and to self-medicate, even if indirectly by pressuring a desired diagnosis and prescription from his doctor (Conrad and Leiter 2008; Ebeling 2011).

Marketing Genetic Diagnostics and the Creation of "Patients-in-Waiting"

Direct-to-consumer genetic diagnostic tests can have an influence on diagnosis by marketing potential risks for developing a disease, even in the absence of any symptoms. In the decade since the Human Genome Project successfully completed a full map of the human genome in 2003, a new industry in personalized medicine and DTC genetic diagnostic testing has sprouted up to take advantage of the plummeting costs and streamlined processes that have made gene sequencing faster and more affordable. Generally these diagnostic tests fall into two broad categories. The first category includes tests that are regulated by the FDA as medical devices, are marketed to medical professionals, and can only be ordered and administered by a doctor or health institution to help designate a diagnosis or treatment plan. Tests that help a doctor optimize the best dosing level for the blood thinner warfarin based on a patient's genetic makeup or the controversial BRACAnalysis test are examples of tests within this class (Boddington 2009).

The second category of tests includes those that are not necessarily regulated by the FDA and are marketed and sold directly to consumers with no intervention by a physician. Some tests are used and marketed for curiosity purposes, such as to investigate genealogical history, while others claim to provide predictive information on diseases ranging from Alzheimer disease and multiple sclerosis to prostate cancer and asthma (Chapman 2008). Companies such as 23andMe Inc. (with financial backing and company leadership connected to Internet behemoth Google), Navigenetics, Pathway Genetics, and Knome market DTC tests that scan a person's genetic makeup to look for markers that purportedly indicate a risk for developing diseases (Parthasarathy 2010; Pollack 2010).

These genetic tests are not diagnostic of a disease; they test for the presence of a genetic marker on the patient's genotype. These tests do not determine how that gene may or may not be expressed in the phenotype. For most diseases, the likelihood of a patient actually developing a condition based on a genetic marker depends on many factors, meaning that a person's genes are not necessarily his destiny. Yet this is how many of the DTC genetic tests are marketed. While industry advocates argue that their tests provide crucial health information that empowers patients to make informed decisions about their health or to take preventative action, many medical professionals are deeply concerned that DTC genetic tests do not provide meaningful health information because there is still scant clinical evidence linking genetic variance and the probability of disease. These tests actually have the potential to harm patients because few individuals are equipped to interpret information about disease probabilities. At issue is that the typical odds ratio of most genome-wide association studies is so low as to be statistically and medically insignificant (Magnus et al. 2009).

A DTC test targeting a gene variant related to cardiovascular disease, for instance, may report results of an increase in risk from 1% to 1.6%. While an increase of 50% or more seems like a clear indication that the chances are high that you will develop the disease, a ratio of 1.6 is in fact inconsequential and prone to be misinterpreted by most patients without guidance (Caulfield and McGuire 2012). There is concern that do-it-yourself personalized genetic testing amplifies weak genetic associations, which may lead to unnecessary procedures or a misdiagnosis, not to mention the unnecessary increase in anxiety and worry on the part of patients. Most DTC genetic tests, however, are promoted on these low odds of genetic prevalence leading to disease.

Genetic diagnostic tests and their marketing can influence diagnosis in radical ways. Until recently, companies could "own" genes, patenting them as intellectual property. They could then develop, control, and market tests for those genes. As one example, Myriad Genetic Laboratories Inc., a Utah-based genetic diagnostics manufacturer, co-owned (with the University of Utah) patents on two genes that have been associated with certain hereditary breast and ovarian cancers, BRCA1 and BRCA2. While these forms of cancer are not as common, their detection in women with family histories of breast or ovarian cancer has clear benefits. And the commercial laboratories are understandably keen for their use to be much wider.

The diagnostic test developed and marketed as BRACAnalysis by Myriad is the only one available and accounts for more than 84% of Myriad's revenues. The marketing website for the test promotes the idea that a personal or family history of nonspecific "cancer" is indication enough for suspicion of the BRCA1 or BRCA2 gene, broadening widely by such an assertion the range of individuals likely to consider themselves at risk of having the genetic mutation. Myriad's mass marketing approach targets all women, rather than the specific (and relatively small; less than 5% of breast cancers are associated with BRCA1 and BRCA2) group of women who are at risk. The marketing narrative casts women as "patients-in-waiting," requiring responsible and early testing (Rajan 2005).

The ownership of the BRCA1 and BRCA2 genes has a profound impact on doctors' ability to confirm the gene marker in patients they suspect have heredity cancer. The genetic tests that could confirm that women carry this gene are only covered by insurance policies issued by companies who have negotiated a contract with Myriad. In the absence of such a contract, or of insurance, the tests cost several thousand dollars, preventing many doctors from using the diagnostic tool their patients require. This concern over access to diagnosis is so great that the American Civil Liberties Union along with geneticists, pathologists, patients, and clinicians filed a class-action suit against Myriad, arguing in part that the patents are denying women access to potentially life-saving diagnostics (Fuchs 2013). In June 2013 the U.S. Supreme Court found in favor of the plaintiffs' claim against Myriad's ownership of BRCA1 and BRCA2, arguing that a naturally occurring human gene is not eligible for patenting (Ledford 2013).

THE CROWDED EXAMINATION ROOM

As illustrated by the cases above, when the patient arrives in the examination room, both she and the clinician have often been primed, often despite their best efforts, to understand disease in ways that have been shaped by commercial interests. The reasons for, results of, and interactions during the visit between patient and doctor are steered by much more than the health and well-being of the individual patient. The examination room is crowded with commercial and marketing interests from pharmaceutical and medical device companies, medical industries, health insurers, policy makers and regulators, health advocacy groups, and the patient.

Diagnosis is a process that does not simply begin and end with the patient but rather is a phenomenon that is shaped along the production pipeline of drugs, devices, and diseases, with each moment upstream and down proffering an opportunity for a marketing intervention. From its earliest history in the late nineteenth century to the present, medical marketing seeks to intervene its construction of diseases and attendant cures into the diagnostic relationship between doctor and patient; to promote the use of self-diagnosis among patients; and to shape the understanding and interpretation of the meaning of symptoms, disease, and how to manage health and illness. Pharmaceutical and medical device companies do this from the very beginning of the creation of a compound or the discovery of a molecule or genetic mutation. These interventions begin in the laboratory and extend recursively through the development pipeline through to the regulatory bodies and medical **institutions** responsible for overseeing the safety of medicine or the defining of diseases and to the direct marketing to consumers or medical professionals. Within this context, physicians in training need to expand their understandings of what roles they play in the diagnostic relationship. It is no longer enough for medical professionals to see themselves as arbiters of a medically understood diagnosis, they must also expand their roles to recognize and, when appropriate, act as critics of diagnosis marketing, providing alternative sources of information and treatment that result in effective patient-centered care.

TAKEAWAY POINTS

- Understanding marketing's influence on diagnosis from the perspective of doctors, patients, clinicians, and administrators is important to successful management of health problems.
- The meaning of diagnosis may be transformed by marketing influence for the individuals involved in the diagnostic process, with nonclinical meanings taking precedence.
- Insurers and other health-care managers can deny, divert, or direct diagnoses, which can determine health outcomes for patients.

DISCUSSION QUESTIONS

1. How can medical marketing serve patients while supporting the industry's interests? What are the conflicts, and how might these be managed?
2. Identify five ways in which pharmaceutical marketing has been visible in your practice, education, or health in the past year.

3. Have you ever received a gift (even a small one) from a pharmaceutical sales representative? What was the brand being promoted? How easy was it for you to recall?

4. Identify four sources of information about a disease or syndrome, a medication it is approved to treat, and how to prescribe it. Compare the information presented by these sources to the information provided in a disease awareness campaign. What are the similarities and differences? How do the sources frame the information differently?

5. Are at-home genetic diagnostic tests empowering to patients or endangering their health? What would you say to a patient who presents you with results of a test that you find of dubious use for their health or future chances of illness?

REFERENCES

Aleccia, JoNel. 2008. "Without TV Ads, Restless Legs May Take a Hike." *NBCNews*, http://www.nbcnews.com/id/24603237/ns/health-health_care/t/without-tv-ads-restless-legs-may-take-hike/, May 14 .

American Medical Association. 1911. *Nostrums and Quackery: Articles on the Nostrum Evil and Quackery Reprinted from the Journal of the American Medical Association.* Chicago: American Medical Association.

Arnold, Matthew. 2012. "Pfizer, Crestor Tops for Global Promotional Spend in 2011." *Medical Marketing and Media*, http://www.mmm-online.com/pfizer-crestor-tops-for-global-promotional-spend-in-2011/article/238922/, May 1.

Boddington, Paula. 2009. "The Ethics and Regulation of Direct-to-Consumer Genetic Testing." *Genome Medicine* 1(7): 71.1–2.

Bok, Edward William. 1921. *The Americanization of Edward Bok: The Autobiography of a Dutch Boy Fifty Years After.* New York: Charles Scribner's Sons.

Bursztajn, Harold J., Lisa Cosgrove, David J. Kupfer, and Darrel A. Regier. 2009. "Toward Credible Conflict of Interest Policies in Clinical Psychiatry." *Psychiatric Times*, http://www.psychiatrictimes.com/articles/toward-credible-conflict-interest-policies-clinical-psychiatry, January 1.

Cassels, Alan. 2012. *Seeking Sickness: Medical Screening and the Misguided Hunt for Disease.* Vancouver: Greystone.

Caulfield, Timothy, and Amy L. McGuire. 2012. "Direct-to-Consumer Genetic Testing: Perceptions, Problems, and Policy Responses." *Annual Review of Medicine* 63(1): 23–33.

Chapman, Audrey. 2008. "DTC Marketing of Genetic Tests: The Perfect Storm." *American Journal of Bioethics* 8(6): 10–12.

Cohen, Kerith. 1994. "Truth & Beauty, Deception & Disfigurement: A Feminist Analysis of Breast Implant Litigation." *William and Mary Journal of Women and the Law* 1(1): 149–82.

Conrad, Peter, and Valerie Leiter. 2008. "From Lydia Pinkham to Queen Levitra: Direct-to-Consumer Advertising and Medicalisation." *Sociology of Health and Illness* 30(6): 825–38.

Curry, Phillip, and Marita O'Brien. 2006. "The Male Heart and the Female Mind: A Study in the Gendering of Antidepressants and Cardiovascular Drugs in Advertisements in Irish Medical Publication." *Social Science and Medicine* 62(8): 1970–77.

Ebeling, Mary. 2011. "'Get with the Program!': Pharmaceutical Marketing, Symptom Checklists and Self-Diagnosis." *Social Science and Medicine* 73(6): 825–32.

Fox, Stephen. 1997. *The Mirror Makers: A History of American Advertising and Its Creators*. Champaign: University of Illinois Press.

Fuchs, Erin. 2013. "Supreme Court Seems Highly Skeptical That Biotech Can 'Patent Nature.'" *Business Insider,* http://www.businessinsider.com/supreme-court-myriad -case-2013-4, April 16.

Fugh-Berman, Adriane J., and Susanna J. Dodgson. 2008. "Ethical Considerations of Publication Planning in the Pharmaceutical Industry." *Open Medicine* 2(4): http:// www.openmedicine.ca/article/view/118/215.

Gagnon, Marc-André, and Joel Lexchin. 2008. "The Cost of Pushing Pills: A New Estimate of Pharmaceutical Promotion Expenditures in the United States." *PLoS Medicine* 5(1): e1, doi:10.1371/journal.pmed.0050001.

Ginsburg, Paul B. 2008. "High and Rising Health Care Costs: Demystifying U.S. Health Care Spending." In *The Synthesis Project*, 1–28. Princeton NJ: Robert Wood Johnson Foundation.

Goodrum, Charles, and Helen Dalrymple. 1990. *Advertising in America: The First 200 Years*. New York: Harry N. Abrams.

Greene, Jeremy A. 2005. "Releasing the Flood Waters: Diuril and the Reshaping of Hypertension." *Bulletin of the History of Medicine* 79(4): 749–94.

———. 2007. *Prescribing by Numbers: Drugs and the Definition of Disease*. Baltimore: Johns Hopkins University Press.

Greene, Jeremy A., and David Herzberg. 2010. "Hidden in Plain Sight." *American Journal of Public Health* 100(5): 793–803.

Kaiser Family Foundation. 2011. "The Uninsured: A Primer." In *The Kaiser Commission on Medicaid and the Uninsured*, 1–39. Washington, DC: Kaiser Family Foundation.

Ledford, Heidi. 2013. "Myriad Ruling Causes Confusion." *Nature* 498: 281–82.

Mack, John. 2012. "Lipitor Holds Key to DTC Ad Spending in 2012." *Pharma Marketing* (blog), http://pharmamkting.blogspot.com/2012/04/lipitor-holds-key-to-dtc-ad-spend ing-in.html, April 15.

Magnus, David, Mildred K. Cho, and Robert Cook-Deegan. 2009. "Direct-to-Consumer Genetic Tests: Beyond Medical Regulation?" *Genome Medicine* 1(2): 17.1–3.

OECD. Organisation for Economic Co-operation and Development. 2008. "Pharmaceutical Pricing Policies in a Global Market." Paris: Organisation for Economic Co-operation and Development.

———. 2012. "OECD Health Data 2012." Paris: Organisation for Economic Co-Operation and Development.

Palumbo, Francis B., and C. Daniel Mullins. 2002. "The Development of Direct-to-Consumer Prescription Drug Advertising Regulation." *Food and Drug Law Journal* 57(3): 423–44.

Parthasarathy, S. 2010. "Assessing the Social Impact of Direct-to-Consumer Genetic Testing: Understanding Sociotechnical Architectures." *Genetics in Medicine* 12(9): 544–47.

Pollack, Andrew. 2010. "F.D.A. Faults Companies on Unapproved Genetic Tests." *New York Times*, June 12, B2.

Rajan, Kaushik Sunder. 2005. "Subjects of Speculation: Emergent Life Sciences and Market Logics in the United States and India." *American Anthropologist* 107(1): 19–30.

Sered, Susan Starr, and Rushika J. Fernandopulle. 2005. *Uninsured in America: Life and Death in the Land of Opportunity*. Berkeley: University of California Press.

Sierles, F. S., A. C. Brodkey, L. M. Cleary, F. A. McCurdy, M. Mintz, J. Frank, D. J. Lynn, J. Chao, B. Z. Morgenstern, W. Shore, and J. L. Woodard. 2005. "Medical Students'

Exposure to and Attitudes about Drug Company Interactions: A National Survey." *JAMA* 294(9): 1034–42.

SK&A. 2012. "One Key Market Insights." Irvine, CA: SK&A.

Spielmans, Glen, and Peter Parry. 2010. "From Evidence-Based Medicine to Marketing-Based Medicine: Evidence from Internal Industry Documents." *Journal of Bioethical Inquiry* 7(1): 13–29.

Story, L. 2007. "Anywhere the Eye Can See, It's Likely to See an Ad." *New York Times*, http://www.nytimes.com/2007/01/15/business/media/15everywhere.html?page wanted=all&_r=0, January 15.

Urbina, Ian. 2012. "DSM Revisions May Sharply Increase Addicition Diagnoses." *New York Times*, May 12, A11.

Ventola, C. Lee. 2011. "Direct-to-Consumer Pharmaceutical Advertising: Therapeutic or Toxic?" *Pharmacy and Therapeutics* 36(10): 681–84.

Welch, H. Gilbert, Lisa M. Schwartz, and Steven Woloshin. 2011. *Overdiagnosed: Making People Sick in the Pursuit of Health*. Boston: Beacon Press.

Let's Send That to the Lab
Technology and Diagnosis

John Gardner

STARTING POINTS

- In contemporary medical practice, clinicians rely on a vast array of diagnostic tools and instruments.
- Clinicians often count on other health professionals such as laboratory technicians and radiographers to help make a diagnosis.
- Technologies can enable clinicians to make more precise diagnoses and therefore reduce uncertainty.
- Diagnostic technologies can help provide an overall coherence to a set of symptoms.

A young man comes to see you. He says that he has been feeling ill: he is tired and feverish, he has lost his appetite, and he has a headache and sore throat. He says that at first he thought it was just the flu, but it's been over two weeks since he got sick, so he decided he had better see a doctor. You check his personal medical history on the computer, ask a few more questions about his symptoms, and take his vital signs. You then auscultate his lungs and heart, and take a look at his throat.

His temperature is elevated, and his throat inflamed. You consider strep throat, mononucleosis, or another viral infection as the most likely causes. A rapid strep test will help confirm the former or infer the latter two possibilities. In his case, strep comes up negative, so you decide to draw some blood. The lab can help you confirm your diagnostic hypothesis of a viral infection. When the results come back, not only do they show an elevated white blood cell count, they reveal atypical lymphocytes. A further monospot test shows Epstein Barr virus antibodies. You contact him to let him know he has infectious mononucleosis.

As this example shows, even relatively routine diagnoses involve a range of technologies. From the simple desktop computer, digital thermometer, and stethoscope to the more specialized automatic hematology analyzer, medicine is saturated with technologies. It may even be accurate to say that modern medicine is the consequence of technologies. Technological advances enable health professionals and laboratory technicians to peer into the body; to identify the presence of pathogens; to extract body fluids and decipher their composition; to develop and administer treatments; and to store, transfer, and share information quickly and efficiently. Throughout much of the twentieth century there has been an exponential growth in medical technologies, and today in contemporary clinical practice instruments and devices have become an indispensible component of diagnosis.

We often think of technology as tools that make our life easier. We use them to carry out tasks quickly and with precision, or to undertake tasks that would otherwise have been impossible. We tend to believe that these tools improve our lives, and that the more medical technologies we have, the better health professionals will become at diagnosing and treating disease. It is this faith that drives a huge medical device industry to invest billions of dollars in researching, producing, and promoting new medical technologies each year. But as discussed in this chapter, technology is far more than just a tool that makes our lives easier. Technologies are **socially embedded**. They exist within a network made up of **professions** and **institutions**, users and citizens, governments and regulatory agencies, and of course commercial industry. This network and its agents shape how and where technologies are used, and they in turn are shaped by the technology.

In this chapter, I provide examples of how diagnostic technologies have been shaped by, and also transformed, the social relations within which they are embedded. Diagnostic technologies have altered the health-care professions; enabled the delineation and creation of new diseases; produced a new, ethically challenging environment for **patients**; and contributed to how individuals understand themselves and those around them. Medicine is made up of **sociotechnical networks**, within which health-care workers, patients, and medical technologies interact, influence, and reshape each other in complex ways that cannot always be predicted. In short, people have designed and produced diagnostic technologies, and these technologies have in turn transformed the social world of people. We can conceptualize diagnosis as a process that involves the formation of a sociotechnical network; humans and technologies are assembled together and interact, each reliant upon the other.

THE POWER OF OBJECTIVITY

Patients are often reliable sources of information about their illness. They describe bodily sensations and provide valuable details about family and personal history, all of which help the clinician make a diagnosis. But patients are emotional: their fears, anxieties, attitudes, and beliefs can hinder their ability to act as reliable observers of their condition. This is not to say that clinicians are any less fallible in their observations, or any less emotional. The pressures of working long days and juggling multiple interests can likewise affect their judgment. Clinicians, too, have attitudes and beliefs, despite their advanced training in pathophysiology and psychology. One reason why we place so much faith in diagnostic technologies is because we think of them as providing us with an objective glimpse of the body and disease free of the complexity of human emotion. While humans occupy a murky subjective world of emotions and interests, we think of machines as operating only within an objective world of facts. Diagnostic technologies provide glimpses of reality, of the body and disease as they "really" are.

Think back to the hypothetical case of infectious mononucleosis above. While you were able to provide a probable diagnosis, it was the diagnostic technology within the laboratory that was the final arbiter of his condition. It could find the truth of the infection in the blood sample and provide confirmation of the diagnosis. In the last fifty years, health professionals have developed what Reiser (1981) referred to as "a marvelous faith" in diagnostic laboratory tests, so much so that they often become the first step in clinical investigation, taking precedence over patient complaints and clinical examinations (Keating and Cambrosio 2003, 44).

Often the results provided by a diagnostic technology, such as a rapid strep test or an automatic hematology analyzer, confirm the opinion of the clinician and explain the patient's symptoms. In such cases, the feeling of certainty provided by diagnostic technology can provide both parties with the confidence to move forward with a particular treatment. In other cases, however, diagnostic technology may provide results that contradict the clinician's initial opinion or fail to verify the patient's account. When this occurs, the result provided by diagnostic technology usually takes precedence, which can be disheartening for patients.

Rhodes et al. (1999) interviewed patients who had undergone diagnostic testing in order to identify the possible cause of their chronic back pain. Diagnostic tests were carried out with visualizing technologies: radiography (X-ray), computer tomography (CT scans), and magnetic resonance imaging (MRI). For some patients, these technologies identified physical abnormality (such as a dislocated disc) as the likely cause of pain. For others, the technology revealed nothing significant. Those patients for whom technology could validate their pain felt a sense of relief: the technology proved their subjective experience. Patients whose diagnostic tests failed to show any abnormalities felt as if their claim of feeling pain had been undermined.* Their experience of pain was not, on its own, considered a reliable indication that something was physically wrong with their body. Patients felt that, in the absence of confirmatory results, their clinician did not take them seriously. Some were told that their pain had no physical cause and must be psychological, and others had the legitimacy of their claims doubted by family members, coworkers, or employers (Rhodes et al. 1999). These patients felt belittled and isolated, adding further psychological and emotional strain to their physical pain. (Interestingly, after pushing for more diagnostic tests, some of these patients later had positive physical findings, thus demonstrating the fallibility of the earlier tests.)

> And then you've got the doctors for four years telling you, "Well, we can't find anything wrong. It's all in your head." And you're going, "no, it's right here. My head ain't down here." (Rhodes et al. 1999)

The example above highlights the authority accorded to diagnostic technologies, particularly those that provide visual representations of the body and its internal spaces. One implication of this faith in technology is that it reduces the im-

---

*These types of diagnostic tests can also show significant abnormalities that have nothing to do with the symptoms that the patient is having.

portance accorded to the patient account, which may lead patients to feel voiceless, adding further strain to their experience of illness.

Yet there are situations where the results of a diagnostic technology are not accorded more authority than the viewpoint of the patient. Diagnostic technologies used to screen for coronary artery disease are often used with suspicion by cardiologists. Electrocardiogram (EKG) stress tests, stress echocardiography, and single-photon emission CT are relatively inexpensive, noninvasive, and widely used, but they are widely known to be inaccurate (Gibbons et al. 2002; Weustink et al. 2010, 630). Rather than provide a definitive diagnosis, such tests results are used in conjunction with a patient's details to calculate their probability (or risk) of having coronary heart disease (Banerjee et al. 2012, 478).*

A study by Gardner et al. (2011) offers an example. The study followed a patient with chest pain as he underwent various diagnostic procedures, including an EKG stress test. At the end of the stress test, the cardiologist told the patient that the EKG indicated that his heart was fine, and that the most likely cause of his chest pain was anxiety. But, the cardiologist added, although the test is useful, it is not 100% accurate: the patient's chest pain could still be caused by heart problems. The cardiologist's response to the results was not to dismiss the patient's claim that he was in pain, but to emphasize the fallibility of the test. He warned the patient that "the treadmill test is just the basic screening test and there is a chance it's wrong . . . If, as you're walking up those steps at home . . . you start finding you do get chest tightness or chest pain, then come back and see us, because there are other more accurate tests we can do to look and see whether this is a problem" (Gardner et al. 2011, 848).

No diagnostic tests, even those involving complex, expensive technologies, are 100% accurate. The diagnostic tests for infectious mononucleosis can produce false positive results, and MRI scans can fail to detect a slipped intervertebral disc. MRI scans are also known to produce false positives; one study found that MRI images revealed substantial spinal column abnormalities (such as a herniated intervertebral discs) in one third of individuals, all of whom were asymptomatic (Boden et al. 1990). It is important for clinicians to remember the limitations of diagnostic technologies, as discussed below.

THE CREATION OF DISEASE

Diagnostic technologies do more than enable us to identify disease. They influence how we understand and manage disease, and they also help identify new diseases. Diagnostic technologies can provide an overall coherence to a set of

---

*To be more precise, clinicians start with a pretest probability of a disease and then use the results of the diagnostic test to arrive at a posttest probability. Diagnostic tests are most useful when the pretest probability is in the 35–65% range. If the pretest probability is low, then even after a positive test the posttest probability will still be low. Similarly, if the pretest probability is high, then it's likely still high after a negative test.

symptoms or bodily features. They let clinicians go inside the body and identify the possible cause of a patient's ailments, shedding light on a pathogen, a genetic abnormality, some sort of sclerosis, or tumorous cell growth. Consequently, diagnostic technologies play a large role in how health professionals come to understand and manage diseases. By giving a set of symptoms and signs an overall coherence, they also aid in providing disease with an identity that guides the clinician and can subsequently structure the lived experience of the patient.

In some cases the emergence of a new diagnostic technology may drastically alter how health professionals and patients perceive an already-identified disease. It may, in other words, re-create the disease. An example is the development of antibody tests for HIV and the changing identity of AIDS (Wailoo 1997). Prior to the HIV antibody test, AIDS was understood as a fragmented collection of what were once rare, opportunistic infections (such as Kaposi sarcoma and pneumocystis pneumonia). With the development of the antibody test and after much debate, AIDS became immunologically defined, and this collection of curiously concurrent ailments became unified as one entity. As Wailoo points out, such identification of the disease has shaped how health professionals think about and manage those afflicted with the condition, in turn framing the experience of those with HIV/AIDS as well as informing social policy (Wailoo 1997).

In this sense, HIV/AIDS as we understand it today has been profoundly influenced by a particular diagnostic technology. Diagnostic technologies such as the HIV antibody test have enabled new treatments to be developed and health outcomes to be improved. As Wailoo (1997) points out, however, in addition to simplifying and resolving our understanding of the body and disease pathology, "technologies have also been constituting, creating and complicating diseases" (2). The technology has also brought about a series of dilemmas associated with diagnosis more generally. For some, the HIV antibody test appropriately identifies potentially dangerous HIV in individuals who have, or will develop, the spectrum of ailments characteristic of AIDS. For others, it has become a potentially intrusive means of stigmatizing and perpetuating social discrimination, a means of assigning insurance liability and assigning assumptions about sexuality (Wailoo 1997).

The emergence of new diagnostic technologies may also enable the delineation of new diseases. Klinefelter syndrome, a condition that affects men and is characterized by the presence of more than one X chromosome, offers an example. It is not life threatening, and although most men will be infertile, the signs and symptoms are relatively mild: men with Klinefelter syndrome are often quite tall, and they may have partial breast formation, small testicles, and learning difficulties (Klinefelter 1986). Some men with Klinefelter syndrome are visibly indistinguishable from other men. Before new diagnostic technologies were developed in the mid-twentieth century that enabled the detection of particular hormonal and genetic abnormalities, Klinefelter syndrome did not exist. Affected men were dispersed throughout the population, and because their physical abnormalities were not debilitating or conspicuous, there was little reason to single them out as being members of a distinct group of afflicted individuals. As the twentieth century progressed and Western societies became increasingly body conscious, men with slightly feminine traits became the subject of medical investigations (Klinefelter et al. 1942). The development of new diagnostic technologies provided an underlying coherence to these feminine traits and enabled affected men to be grouped together as having the same type of genetic abnormality. Now, men diagnosed as having more than one X chromosome may be offered testosterone therapy in order to induce the formation of a more masculine physique.

It is in this way that diagnostic technologies contribute to the creation of diseases. It is how diagnostic technologies have contributed to the rise in what Armstrong (1995) has referred to as the "problematisation of the normal." As the twentieth century progressed and more of the populations in developed countries were subject to an expanding network of diagnostic and information technologies, a host of new diseases were identified and delineated. Many of these diseases were not causing deadly, debilitating, or bed-confining ailments; rather, like Klinefelter syndrome, they referred to physical or behavioral aberrations within a population.

PATIENT SELF-AWARENESS

Diagnostic technologies can also encourage patients to think differently about themselves. Chapter 5 discusses how a diagnosis of an illness or condition can have a transformative effect on a patient. It can present them with information that makes them see themselves in a completely different light, maybe causing them to reassess their life goals or their values, or perhaps prompting them to change how they relate to others. Let's look briefly at how a patient's interaction with diagnostic technology can influence the way they think about themselves and those around them.

In the process of providing overall coherence to a set of symptoms and bodily features, diagnostic technologies have provided new ways for individuals to understand who they are. In effect, diagnostic technologies open up the body, exposing its inner parts and processes to the scrutiny of clinicians and the awareness of patients. In many cases, a patient's new awareness of a genetic abnormality or the presence of a pathogen, for example, will have little effect upon them. They may quickly forget this new knowledge, or it may be completely irrelevant to their day-to-day living. In some cases, however, diagnostic technologies have provided individuals with information that has had a major effect on how they think about themselves and how they relate to others. A good example is the way in which the diagnosis of a genetic condition can affect the way a person sees himself. Again, Klinefelter syndrome is an illustrative example. Now that diagnostic tests have been developed to determine the presence of an extra X chromosome, affected men can think of themselves as having Klinefelter syndrome or as "being XXY," and they can choose to associate and interact with others who identify themselves the same way. In many countries around the world, Klinefelter syndrome support groups have been established. These groups promote awareness of Klinefelter syndrome, bring together affected individuals, organize conferences, and circulate advice on how to manage the condition (Bock 1993). So although individuals with Klinefelter syndrome can live relatively normal lives and have varying degrees of signs and symptoms, for many, their knowledge of a shared genetic abnormality has created a community. It has provided them with a means of self-identification and it has encouraged them to form social networks with other affected men.

In a sense, diagnostic technologies have enabled biological or biochemical components of the body to acquire a social dimension: by making the internal components of the body visible, it has enabled them to have an influence that is not restricted to the biological body. As the Klinefelter syndrome example illustrates, a genetic mutation can become the basis for a patient's self-identification or the basis for the formation of a new social group. The anthropologist Paul Rabinow (1996) refers to this as **biosociality**. New medical technologies have brought about an environment where individuals can conceptualize themselves, and associate with others, according to particular genetic abnormalities. Diagnostic technologies have multiplied the attributes we can use to make sense of ourselves.

INSTITUTIONAL BATTLES

As diagnostic technologies become more common and complex, clinicians become increasingly reliant on a network of other health professionals and technicians to make a diagnosis. As the imaginary case of infectious mononucleosis diagnosis above illustrates, many diagnostic tests are carried out by laboratory technicians. Training to become a lab technician requires becoming a competent operator of an assortment of diagnostic machines and devices and can take several years. Despite many years of training, it would be unrealistic to expect a family physician to know how to use the many laboratory techniques and machines commonly used in diagnosis. So there is a division of labor and a wide range of professions involved in the diagnostic process. Keating and Cambrosio (2003) argue that division of labor is part of a long-term transformation of medicine into biomedicine, in which health professionals rely heavily on the ability of technology to detect an expanding number of biological and molecular markers before making a diagnosis. As a result, diagnosis is no longer something that happens only inside the consultation room; it can now involve many specialists in several different physical locations. Much of a clinician's authority derives not so much from their ability to make a diagnosis on their own, but from their ability to utilize this network of specialists.

There is much to gain from being part of this network of specialists. As a consequence, diagnostic technology can become the focus of conflict. Different groups may battle to establish themselves as the expert of a particular technology and thus control access to it. This was certainly the case with X-ray technology when it was first introduced, and later MRI technology. When X-ray technology emerged in the late nineteenth century, there was little understanding among health professionals as to what a useful X-ray should look like, or even how it could be used in diagnosis (Pasveer 1989). Potentially anyone who was interested (physicists, engineers, electricians, photographers) could use the new technology. At the turn of the century in Europe and North America, groups of individuals banded together to form official radiological societies. Members of these societies set about establishing formal standards dictating how the technology should be used, so that the resulting images would consistently be of a sufficient quality that they could be useful in clinical practice. In order to protect this standard, radiological societies had to ensure that only their own, sufficiently trained members could use the technology. In order to join a society, recruits had to pass specific entrance criteria (such as obtain a diploma in radiology) and abide by their rules (Pasveer 1989). In 1917, a group of leading radiologists in Britain formed the British Association of Radiology and Physiology. Their goal was to promote and protect the status of radiologists, which they accomplished by establishing the Cambridge Diploma in 1920, which "soon came to be demanded from anyone applying for a radiological post in a hospital. Radiology had become a qualified specialism" (Pasveer 1989, 367). As the twentieth century progressed, clinicians recognized just how valuable the standardized and high-quality X-ray images could be, and subsequently radiography departments became commonplace in most hospitals. By developing standards and restricting X-ray access, radiological societies were able to ensure that only their members could enjoy the privileges that went with managing an important diagnostic technology.

Throughout the twentieth century, professional radiography societies have managed to assert themselves as the experts in producing and interpreting images of the body. In the 1980s, however, this privileged position was threatened with the introduction of a powerful new diagnostic imaging tool: magnetic resonance imaging, or MRI. (MRI was initially called "nuclear magnetic resonance," but the name was changed because it was thought that the word "nuclear" would discourage patients.)

With regard to the interpretation of radiograms, there will be general sympathy with Dr. Arthur and his colleague when they insist that only men of sound medical training and experience should be allowed to control the X-ray tube and interpret its results. For the non-professional operator to offer medical opinion upon a radiogram is sheer impertinence. ("Reviews," *British Medical Journal*, February 6, 1909)

When MRI was first introduced into clinical practice, there were debates over which particular medical specialty should control the technology (Joyce 2006).

The results produced by MRI could be represented as either numbers or images. Scientists felt that some of the important diagnostic information would be lost if it were displayed as images. Some commentators argued that nuclear medicine physicians should control MRI devices, since their training would enable them to understand what the findings meant (Joyce 2006). If nuclear medicine physicians assumed responsibility for MRI devices, radiographers would lose their monopoly over diagnostic imaging technologies, threatening their access to work, research funding, and other resources. But by this time, ultrasound and computerized axial tomography technology had been introduced into clinical practice, and health professionals and patients had become accustomed to dealing with images. Because radiographers had already established themselves as experts in producing and interpreting such images of the body, they were granted control of

MRI (Joyce 2006), giving them reign over the technology that initially had threatened their privileged position. As MRI technology was further developed for diagnostic use, radiographers influenced its design. At first MRI produced colored images of the body, but they were soon changed to gray scale because radiographers were accustomed to interpreting black-and-white X-ray images.

The cost (expensive) and size (large) of MRI technology also restricted who could use it. A hospital could purchase an MRI device and put it in the radiography department, but a private clinician would have neither the money nor the space to run it (Joyce 2006, 13). Today MRI technology is considered to be the **gold standard** in imaging diagnostics. Radiographers have managed to retain control of this vital technology, firmly establishing themselves as an important component of many diagnostic processes. And the skills of radiographers continue to be in high demand. In the United States, clinicians' ongoing reliance on images and a growing patient population has brought about exponential growth in imaging procedures such as MRI and CT for much of the last twenty years.

As these examples of imaging diagnostic technologies illustrate, a network of health professionals in different locations may be involved in a diagnosis. They also illustrate that diagnostic technologies are valuable resources, and that different groups may dispute who should control them and who should be part of the diagnostic network. In some cases, a new group may form and take control of a technology, establishing themselves as experts. These disputes influence how a technology is used and by whom.

NEW ETHICAL CHALLENGES

Diagnostic technologies are not infallible. The rapid strep test, the automatic hematology analyzer, and the EKG stress test can all produce misleading results. Nevertheless, we tend to think that if a diagnosis that has been made with a complex, expensive technology, it is likely to be accurate. As noted in chapter 3, resolving uncertainty is one of the primary purposes of diagnosis. If clinicians and patients are convinced that an accurate diagnosis has been made, they will have confidence to move forward with a particular course of action, like a treatment plan for example. Diagnostic technologies should provide information that makes it easier for clinicians and patients to make decisions about what to do next.

But the diagnostic technologies involved in many types of screening convey information that is based on probability rather than certainty. This is the case with technologies used in prenatal screening, as illustrated by Williams (2006). Antenatal ultrasound screening, for example, can indicate that something might be wrong with the developing fetus rather than provide clinicians and their patients with a definitive diagnosis. Many women feel as though it is their duty as a mother to undergo antenatal diagnostic screening tests and to do whatever they can to ensure their child will be healthy, even if it involves risky experimental fetal surgery (Williams 2006). The development of technology that enables these tests means that mothers may now have to make decisions that can be emotionally challenging and can have severe repercussions for their family's life. A burden of responsibility for the child's health is placed on a woman even before her child is born. Anthropologist Rayna Rapp (1999) has referred to women as **moral philosophers of the private**—they are forced to make difficult ethical decisions, often using probability-based information, while having to reflect on complex issues such as the appropriateness of abortion and whether an intellectual or physical impairment will prevent a child from having a fulfilling and meaningful life.

A good example is parents we see at 20 weeks [into pregnancy] where there is a mild dilatation of the cerebral ventricles where we could say, "look, there is something like an 85–90 per cent chance that this fetus is going to be OK" . . . if they are unlucky they will have a baby that's going to be mentally handicapped. Most couples, given the odds of 10 per cent that the baby is going to be handicapped, most will take a risk, but they would be very, very anxious obviously. (Williams 2006)

Diagnostic technologies can create an environment where patients have to make ethically challenging decisions.

As Webster (2002) states, high-tech medicine can generate forms of diagnosis based on risk and probability rather than clear causality. This is particularly true in the realm of genetic diagnostics, where presymptomatic patients are told they might develop a disease in the future, a situation that occurs when the disease is multigenetic. Such information does not necessarily provide guidance on how to act in the present (Brown and Webster 2004). So while many diagnostic technologies can make decision making easier, some have brought about an environment that is more challenging and potentially more stressful for patients.

SOCIALLY EMBEDDED DIAGNOSTIC TECHNOLOGIES

Diagnostic technologies, like all technologies, can change our world in ways that we never intended or envisaged; diagnostic technologies are developed and produced with the intention of overcoming particular challenges, and in the process of achieving this aim they create for us a whole new set of challenges and opportunities. As Brown and Webster (2004) put it: "Medical technologies act in a multivalent way *at the same time*; advanced techniques used to gain a more sophisticated understanding of the body (or mind) can, simultaneously, open up new and quite different questions (and answers), not only for medicine, but also for other social actors—such as lay people, bioethicists, non-medical sciences, regulators" (53).

Diagnostic technologies are therefore more than just tools. Tools are developed by humans to facilitate human actions. They are used to help people solve a problem or to achieve some preidentified goal. While diagnostic technologies certainly enable health professionals to provide quicker and more accurate diagnoses, they do far more than just facilitate human action.

As discussed above, a reliance on complex diagnostic technologies means that diagnosis is no longer restricted to the consultation room; the clinician will often delegate diagnostic work to a range of specialists working in different locations, such as a laboratory or radiology department. Diagnosis, then, often involves a network of trained specialists and diagnostic technology. In the process of adopting, molding, and accommodating diagnostic technologies, actors are often prompted to adjust and transform. As with the introduction of X-ray technology and the development of radiography societies, new professional groups can arise. Professional groups may also modify themselves and jostle with others in order to take control of a new lucrative technology such as MRI. (Or professional groups may modify the technology in order to consolidate their control.) In some cases, diagnostic technologies have brought about the delineation and creation of new diseases. As illustrated in the example of chronic back pain, the use of diagnostic technologies can make patients feel alienated, worsening their experience of illness, especially when clinicians assume that technologies provide an infallible, objective view of the body and disease. Diagnostic technologies can also create novel, difficult ethical dilemmas for patients and clinicians. As the example of antenatal screening shows, patients can be forced into becoming "moral philosophers," where they must scrutinize their beliefs and decide what is the most "ethical" course of action. And diagnostic technologies can provide individuals with a new awareness of themselves, as with Klinefelter syndrome, prompting patients to reassess their identity and encouraging them to establish new social networks. As the above examples illustrate, diagnostic technologies are socially embedded; they shape, and are shaped by, a network of actors each with their own goals and interests.

Health professionals rely on an assortment of technologies to do their job, from the basic thermometer and stethoscope to the more complicated X-ray and MRI. Indeed, modern medicine would not exist without technology. In contemporary medical practice, we can conceptualize diagnosis as a process that involves the formation of a sociotechnical network; humans and technologies are assembled together and interact, each reliant upon and shaping the other. A diagnosis emerges from these interactions and cannot be attributed solely to the activities of humans, or solely to the activities of diagnostic technologies.

IMPLICATIONS FOR CLINICAL PRACTICE

Should this understanding of diagnostic technology as being socially embedded influence how health professionals use such technologies? What are the practical implications of viewing medicine as being composed of sociotechnical networks? Seeing diagnostic technology as being socially embedded can help health professionals to become more comfortable working within an environment that is plagued by uncertainties. A degree of uncertainty and ambiguity is to be expected during diagnostic processes, not because something has gone wrong, but rather because all diagnostic procedures, whether they rely on complex technology or a physician's clinical skills, can only ever provide a partial, selective view of the body and disease.

As Haraway (1991) argues, we assume that technology can provide us with what she calls a god's-eye view of the world around us; an objective view of the world as it really is, untainted by human bias. From the images produced by an electron microscope of tiny virus particles to those of huge, distant, colorful galaxies captured by the Hubble telescope, it's as if technology enables us to see everything, unhindered by the specificities of location. But as Haraway (1991) adds, there is no such thing as an omniscient view that sees "everything from nowhere equally and fully" (191). The electron microscope and the Hubble telescope, for instance, do not present things as they really are. They produce carefully prepared visual renditions, using complex algorithms to transform visually indiscernible data into accessible and impressive pictures. Data are strategically manipulated into an easily digestible form, digestible because it corresponds to our expectations of what such entities should look like. (The grayscale images of the brain produced by MRI are another good example of this transformation of data into an accessible and useful form.) Diagnostic technologies, then, are designed so that they incorporate and reproduce specific ways of seeing, or ways of understanding the body and disease. Rather than enabling a passive, unmediated vision, they produce partial, but often wonderfully detailed, representations.

There are two consequences of renouncing the belief that a "god's-eye view" is possible. First, it encourages us to maintain a healthy skepticism toward the results provided by diagnostic technologies. While diagnostic technologies are undoubtedly useful, they do not provide a window into things as they really are. This fact is illustrated with the earlier example of the EKG stress test. Even if the test result indicated that the heart was healthy, the cardiologist refused to rule out the possibility of heart disease in a patient with chest pain. The cardiologist recognized that the stress test is fallible. If we compare this example to one of back pain, we can see that inconsistency is not necessarily a bad thing. In the back pain example, clinicians placed (or misplaced, as it turned out) so much faith in the results of diagnostic technology that they completely overlooked the viewpoint of their patients, who as a consequence felt alienated and distressed. A lack of certainty can provide patients with a space to have their viewpoints heard.

This brings us to the second consequence: we should expect that test results and clinical findings will not always neatly align and confirm one another. In order to make a diagnosis, a clinician will often have to coordinate the findings of a clinical examination, the patient's narrative, and perhaps several diagnostic tests. Ideally, the findings of each of these will neatly cohere, enabling the clinician to give a clear diagnosis. In textbook cases, specific clinical signs point toward a particular illness, subsequently confirmed by clear diagnostic results. But the reality of day-to-day medical practice is seldom as clear-cut. As Mol (2002) has illustrated, clinical signs and the findings from diagnostic tests often do not form a coherent, unified picture. Instead, clinicians have to patch together accounts, results, and findings that don't neatly align or confirm one another. The fact that such accounts, results, and findings do not neatly align is not evidence that something has gone wrong. Rather, it is because each is a mediated, partial, and actively produced rendering, and not the product of having an omniscient view. A degree of ambiguity, even incoherence, will be unavoidable. Learning how to manage this incoherence, how to patch together accounts, findings, and results, is a skill that clinicians and health professionals probably acquire best by first-hand experience in a busy and messy, everyday clinical atmosphere.

TAKEAWAY POINTS

- Diagnostic technologies are credited with much authority, and often trump the patient's account of illness, adding strain to the patient's experience.
- The emergence of new diagnostic technologies has led to the delineation of new diseases, contributing to the "problematization of the normal."
- Professional groups often tightly control diagnostic technologies.
- Diagnostic technologies are designed and produced by people, and they in turn transform their social world.
- While not infallible, diagnostic technology may be seen as more objective and robust than other forms of diagnostic generation, leading to overreliance of technology and overdiagnosis.

DISCUSSION QUESTIONS

1. Imagine that you are experiencing some sort of pain and diagnostic tests have failed to find any cause. How would this make you feel? What would you do next?
2. Make a list of some of the technologies that you use every day. What specific goals do these technologies enable you to achieve? In what ways do you think these technologies may have unintentionally altered your behavior?
3. Imagine that you were offered a diagnostic test that would determine your chances of developing a debilitating illness in the future. Would you take the test, or would you prefer not to know? Why?
4. Make a list of some technologies that are carefully controlled by groups or professional organizations. How might these groups limit access to the technology? What advantages do they gain from controlling these technologies?

REFERENCES

Armstrong, David. 1995. "The Rise of Surveillance Medicine." *Sociology of Health and Illness* 17(3): 393–404.

Banerjee, Amitava, Daniel R. Newman, Anne Van den Bruel, and Carl Heneghan. 2012. "Diagnostic Accuracy of Exercise Stress Testing for Coronary Artery Disease: A Systematic Review and Meta-Analysis of Prospective Studies." *International Journal of Clinical Practice* 66(5): 477–92.

Bock, Robert. 1993. "Understanding Klinefelter Syndrome: A Guide for XXY Males and Their Families." *National Institutes of Health*, www.nichd.nih.gov/publications/pubs /klinefelter.cfm#xwhat.

Boden, Scott, David Davis, Thomas Dina, Nicholas Patronas, and Sam Wiesel. 1990. "Abnormal Magnetic-Resonance Scans of the Lumbar Spine in Asymptomatic Subjects." *Journal of Bone and Joint Surgery* 72: 403–8.

Brown, Nik, and Andrew Webster. 2004. *New Medical Technologies and Society: Reordering Life*. Cambridge: Polity.

Gardner, John, Kevin Dew, Maria Stubbe, Anthony C. Dowell, and Lindsay MacDonald. 2011. "Patchwork Diagnoses: The Production of Coherence, Uncertainty, and Manageable Bodies." *Social Science and Medicine* 73(6): 843–50.

Gibbons, Raymond J., Gary J. Balady, J. Timothy Bricker, Bernard R. Chaitman, Gerald F. Fletcher, Victor F. Froelicher, Daniel B. Mark, Ben D. McCallister, Aryan N. Mooss, Michael G. O'Reilly, William L. Winters Jr., Elliott M. Antman, Joseph S. Alpert, David P. Faxon, Valentin Fuster, Gabriel Gregoratos, Loren F. Hiratzka, Alice K. Jacobs, Richard O. Russell, and Sidney C. Smith Jr. 2002. "ACC/AHA 2002 Guideline Update for Exercise Testing: Summary Article: A Report of the American College of Cardiology/American Heart Association Task Force on Practice Guidelines (Committee to Update the 1997 Exercise Testing Guidelines)." *Circulation* 106: 883–1892.

Haraway, Donna. 1991. "Situated Knowledges: The Science Question in Feminism and the Privilege of Partial Perspective." In *Simians, Cyborgs, and Women: The Reinvention of Nature*. London: Free Association.

Joyce, Kelly A. 2006. "From Numbers to Pictures: The Development of Magnetic Resonance Imaging and the Visual Turn in Medicine." *Science as Culture* 15(1): 1–22.

Keating, Peter, and Aberto Cambrosio. 2003. *Biomedical Platforms: Realigning the Normal and the Pathological in Late-Twentieth-Century Medicine*. Cambridge, MA: MIT Press.

Klinefelter, Harry. 1986. "Klinefelter's Syndrome: Historical Background and Development." *Southern Medical Journal* 79(9): 1089–93.

Klinefelter, Harry, Edward C. Reifenstein Jr., and Fuller Albright. 1942. "A Syndrome Characterized by Gynecomastia, Aspermatogenesis without Aleydigism, and Increased Excretion of Follicle Stimulating Hormone." *Journal of Endocrinology* 2: 615–27.

Mol, Annemarie. 2002. *The Body Multiple*. Durham, NC: Duke University Press.

Pasveer, Bernike. 1989. "Knowledge of Shadows: The Introduction of X-Ray Images in Medicine." *Sociology of Health and Illness* 11(4): 360–81.

Rabinow, Paul. 1996. *Essays on the Anthropology of Reason*. Princeton, NJ: Princeton University Press.

Rapp, Rayna. 1999. *Testing Women, Testing the Fetus*. London: Routledge.

Reiser, Stanley J. 1981. *Medicine and the Reign of Technology*. Cambridge: Cambridge University Press.

"Reviews: Radiography and Diagnosis." 1909. *British Medical Journal* 1: 339.

Rhodes, Lorna A., Carol A. McPhillips-Tangum, Christine Markham, and Rebecca Klenk. 1999. "The Power of the Visible: The Meaning of Diagnostic Tests in Chronic Back Pain." *Social Science and Medicine* 48(9): 1189–203.

Wailoo, Keith. 1997. *Drawing Blood: Technology and Disease Identity in Twentieth-America*. Baltimore: John Hopkins University Press.

Webster, Andrew. 2002. "Risk and Innovative Health Technologies: Calculation, Interpretation and Regulation." *Health, Risk and Society* 4(3): 221–26.

Weustink, Annick C., Nico R. Mollet, Lisan A. Neefjes, W. Bob Meijboom, Tjebbe W. Galema, Carlos A. van Mieghem, Stamatis Kyrzopoulous, Rick Neoh Eu, Koen Nieman, Filippo Cademartiri, Robert-Jan van Geuns, Eric Boersma, Gabriel P. Krestin, and Pim J. de Feyter. 2010. "Diagnostic Accuracy and Clinical Utility of Noninvasive Testing for Coronary Artery Disease." *Annals of Internal Medicine* 152(10): 630–39.

Williams, Clare. 2006. "Dilemmas in Fetal Medicine: Premature Application of Technology or Responding to Women's Choice?" *Sociology of Health and Illness* 28(1): 1–20.

Fighting to Be Heard
Contested Diagnoses

Catherine Trundle, Ilina Singh, and Christian Bröer

STARTING POINTS

- Despite its explanatory power, the diagnostic process does not provide explanations for all patient complaints.
- Patients sometimes challenge the diagnoses they receive and argue for alternative explanations for their illnesses.
- In situations of contested diagnosis, medical experts often juggle two competing motivations: the desire to explain illness within the bounds of scientific certainty and the need to treat the patient and offer a pathway back to health.
- Medical experts vary in their approach to diagnosing contested illness: some see them as the product of misdiagnosis, some believe they are psychosomatic, and others seek to legitimate them biomedically.

Previous chapters have highlighted places where there is potential for conflict; this chapter explores how diagnoses can become sites of contest, rather than of agreement. Conflict can arise when illness refuses to yield the level of proof that epidemiology, clinical medicine, and toxicology require, or its existence is doubted within mainstream medicine. Other forms of contest take place when doctor and **patient** disagree on the symptoms of an illness, its exact etiology, or its treatment. This chapter explores core features of contested diagnoses and provides case studies to demonstrate the social dynamics that can occur when diagnostic processes create conflicts and disagreements.

We begin by examining the often-fraught diagnostic processes that surround unexplained physical symptoms, providing a case study that illustrates the difficulties medical experts face when confronted with unexplained symptoms and the disagreements that can ensue. This chapter then traces patient experiences of, and responses to, a contested diagnosis, as well as the psychological effects that the absence of an illness label produces.

We examine two major domains of diagnostic contest. First, we chart the contests surrounding environmental illnesses, demonstrating the challenges they pose to medical notions of proof. Such illness claims also expose how social factors such as class, gender, and ethnicity curtail access to diagnostic processes and the medical information crucial to crafting a diagnosis. A case study of nuclear bomb test veterans illustrates how structures of power and social practices can limit patients' abilities to seek an accurate diagnosis and gain recognition. We also detail the rising influence of **environmental health movements** that challenge conventional medical explanations of environmental illness. We show how activists shape the labeling of disease and political responses to risk, and reveal the tensions and dialogues between expert authority and patient experience.

Next we examine attempts to medicalize and demedicalize certain mental illnesses, taking attention deficit hyperactivity disorder (ADHD) as an extended case study. Finally, while outlining some of the problems with the category "contested diagnosis," we demonstrate the importance of understanding the social, cultural, and political factors that shape conflicts within the diagnostic process.

WHAT IS A CONTESTED DIAGNOSIS?

Contested diagnoses commonly occur because the illnesses themselves are highly contested. According to Joseph Dumit (2006), contested illnesses have five key features. First, they are often chronic, not easily fitting mainstream understandings of acute disease and its treatment. Second, their symptoms are "biomental"; doctors cannot determine if they are caused by mental or physical ailments or whether they are the result of genetic, toxic, or social factors. Third, their treatments include a wide range of conventional and alternative options. Fourth, they have "fuzzy boundaries": they can be attributed to comorbid conditions, linked to other illnesses with similar symptoms, or classified as a mistaken diagnosis. And, fifth, they are "legally explosive." Sufferers find it difficult to gain disability status, often using litigation in order to gain recognition and challenge illness categories.

Dumit's definition does not fully encapsulate contested diagnosis, however. Diseases that are accepted by biomedicine and society, which have a clear biological explanation, and that are medically uncontroversial can still generate considerable contests in the diagnostic process. Patients, doctors, and their families can disagree over the type of treatment, access to medical information, decision-making processes, or the role played by social, economic, and political factors in shaping disease rates and health outcomes. We define contested diagnosis to incorporate all of the contests, challenges, and disagreements that occur during the diagnostic process.

CONTESTS OVER THE MEANING OF UNEXPLAINED PHYSICAL SYMPTOMS

Many contested diagnostic processes center on a patient's experiences of medically unexplained physical symptoms. If medical practitioners attempt to make a diagnosis in such cases, they do so in the face of no observable organic disruption or pathology, relying instead on the troubling symptoms that patients report. Examples of illnesses with unexplained symptoms include chronic fatigue syndrome,

Gulf War syndrome, fibromyalgia (chronic pain), and multiple chemical sensitivities. Even the term "contested illness" can be contested, as some might hold the view that chronic fatigue syndrome and these other "conditions" can only be described as a collection of unexplained symptoms. Because doctors cannot observe the causes of these symptoms using established diagnostic tests, many respond with skepticism and disbelief. Often experienced as chronic and debilitating, symptoms for these conditions tend to be multiple and complex, with non-localized or shifting symptoms like pain, muscle aches, stomach problems, headaches, and fatigue. Furthermore, patients of contested illness with unexplained symptoms usually do not respond well to conventional medical treatments. This is evident within diagnoses of fibromyalgia, in which biomedical tests typically reveal no observable pathology, patients suffer a range of persisting and shifting symptoms, and treatment usually consists of reactive symptom management. At the heart of many medical debates about contested illnesses is the question of whether these illnesses are "real" in a somatic sense or "just psychological" or psychosomatic (Nettleton 2005; Shriver 2006; Ware 1992). The first case study below, of multiple chemical sensitivities, provides a clear example of the key features of disease discovery for physically unexplained symptoms, expert skepticism, the patient's experience of such conditions, and the medical and legal conflicts that can ensue.

Multiple Chemical Sensitivities

Mark Cullen (1987) coined the diagnostic label multiple chemical sensitivities (MCS) when he noticed adverse sensitivity to household chemicals among his patients. Symptoms reported included headaches, drowsiness, joint aches, upset stomach, and irritated eyes, nose, and throat. Since Cullen's observations, medical researchers have conducted a significant number of studies on MCS, producing conflicting results; many medical specialists claim that these studies do not prove the existence of the disorder. Tests conducted on patients do not usually reveal detectable levels of toxic chemicals, and MCS symptoms are wide ranging and difficult to measure using standard biomedical models and tests.

Many medical specialists believe that a diagnosis of MCS is often a misdiagnosis, and that hay fever, lupus, migraines, or anxiety disorders are more likely to provide an explanation for the patients' ailments. Others believe that many MCS patients have both mental illnesses and irrational anxieties regarding chemicals, which together produce a psychosomatic reaction. Yet another group of medical specialists disagree, arguing that MCS is a physiological disorder that affects the nervous system (e.g., Winder 2002), or that certain patients have a genetic predisposition to develop extreme chemical intolerance (e.g., Ashford and Miller 1998). As a consequence, different medical and public bodies and legal rulings offer uneven levels of recognition and opportunities for disability support. For example, while many national and international medical bodies have produced documents stating that there is insufficient proof of MCS, lawsuits in some countries such as Austria and the United States have paved the way for legal recognition of MCS (Phillips 2010b).

Since the 1980s, federal agencies and state government authorities in the United States have begun to formally accept the existence of MCS (Donnay 1999). Yet this recognition remains patchy, and increased legal, political, and bureaucratic recognition does not necessarily translate into increased acceptance in the medical sphere.

Diagnosis provides the recognition necessary for patients to gain resources. MCS patients often have difficulty gaining access to disability entitlements, which might support them to regain health. Without a legitimate disease label, patients often struggle to maintain employment or fail to access adequate support within the workplace (Phillips 2010b). Lacking a definitive diagnosis, the patient often struggles to assume a recognized **sick role** and **identity** in a range of social settings (Lipson 2004).

Not having a diagnosis can result in negative patient experiences, even when the doctor takes the symptoms seriously. Patients complain of trivialization by their doctors (Ware 1992). They may also report experiencing blame. If their symptoms are not caused by a physical condition, medical specialists infer, then they must be mentally produced, and caused by a psychological disturbance such as stress or depression (Ware 1992). They may experience a devastating sense of self-doubt in the face of medically unexplained symptoms. Some patients complain that they begin to feel "crazy" when engaging with doctors and begin to question their own interpretations of their bodily experiences and sensations (Bell 2012). Finally, patients of contested illnesses with medically unexplained symptoms have reported feeling senses of betrayal by their doctors, who they believe refuse to listen to them and take their complaints seriously. All of these experiences have the effect of delegitimizing the patient's understanding, interpretation, and experience of sickness.

Doctors can also experience personal and professional difficulties when diagnosing contested illness. Tarryn Phillips (2010a) illustrates this point in her research on MCS. Some medical practitioners act as expert witnesses in lawsuits for plaintiffs claiming to suffer from MCS due to workplace exposure. In asserting that MCS is an organic, physical condition, these medical practitioners go against mainstream medical opinion and can be viewed as being beyond the bounds of what is acceptable to a medical worldview. In response to their public and legal support of MCS sufferers, these doctors reported experiencing professional isolation, disillusionment, emotional drain, and peer pressure. Because the legal system is by its very nature adversarial, the differing medical opinions that exist between skeptical and supportive doctors are polarized into opposing, simplified positions. This works against increased dialogue, understanding, and collaboration between these medical perspectives (Phillips 2010b). It also demonstrates that debates about contested illnesses within medical spheres can generate strong, heated disagreements; the medical profession is far from reaching any clear consensus in diagnosing such illnesses; and medical practitioners also face their own battles of social legitimacy when faced with the task of diagnosing contested illnesses.

PATIENT RESPONSES TO A CONTESTED DIAGNOSIS

Without a medically accepted diagnosis, patients often struggle to gain support and sympathy from friends and family. They experience **stigma**, a form of social shame in which they are made to feel that their experiences do not match acceptable definitions of illness and disability. They may resort to secrecy, choosing to hide their illness from others, including family, friends, work colleagues, and doctors. This secrecy can be a great burden for sufferers of contested illnesses, as without a diagnosis they cannot find an appropriate treatment and plan for regaining health. Here the diagnosis is in conflict with the patient's own bodily experience, even if this conflict is not outwardly articulated (Ware 1992).

Conversely, patients may contest the diagnosis with doctors and in other social settings, seeking alternative explanations and diagnoses from other doctors or alternative practitioners—in effect "shopping around" (Bell 2012)—until they receive a diagnosis that fits their own experiences and understandings of their bodies and illness. In this process they often assert that their illness is a physical reality at the same time that they reject psychological explanations (Ware 1992).

> The perception of pain is an entirely subjective experience. Acknowledging this, the pain of a person cannot be contested. Yet, interpreting the meaning of bodily pain is a common component of discussion, negotiation, and conflicts in clinical practice. (Malterud 2002, 376)

DIAGNOSING ENVIRONMENTAL CONTESTED ILLNESSES

Advocates for sufferers of many contested illnesses, including MCS, assert that these conditions result from harmful environmental toxins. Engineered chemicals and compounds such as pesticides, insecticides, and air pollutants are now found in many of the environments in which we live and work. Ours is also an era in which public concerns and anxieties regarding the health of the environment are widespread. As Brown et al. (2000) note, "Virtually all diseases and conditions that can be attributed to environmental causes are highly contested and the source of considerable confusion, anger and resentment" (9). They argue that there is a link between these diseases and production and consumption practices, and therefore that interventions require political action, not just medical intervention. As a consequence of such concerns, environmental health movements and **health social movements** have emerged that challenge biomedicine's skepticism toward such illnesses.

One reason that contested environmental illnesses generate such debate relates to the continuing uncertainties that surround toxicological and epidemiological knowledge, and the powerful influence of the large corporations that often influence the science. The causal pathways between low-level environmental toxins and health are complex and still only tentatively understood (Engel et al. 2002). Normal clinical and epidemiological models and techniques struggle to map low-dose exposure and response and do not adequately reveal these pathways. Even if epidemiological studies reveal elevated levels of illness, they are unlikely to be able to distinguish causally between exposure to toxins and other factors such as lifestyle behavior or hereditary predisposition (Dew 2002).

Proponents of social health movements argue, however, that many of the uncertainties and social conflicts surrounding contested environmental illnesses are socially generated. They reflect not just gaps in our scientific knowledge, but also wider social values and practices that make these illnesses more unknowable and conflict riven. Environmental health movements note that one key issue is the types of health information that is recorded or left out of the medical file (Brown et al. 2000). Most environmental toxin exposure rates are rarely recorded and are thus difficult to gauge. Standard medical care does not tend to record an individual's exposure to potentially hazardous chemical and toxic compounds (Brown et al. 2000)

The medical record of a mother who disinfects her house with monoethanolaimine, commonly found in "Easy Off," kills weeds with diazonon, found in most herbicides, and lives down the road from a petroleum cracking factory is likely to be written as if these environments are not health related. (Brown et al. 2000, 10)

In a similar vein, environmental health advocates argue that routine environmental surveillance of toxin levels by scientists or government regulators is often lax or nonexistent. A lack of medical attention to potential environmental exposure reflects not only the limits of science and the clinical difficulties in determining dose-response relationships, but also political and social priorities and debates.

Yet it is not just a question of the significance society and medicine give to recording data and tracking toxins' effects. Some groups are more at risk of toxin exposure, as chemicals are not evenly distributed throughout the environment. Those who are most highly exposed to potentially hazardous chemicals often belong to lower socioeconomic groups and in many cases are ethnic minorities, demonstrating how socially vulnerable groups live and work in environments with high potential burdens on their health. In the United States, for example, low-income African American families are more likely to live in older, substandard housing that exposes them to higher concentrations of lead paint than other social groups (Markowitz and Rosner 2013).

Because of their marginalized status, minority and low-income groups may have less access to medical care and less social power and political leverage to influence industrial practices, governmental regulation, and scientific research, as well as to effect changes in their environments or demand medical support, all of which affect the diagnostic process (Brown et al. 2000). Certain institutional settings and political structures thus create differential social levels of toxic exposure and access to crucial medical evidence. One contemporary example is military service personnel, and the following case study of nuclear test veterans provides an illustration of the particularly difficult struggles that some groups face in gaining an adequate diagnosis for environmental illnesses.

Diagnosing Contested Environmental Illness among Military Personnel

Military service personnel are often exposed to a range of toxic hazards, including Agent Orange, depleted uranium, toxic oil fire fumes, experimental vaccines, and radiation (Scott 1988; Shriver 2001, 2006; Trundle 2011b). In all these cases governments have, at least initially, denied that the ill health of service members can be linked to their time in the armed forces, and medical experts remain divided as to the exact causes of their illnesses.

The diagnostic processes that such service members face reflect social, political, and cultural dynamics that limit their power and **agency** to seek a legitimate diagnosis. These issues can be seen among the British servicemen who participated in the United Kingdom's nuclear testing program in Australia and the Pacific in the 1950s (Trundle 2011b). Today, many of these veterans claim to suffer from illnesses such as blood cancers; skin, eye, and stomach problems; and fatigue, which they blame on radiation exposure. In seeking diagnoses they encountered many barriers.

The culture of secrecy surrounding military organizations and operations means that accessing medical records and information like exposure rates can be a difficult, lengthy process (Trundle 2011a). When veterans requested their military service medical files, some were told by the state that the documents did not exist, had been lost, or had been destroyed. Those who did receive their medical files reported that records of particular medical consultations during service were missing or had been removed from their files. Moreover, requests for information on the radiation readings from the testing sites were commonly withheld in the name of national security.

Gendered ideas about masculinity within the military also limited the servicemen's engagements with medical systems. During the nuclear testing program, servicemen who went to the sickbay too often were taunted or harassed by fellow servicemen, who called them "sick bay rangers." In such a context, medics could not accurately record many of the men's complaints following potential exposure to nuclear testing. Furthermore, on returning home to the United Kingdom, many widows reported that their late husbands had refused to link their illnesses to the nuclear testing program out of loyalty to the armed forces.

These barriers prevented many veterans from accessing the crucial information that might link their symptoms and physical complaints to the nuclear testing program. Seeking proof of exposure to radiation was crucial to gaining a diagnosis, to identifying who was to blame, and to gaining access to military pensions and medical support. These issues demonstrate how diagnosis is embedded within wider structures of power that limit and enable the flow of information.

HOW DOES THE DIAGNOSTIC PROCESS WORK FOR CONTESTED ENVIRONMENTAL ILLNESSES?

Lay groups often shape the emergence and definitions of contested illnesses, initiating the diagnostic process. Individuals notice reoccurring illnesses and symptoms within and across their social networks. Anecdotal evidence begins to circulate that these symptoms are shared and localized within a particular neighborhood, workplace, or community, raising wider fears and awareness. Disease discovery here is often based on an intuitive experiential sense that something is wrong as well as an iterative experience. Community groups, social collectives, or worker unions often then raise public concerns, propose potential environmental causes, and demand action from government, industry, or scientific groups.

As Phil Brown (2007) reports, governments and scientific communities are often slow and cautious in responding to lay concerns. They commonly regard the evidence as unscientific and thus unpersuasive, and require evidence of a "plausible risk" before acting, placing the burden of proof on those claiming to suffer from environmental illness. Moreover, the industries producing these toxins are often swift to respond against "unsubstantiated claims," are backed by significant financial resources to support such counterclaims, and are able to publicly mobilize scientific opinions that declare their products safe. In industrial workplace situations, occupational health physicians charged with ensuring worker safety can experience a conflict of interest between the workers they treat and the employers on whom they are often financially dependent. Governments that rely on such industries for tax revenue, jobs, and investment are also often reluctant to take swift actions against them. It took decades after the scientific evidence became compelling that both tobacco and lead were deleterious to health before the U.S. government took action to recognize the link, partially because of the strong influence of industry lobbies and industry-sponsored scientists (Markowitz and Rosner 2013; Oreskes and Conway 2010). These political and economic imperatives can delay the accumulation of appropriate scientific data, hinder policy action, and often lead communities to initiate their own epidemiological and lay studies as they search for answers.

In response to this process, social movements and public groups often lose faith and trust in governments, the medical sphere, and industries (Brown 2007), leading to a sometimes adversarial relationship between the parties and, for lay groups, a cynical, suspicious attitude toward official attempts to solve and respond to their health concerns. Claiming contested illnesses can thus become a polarized and fraught process of conflict, and many contested illnesses claims have resulted in litigation (Phillips 2010a), where questions of proof, responsibility, and culpability can be tested. Here medical expertise is often not the driving force of contested illness claims; rather, social movements, lawsuits, public opinion, and political processes drive the labeling, diagnosis, and treatment of many contested illnesses, mobilizing medical knowledge in the process.

LAY KNOWLEDGE AND HEALTH SOCIAL MOVEMENTS

The term **health social movement** refers to "collective challenges to medical policy, public health policy and politics, belief systems, [and] research and practice which include an array of formal and informal organizations, supporters, networks of co-operation and media" (Brown and Zavestoski 2004, 679). Health social movements emerged with the Industrial Revolution as workers groups, unions, and sympathetic scientists sought to improve industrial health. Health social movements became a more diverse and visible social phenomenon from the 1980s, mobilizing a range of lay activists, scientific experts, political forces, journalists, and groups of sufferers into powerful health lobbies. These developments reflect several wider social shifts. First, several high-profile incidents, including the nuclear disasters of Chernobyl in the Soviet Union in 1986 and Three Mile Island in the United States in 1979, shook widespread faith in the advances of science. Second, the increasingly visible adverse effects of certain chemicals—such as DDT, asbestos, cigarette smoke, and lead, which medical authorities had previously assured their citizens were safe—undermined faith in medical authority, and led many to conclude that modern scientific advancements were resulting in an increasingly unpredictable, dangerous world (Kroll-Smith and Floyd 1997).

Third, and as a consequence of such health scares, by the 1980s many people were challenging the authority of medical and technological expertise, questioning who gets to decide what knowledge is legitimate and demanding more democratic modes of "citizenry knowledge." Shifts toward a more democratic approach to knowledge production also reflect the legacies of feminism, civil rights, and indigenous rights, all of which challenged academic knowledge, its power structures, and the **epistemological** assumptions within it. These shifts reflect the fact that democratization in Western countries has become more direct, deliberative, interactive, participative, and issue-specific. It is not just a reaction to citizens' demands but also a call on citizens to make demands. In demanding a more democratic mode of engagement with scientific knowledge, health social movements are "separating the physician from their language and shifting the site of biomedical theorizing from hospitals, clinics, and offices to kitchen tables, living rooms and patios" (Kroll-Smith and Floyd 1997, 7). These health activists are thus "not abandoning expert knowledge but they are moving away from the expert system" (7), refusing to allow health professionals to determine the rules of diagnostic debates.

Fourth, new social media and the Internet have opened up novel and powerful opportunities for social health movements to coordinate action, disseminate knowledge democratically, and support fellow sufferers. The Internet plays an important role in acknowledging suffering, raising collective awareness, and empowering patients in the use of medical knowledge (Dumit 2006). Through the Internet, health social movements transform patients into lay experts who engage proactively with the medical sphere. As has been well rehearsed in arguments about its role, the Internet can also be a source of misinformation.

> Discussion groups regularly cite the media, keeping each other informed as to the public status of their condition, honing arguments in response, and celebrating victories when they occur . . . these provide a forum where self-redescription can take place . . . Another response of many sufferers is to attempt to educate others, including their doctors through facts. They use the internet to share tips, medical articles, and strategies for making their doctors understand their condition. (Dumit 2006, 584)

A good example of the influence of social movements on diagnostic processes can be seen in contests over the illness label "electrohypersensitivity." Debates over electrohypersensitivity reveal how governments must juggle competing demands between science, commercial interests, and health social movements.

Electrohypersensitivity

Electrohypersensitivity (EHS) is a contested diagnosis tied to the perceived effects of common technical devices, like power lines and mobile phones, that produce electromagnetic fields (EMFs). Whereas the ill effects of ionizing EMFs (e.g., X-rays) are well known and accepted, the effects of nonionizing EMFs (e.g., radio waves) are less clear. Electromagnetic fields can heat human tissue, and most regulations concerning human exposure are meant to avoid this thermal effect. A number of people, sometimes organized into activist groups, report health complaints due to EMFs. Complaints include skin irritation, fatigue, headache, dizziness, and pain (Eltiti et al. 2007).

Research so far reveals that certain biological effects can be recognized, but they do not indicate health effects (e.g., Hardell et al. 2008; Johansson 2006; Kan et al. 2008; Regel et al. 2006; Röösli et al. 2007). These results have led the World Health Organization (WHO) to define electrohypersensitivity as an idiopathic environmental intolerance attributed to EMFs, or IEI-EMF (Hillert et al. 2006). In other words, there is an illness, but it is psychosomatic, caused by EMFs only in the minds of self-declared sensitive individuals. This interpretation is backed by provocation studies in which sensitive individuals were unable to detect EMF exposure (Rubin et al. 2010). In return, these studies have been criticized for not matching the effects of real-life exposure.

The contestation surrounding EHS first concerns the categories and concepts used to describe it. The lack of agreement on the relation between EMFs and EHS is visible in the range of names for the condition: "electrostress," "electrosensitivity," "electromagnetic oversensitivity," "electrohypersensitivity," "microwave sickness," "microwave syndrome," "radiation sickness," or IEI-EMF. To overcome these diagnostic uncertainties, health activists and sufferers use particular framing devices. Using the acronym EHS itself mimics medical practice (e.g., coronary heart disease, or CHD, and chronic obstructive pulmonary disease, or COPD) and suggests an entity rather than diverse sensations. Calling the proposed condition EHS makes it resemble similar disorders; for example, MCS or chronic fatigue syndrome. EHS sufferers furthermore suggest that one day the link between their condition and EMF will become evident, with references to well-known "triggers" like asbestos or smoking. Activists and sufferers also exploit scientific uncertainty: by stating that negative effects cannot be ruled out, they imply that current illnesses might very well be related to EMF. Finally, EHS sufferers reframe their suffering as a warning sign. As the proverbial "canary in a coal mine" (De Graaff and Bröer 2012), they perceive their suffering as relevant to the whole population. Through contests over framing, health activists seek to establish the diagnostic category by way of mobilization, lobbying, and raising awareness.

Despite scientific refutation and skepticism, the public activism of environmental health movements and patient groups has helped to secure a precautionary approach to EMF. Power lines and MRI equipment are accepted as potential sources of carcinogenic effects. The Council of Europe has advised banning the use of mobile phones and wireless networks in schools, and recommended adherence to the "as low as reasonably achievable" principles for EMF exposure (Huss 2011). On May 31, 2011, the WHO (2011) reclassified mobile phones as "possibly carcinogenic." The political attempts to develop EHS-related policy demonstrate the power of environmental health movements to shape policy and public debate surrounding disease labeling.

The case of EHS is typical of risk society (Beck 1992). Rapid technological advances, unintended side effects, vested commercial interests, and active citizen groups demanding a precautionary approach all influence policy making, risk communication, and epidemiological research. Governments try to balance these various pressures. Without questioning the "roll-out" of mobile phone technology and other EMF equipment, many countries have adopted limited precautionary policies for EMF. Such policies in combination with research on the health effects of EMF keep alive the possibility of a causal relation between EMF and physical distress. Uncertainty regarding the long-term effects legitimizes the research, which organized sufferers interpret as taking their claims seriously. This also translates into different approaches of precaution itself. While governmental policies are limiting exposure after the rollout of the technology, activists have, from early on, pleaded for more research before implementing the technology.

In the case of EHS, sufferers fuse a range of symptoms and explanations into a diagnosis to which their own suffering testifies. Through the lens of risk, they project their condition onto a wider public. Presented in this way, the contestation and uncertainty over the diagnosis prevents governmental action. To the contrary, presenting EHS as a risk triggers governmental responses that are common for risk society: the use of research to take the heat out of the debate at the level of politics (depoliticization), the political activity of social movement participants who are not office holders in the political sphere (subpoliticization) or in stakeholder activities, and attempts to manage perception through communication.

From the point of view of citizens in risk society, expert knowledge and political authority are contested themselves for their role in producing risks. At the same time, these authorities are called upon. Particularly, we witness a tension between increasing demands for expert authority and the recognition of experiential truth of sufferers. With regard to EHS, the question whose diagnosis of illness holds is not yet decided.

THE QUEST FOR DEMEDICALIZATION AND DESTIGMATIZATION

In the contested illnesses discussed above, patients have in many circumstances sought to medicalize their conditions; that is, to gain a legitimate illness label. By contrast, other contested illnesses have provoked attempts to demedicalize and destigmatize the illness label. For example, some advocates and communities for the deaf have in the last decades sought to reclassify deafness from a disability to a differently abled group with rights to maintain their own culture and gain resources to live well without hearing. Deaf advocates see sign language as a legitimate and expressive language in its own right, and believe that the social and cultural worlds that develop in Deaf communities are richly rewarding modes or existence for their participants (Lane 1992). How deafness is labeled (impairment or healthy state) has profound social consequences. It determines whether treatments should be sought or imposed, cochlear implants provided, or deaf schools resourced. Seeking **demedicalization** is thus often an attempt to contest stigmatized identities that deviate from social **norms** to craft new, acceptable social norms, and to access resources.

Many calls for demedicalization challenge mental illness labels, and the medical classification of certain behaviors and thought processes as mentally deviant.* For example, some medical scholars have challenged the globally rising rates of depression diagnoses (see chap. 8). These issues can also be seen in the growing diagnoses of ADHD, an illness label that reveals contests over changing social norms, transforming ideas about childhood and gender and the role of commercial interests in disease diagnosis.

Attention Deficit Hyperactivity Disorder

Attention deficit hyperactivity disorder is a highly contested disorder because it is diagnostically ambiguous, is often treated with stimulant drugs like Ritalin and Adderall, and is so closely linked with boundary setting and determining what constitutes normal childhood behavior. ADHD is usually diagnosed in childhood, and approximately 75–80% of children diagnosed are boys. There is growing awareness of adult ADHD, with services for adults rapidly growing in the United Kingdom, United States, and elsewhere. ADHD diagnoses generally are increasing in many countries, alongside a rise in consumption of stimulant drugs. An estimate of global prevalence of ADHD suggests that 5% of school-age children meet criteria for a clinical diagnosis; however, there is variation across geographic areas (Polanczyk et al. 2007).

Within large, heterogeneous countries such as the United States, there is also within-country variation in ADHD diagnosis. In the United States, there are school districts in which ADHD diagnosis prevalence is extremely high, such as in some middle-upper-class East Coast school districts, as well as school districts in which ADHD is underdiagnosed, such as in parts of rural West Virginia (Costello et al. 2001).

Although the United States is still the largest consumer of methylphenidate, a key ingredient in the drug used to treat ADHD, consumption in other countries is growing. Ten years ago, the United States consumed over 80% of the world's meth-

*Homosexuality is one prominent example; it was removed from the *Diagnostic and Statistical Manual of Mental Disorders* in 1973 after intense political debate (see Kirk and Kuchins 1992).

ylphenidate; in 2009 the International Narcotics Control Board estimated that the global share of U.S. consumption of methylphenidate had dropped to under 75% (International Narcotics Control Board 2009).

The obvious ambiguity in the ADHD diagnosis, as well as increases in diagnosis and drug treatments, has given rise to public and intellectual concerns about the legitimacy of ADHD. A key argument in the contestation around ADHD is that it *medicalizes* normal childhood behaviors—specifically, normal boyhood behaviors (Conrad 1976; Conrad and Potter 2000).

Rather than diagnosis representing disease or pathology, an ADHD diagnosis is thought to reflect institutional or political interests in children's performance and achievement. Political interests focus on children's futures as socially and economically productive citizens, while institutional interests, such as schools, may be interested in shaping children who are willing to learn and to perform. High-achieving students reflect well on the school, which achieves power, influence, and funding on the basis of its performing children.

Governmental and institutional techniques for shaping their citizens are sometimes referred to as forms of **biopower**—knowledge, practices, and forms of control that shape citizens' bodies and minds. These forms of control are seen to have hegemonic effects, meaning that they exert an oppressive power over the individual. As a result, the individual is made to be "docile" and supplicant in his relation to power.

Another basis for contestation around the ADHD diagnosis focuses on the benefits linked to the diagnosis. For example, in many countries the label "ADHD" defines a disability category, and this category in turn shapes children's educational paths and their potential futures. It is not just high-level institutional interests that organize to manage, define, and treat a child's behavior; parents can also have a vested interest in ADHD diagnosis, especially in conditions where substantive educational services for children with different learning styles are lacking (Mayes et al. 2008). Adding to the doubts about ADHD as a diagnosis, some doctors have admitted that while they question its legitimacy, they use the diagnosis and its treatment to help low-income children manage the conditions in impoverished and underresourced schools (Schwartz 2012).

A further source of controversy is the role of the pharmaceutical industry. Historically the developmental paths of Ritalin, a key drug treatment for ADHD, and of the diagnosis itself are intertwined in complicated ways. Ritalin was not invented to treat ADHD, and ADHD was not invented as a reason to use Ritalin, but the diagnosis and the drug can be said to have co-evolved symbiotically since the late 1950s. Ritalin advertising initially played an important role in educating physicians both about the effects of Ritalin on behavioral problems in children, and about the psychiatric diagnoses under which those behavioral problems were subsumed. And while the advent of **direct-to-consumer** advertising of drugs in the 1980s in some countries shifted the marketing focus from the physician to parents, marketing the diagnosis to parents and teachers had already started in the 1970s (Schrag and Divoky 1975). Contemporary advertisements for stimulant drugs sell a lifestyle and a set of ideal family relationships; in many advertisements there is no mention of

ADHD symptoms. Rather, what is depicted is the putative result of treatment: joyful or peaceful mothers and sons—or, more rarely, fathers and sons (Singh 2007). The consumer advertisements, and the debate surrounding their role in increased diagnosis of ADHD, indicate that ADHD has come to embody contemporary anxieties about children, schooling, parenting, and the proliferation of psychiatric explanations and treatments for a population subgroup that was called, some decades ago, the "worried well."

A final important point about the debates over ADHD is that they rarely involve substantive engagement with children themselves. An interview study with over 150 children between the ages of nine and fourteen in the United States and United Kingdom revealed that diagnostic process had not involved an in-depth discussion with the child, nor had the diagnosis been explained in a way that ensured the child's understanding. Following the diagnosis, children felt that clinic visits were simply wellness checks in which they got weighed and measured as a precaution against unwanted side effects (Singh 2012).

WHAT IS PROBLEMATIC ABOUT A "CONTESTED DIAGNOSIS"?

While the terms "contested illness" and "contested diagnosis" are useful in highlighting a range of patient experiences, they are also problematic. Significantly, these terms tend to differentiate too sharply between "medically unexplained" or "socially constructed" disorders and "normal," uncontested biological illness categories. In reality, all illnesses and diagnostic labels are at times open to contest. Even if a medical condition's etiology and symptoms are biologically explained, the diagnostic process might still be contested in a range of ways.

Studies of asthma activism, in which patient activist groups seek to shift attention in the diagnostic setting, offer an example. These activists resist doctors' attempts to emphasize the importance of medication adherence and monitoring regimes, which individualizes the disease and blames the patient for worsening health, when they feel their problems result not from compliance to medical treatment but from industrial contamination and lax government regulation of air pollution (Brown 2007).

In a similar vein, cancer sufferers can dispute their doctors' explanations of the potential aggravators or causes of their illness. They may question whether the factors that matter are lifestyle choices over which sufferers are expected to bear individual responsibility, or environmental toxins in their communities over which they have little control and which would involve governmental regulations (e.g., Balshem 1993; Brown 2007).

These examples illustrate how even medically legitimized illnesses with agreed-upon biological etiologies can be hotly contested in the diagnostic process. Diagnosis is not simply about explaining a biological disease process. It also involves explaining how a patient came to be sick and the role of social, political, or economic factors that shape the emergence, trajectory, or treatment of an illness.

Diagnosis is a crucial process in determining how patients not only interpret the physical cause of their sickness, but also understand how they came to be sick, who might be to blame, and what steps are required in order to regain health. At every step there is space for contested meaning.

THE SHAPE OF CONFLICT

Conflict can arise in many phases of the diagnostic process. It sometimes reflects the limits of diagnostic models, tests, and knowledge, as well as the varied medical opinions that continue to surround some uncertain disease categories. Yet conflict also reflects shifting social, cultural, political, and historical norms and ideas. Disease labels do not simply account for biological processes but are classificatory tools that define the abnormal and deviant body. Our classificatory systems are shaped by our cultural ideas such as gender, ideas about childhood, or correct emotional states. They may reflect economic imperatives now evident within commercial healthcare regimes, the power of the state, or class dynamics and systems of inequality.

The effects of a contested diagnosis on a patient can be profound and often psychologically troubling. When medicine cannot provide certainty, patients may become actively involved in seeking alternative knowledge regimes, building health social movements, or calling for destigmatization. All of these processes underscore the importance of understanding the range of actors who are invested in defining illness and its treatment, and the wide-ranging social and cultural factors that shape conflicts in the diagnostic realm.

TAKEAWAY POINTS

- Not receiving a diagnosis can be a troubling experience for a patient. It can lead to social stigma and can hinder a patient's access to the resources required to regain health.
- Political, economic, and social factors such as gender, inequality, or commercial interest shape access to and contests over diagnosis.
- Health social movements have become actively involved in the diagnostic process, along the way challenging medical, scientific, and political authority.
- Contests over diagnosis can involve attempts to destigmatize or demedicalize a condition or illness community.

DISCUSSION QUESTIONS

1. Think of a situation in which you were a patient and disagreed with a medical specialist's diagnosis. What was your response? How did the disagreement affect your sense of judgment and approach to diagnosis?
2. Think of a disease for which social attitudes and medical opinions have shifted within your own lifetime. What social and cultural factors shaped these changing attitudes?

3. What are some ways that medical specialists could lessen the sense of shame, self-doubt, and trivialization that some patients experience when seeking a diagnosis for a contested illness?

4. Are the goals of patients and medical specialist always the same? How might they differ? What conflicts might these differences create?

REFERENCES

Ashford, Nicolas, and Claudia Miller. 1998. *Chemical Exposures: Low Levels and High Stakes*. New York: Van Nostrand Reinhold.

Balshem, Martha. 1993. *Cancer in the Community: Class and Medical Authority*. Washington, DC: Smithsonian Institution Press.

Beck, Ulrich. 1992. *Risk Society: Towards a New Modernity*. London: Sage.

Bell, Lara. 2012. "The Disrupted and Realigned Self: Exploring the Narrative of New Zealanders with Chronic Fatigue Syndrome/Myalgic Encephalomyelitis." PhD diss., Victoria University of Wellington.

Brown, Phil. 2007. *Toxic Exposures: Contested Illnesses and the Environmental Health Movement*. New York: Columbia University Press.

Brown, Phil, Steve Kroll-Smith, and Valerie J. Gunter, eds. 2000. "Knowledge, Citizens and Organisations: An Overview of Environments, Diseases, and Social Conflict." In *Illness and the Environment: A Reader in Contested Medicine*, 9–25 New York: New York University Press.

Brown, Phil, and Stephen Zavestoski. 2004. "Social Movements in Health: An Introduction." *Sociology of Health and Illness* 26: 679–94.

Conrad, Peter. 1976. *Identifying Hyperactive Children: The Medicalization of Deviant Behavior*. Lexington, MA: Lexington.

Conrad, Peter, and D. Potter. 2000. "From Hyperactive Children to ADHD Adults: Observations on the Expansion of Medical Categories." *Social Problems* 47(4): 559–82.

Costello, E. J., A. Angold, and G. P. Keeler. 2001. "Poverty, Race and Psychiatric Disorder: A Study of Rural Children." *American Journal of Public Health* 91: 1494–98.

Cullen, Mark. 1987. "The Worker with Multiple Chemical Sensitivities: An Overview." *Occupational Medicine* 2: 655–61.

De Graaff, Bert, and Christian Bröer. 2012. "'We Are the Canary in a Coal Mine': Establishing a Disease Category and a New Health Risk." *Health Risk and Society* 14(2): 129–47.

Dew, K. 2002. "Accident Insurance, Sickness, and Science: New Zealand's No-Fault System." *International Journal of Health Services* 32(1): 163–78.

Donnay, A. H. 1999. "On the Recognition of Multiple Chemical Sensitivity in Medical Literature and Government Policy." *International Journal of Toxicology* 18(6): 383–92.

Dumit, J. 2006. "Illnesses You Have to Fight to Get: Facts as Forces in Uncertain, Emergent Illnesses." *Social Science and Medicine*, 62(3): 577–90.

Eltiti, S., D. Wallace, K. Zougkou, R. Russo, S. Joseph, P. Rasor, and E. Fox. 2007. "Development and Evaluation of the Electromagnetic Hypersensitivity Questionnaire." *Bioelectromagnetics* 28(2): 137–51.

Engel, Charles C., Joyce A. Adkins, and David N. Cowan. 2002. "Caring for Medically Unexplained Physical Symptoms after Toxic Environmental Exposures: Effects of Contested Causation." *Environmental Health Perspectives* 110(4): 641–47.

Hardell, L., M. Carlberg, F. Söderqvist, and K. Hansson Mild. 2008. "Meta-Analysis of Long-Term Mobile Phone Use and the Association with Brain Tumours." *International Journal of Oncology* 32: 1097–103.

Hillert, L., N. Leitgeb, and J. Meara. 2006. "Working Group Report." In *Electromagnetic Hypersensitivity: Proceedings of the International Workshop on EMF Hypersensitivity*, edited by K. Hansson Mild, 15–26. Prague: World Health Organization.

Huss, J. 2011. "The Potential Dangers of Electromagnetic Fields and Their Effect on the Environment." Doc. 12608. Council of Europe Parliamentary Assembly, Strasbourg, May 6.

International Narcotics Control Board. 2009. "Psychotropic Substances." http://www.incb.org/documents/Psychotropics/technical-publications/2009/Psychotropic_Report_2009.pdf

Johansson, O. 2006. "Electrohypersensitivity: State-of-the-Art of a Functional Impairment." *Electromagnetic Biology and Medicine* 25(4): 245–58.

Kan, P., S. E. Simonsen, J. L. Lyon, and J. R. Kestle. 2008. "Cellular Phone Use and Brain Tumor: A Meta-Analysis." *Journal of Neurooncology* 86: 71–78.

Kirk, S. A., and H. Kutchins. 1992. *The Selling of DSM: The Rhetoric of Science in Psychiatry*. New York: Aldine de Gruyter.

Kroll-Smith, S., and H. Floyd. 1997. *Bodies in Protest: Environmental Illness and the Struggle over Medical Knowledge*. New York: New York University Press.

Lane, Harlan. 1992. *The Mask of Benevolence: Disabling the Deaf Community*. San Diego: Dawn Singer.

Lipson, Juliene G. 2004. "Multiple Chemical Sensitivities: Stigma and Social Experiences." *Medical Anthropology Quarterly* 18(2): 200–213.

Malterud, K. 2002. "Understanding the Patient with Medically Unexplained Disorders: A Patient-Centred Approach." *New Zealand Journal of Family Practice* 29(6): 374–79.

Markowitz, G., and D. Rosner. 2013. *Lead Wars: The Politics of Science and the Fate of America's Children*. Berkeley: University of California Press.

Mayes, R., C. Bagwell, and J. Erkulwater. 2008. *Medicating Children: ADHD and Pediatric Mental Health*. Cambridge, MA: Harvard University Press.

Nettleton, Sarah. 2005. "'I Just Want Permission to Be Ill': Towards a Sociology of Medically Unexplained Symptoms." *Social Science and Medicine* 62: 1167–78.

Oreskes, N., and E. M. M. Conway. 2010. *Merchants of Doubt: How a Handful of Scientists Obscured the Truth on Issues from Tobacco Smoke to Global Warming*. New York: Bloomsbury.

Phillips, Tarryn. 2010a. "'I Never Wanted to Be a Quack!' The Professional Deviance of Plaintiff Experts in Contested Illness Lawsuits: The Case of Multiple Chemical Sensitivities." *Medical Anthropology Quarterly* 24(2): 182–98.

———. 2010b. "Debating the Legitimacy of a Contested Environmental Illness: A Case Study of Multiple Chemical Sensitivities (MCS)." *Sociology of Health and Illness* 32(7): 1026–40.

Polanczyk, G., M. S. de Lima, B. L. Horta, J. Biederman, and L. A. Rohde. 2007. "The Worldwide Prevalence of ADHD: A Systematic Review and Metaregression Analysis." *American Journal of Psychiatry* 164: 942–48.

Regel, S. J., S. Negovetic, M. Röösli, V. Berdiñas, J. Schuderer, A. Huss, U. Lott, N. Kuster, and P. Achermann. 2006. "UMTS Base Station-Like Exposure, Well-Being, and Cognitive Performance." *Environmental Health Perspectives* 114(8): 1270–75.

Röösli, M., M. Lörtscher, M. Egger, D. Pfluger, N. Schreier, E. Lörtscher, P. Locher, A. Spoerri, and C. Minder. 2007. "Mortality from Neurodegenerative Disease and Exposure to Extremely Low-Frequency Magnetic Fields: 31 Years of Observations on Swiss Railway Employees." *Neuroepidemiology* 28: 197–206.

Rubin, G. J., R. Nieto-Hernandez, and S. Wessely. 2010. "Review: Idiopathic Environmental Intolerance Attributed to Electromagnetic Fields (Formerly 'Electromagnetic

Hypersensitivity'): An Updated Systematic Review of Provocation Studies." *Bioelectromagnetics* 31: 1–11.

Schrag, P., and D. Divoky. 1975. *The Myth of the Hyperactive Child and Other Means of Child Control.* New York: Pantheon.

Schwartz, A. 2012. "Attention Disorder or Not, Pills to Help in School." *New York Times*, http://www.nytimes.com/2012/10/09/health/attention-disorder-or-not-children-prescribed-pills-to-help-in-school.html?pagewanted=all, October 9.

Scott, Wilber, J. 1988. "Competing Paradigms in the Assessment of Latent Disorders: The Case of Agent Orange." *Social Problems* 35(2): 145–61.

Shriver, Thomas E. 2001. "Environmental Hazards and Veterans' Framing of Gulf War Illness." *Sociological Inquiry* 71(4): 403–20.

———. 2006. "Managing the Uncertainties of Gulf War Illness: The Challenges of Living with Contested Illness." *Symbolic Interaction* 29(4): 465–86.

Singh, Ilina. 2007. "Not Just Naughty: 50 Years of Stimulant Drug Advertising." In *Medicating Modern America*, edited by A. Toon and E. Watkins, 131–55. New York: New York University Press.

———. 2012. "Not Robots: Children's Perspectives on Authenticity, Moral Agency and Stimulant Drug Treatments." *Journal of Medical Ethics* 39(6): 359–66, doi:10.1136/medethics-2011-100224.

Trundle, C. 2011a. "Searching for Culpability in the Archives: Commonwealth Nuclear Test Veterans' Claims for Compensation." *History and Anthropology* 22(4): 497–511.

———. 2011b. "Biopolitical Endpoints: Diagnosing a Deserving British Nuclear Test Veteran." *Social Science and Medicine* 73: 882–88.

Ware, Norma C. 1992. "Suffering and the Social Construction of Illness: The Delegitimation of Illness Experiences in Chronic Fatigue Syndrome." *Medical Anthropology Quarterly* 6(4): 347–61.

WHO. World Health Organization. 2011. "IARC Classifies Radiofrequency Electromagnetic Felds as Possibly Carcinogenic to Humans." Press Release No. 208. World Health Organization International Agency for Research on Cancer, Geneva, May 31.

Winder, C. 2002. "Mechanisms of Multiple Chemical Sensitivity." *Toxicology Letters* 128(1–3): 85–97.

Lay Diagnosis
An Oxymoron?

Lindsay Prior

STARTING POINTS

- Laypeople as well as doctors diagnose disease and illness.
- Lay diagnosis can be an important trigger for help-seeking behavior, and for shaping views about treatment.
- Lay diagnosis is firmly based in the lives and worlds of patients, and connects for each one the individual personal history, biography, and bodily symptoms, often in complex ways.
- To understand the basis of lay diagnosis, it is usually necessary to engage with the illness narratives that patients ordinarily bring to medical encounters.

Wittgenstein (1958) opens *Blue and Brown Books* with the question, "what is the meaning of a word?" (1), and in the pages that follow he advances slowly but surely toward a simple answer—that the meaning of a word is essentially its use in the language. This elementary strategy of focusing on a use of a word in the language can serve us equally well when we ask questions about the meaning of "diagnosis" and "lay diagnosis." In the latter case, our field of attention is on the deployment of language in everyday rather than professional (medical) discourse. Everyday discourse provides the basis for analysis and discussion in this chapter.

As discussed throughout this book, one of the functions or uses of the term "diagnosis" is to name things—illnesses, diseases, pathologies, and syndromes. Naming implies classification and differentiation, of distinguishing one set of things from another, so lay diagnosis implies the existence of lay nosologies and other forms of taxonomy (see chap. 1). This is perhaps not so different from what occurs in professional (medical) diagnosis of disease, except that professionals often codify and solidify their forms of thinking in various kinds of master texts, such as the *International Classification of Diseases* (ICD; World Health Organization 2008) and the *Diagnostic and Statistical Manual of Mental Disorders* (DSM; American Psychiatric Association 1995), in a way that lay populations do not. Diagnosis also enables both laypeople and professionals to collect an array of observations (about symptoms) in one place and to understand how different symptoms might be connected. And there are other parallels that can be drawn between the worlds of laypeople and professionals with respect to diagnosis—one is that diagnosis plays a pivotal role in narratives of illness and disease.

This chapter explores the connections between diagnosis, symptoms, and narrative. Through these connections we can understand how laypeople make sense of the afflictions that they encounter, not least because the manner in which laypeople classify and diagnose illness is linked to the everyday strategies that they use for treating and managing bodily dis-ease, their willingness to seek professional medical care, and the extent to which they are willing to follow medical advice in managing their ailments (concordance).

Although the ways in which laypeople diagnose pathology have many parallels with the ways that medical professionals do, there are differences. Professionals might be tempted to suggest that lay diagnosis is inferior to professional diagnosis, and in many respects that is true. Laypeople have far fewer technical resources for diagnosis of disease and they rely in the main on experiential more than on standard textbook or theoretical understandings of disease processes. This chapter does not highlight the deficiencies or otherwise of alternative ways of thinking, but instead explores the role that diagnosis plays in the experience of illness. As a reader you may already be convinced that diagnosis is a matter of professional concern alone, that only doctors can truly diagnose disease, and that the act of diagnosis is something reserved for the work of medical professionals. Jutel (2011), for example, suggests that "diagnosis provides a mechanism for discerning the lay from the professional" (7). Gill et al. (2010) argue along similar lines. Nevertheless, there are good grounds for arguing that laypeople are also accomplished diagnosticians (cf. Frankel 2001).

There have been times when, under the banner of "labeling," lay diagnosis has been regarded as a highly influential and powerful process capable of producing the very symptoms and illnesses to which the label (i.e., diagnosis) makes reference (see, e.g., Scheff 1984). Furthermore, across the globe laypeople are increasingly encouraged to take responsibility for their health and well-being, and in some cases are even regarded as "expert" in understanding and managing illness. The UK National Health Service, for example, has an expert **patient** program aimed at facilitating and improving lay expertise (Donaldson 2003). In that context it is not surprising that nonmedical professionals often regard themselves as capable of both diagnosis and managing disease. It is a trend that has no doubt been given additional impetus by the availability of advice on the Internet, and the capacity for anyone who can afford it to submit biological samples for laboratory assay (cf. Copelton and Valle 2009).

In exploring the connections between diagnosis, symptoms, and narrative, this chapter presents three examples. In the first example, laypeople employ a system of differential diagnosis, at least for common illnesses such as cold and flu. The second example shows what can happen when things are not so clear-cut and the nature of the symptom pattern is ambiguous. The third and final example highlights the role that diagnosis "plays in the language" and why, for laypeople as well as medical professionals, diagnosis is so central to the experience of illness.

USING THE LANGUAGE: DIAGNOSING COLDS AND FLU

Some of the most common illnesses that people experience are colds and flu. Both are consequences of viral infections; over two hundred different viruses have been associated with the common cold alone. Around 30–50% of all colds are said to be caused by rhinoviruses, followed by coronaviruses (10–15% of all colds) and influenza viruses (5–15%) (Heikkinen and Järvinen 2003; McChlery et al. 2009). In contemporary biomedical literature, however, cold and flu are regarded as syndromes rather than as well-defined and firmly bounded categories. The preferred clinical designation in the United Kingdom is upper respiratory tract infection, and in the United States it is called an influenza-like illness. Although colds and flu are diagnosed clinically, laboratory findings are regarded as necessary for the confirmation of any diagnosis.

Even in the medical literature, the symptom pattern for colds and flu is far from agreed, so it is not surprising that there are variations between lay ideas about their symptoms and textbook descriptions of the symptom pattern. What is clear is that laypeople can and do undertake differential diagnosis with respect to the two pathologies, as evident in a study of a predominantly white and elderly population (aged over 65) in South Wales concerning diagnosis of cold and flu. The original research was aimed at trying to understand why some elderly people refused to accept a free inoculation against seasonal flu (Evans et al. 2007; Prior et al. 2011)—that is, to take preventative measures—rather than understanding how people sought to deal with symptoms once symptoms had appeared (e.g., by requesting antibiotics). In this chapter the focus is solely on the kinds of factors that influenced how respondents distinguished cold from flu.

The diagnosis of colds and flu in the lay population concentrates, as one might expect, on the symptom pattern; access to laboratory findings is regarded as unnecessary and is in most cases unavailable.* Research that correlated people's self-diagnosis of flu with laboratory tests for influenza virus found that less than a quarter of those who thought they had flu actually had evidence of the virus, even among health professionals who self-diagnosed (Jutel et al. 2011). In any event, laypeople commonly focus on symptoms relating to the body (especially the head), but they also consider behavioral correlates—and to a lesser extent some psychological factors—in arriving at a diagnosis. In addition, laypeople mention symptoms that are not ordinarily associated with flu in the medical literature, and they also link the body to colds and flu in ways that can run counter to a prevailing Western medical cosmology that seeks to connect pathology to specific anatomical sites.

Figure 12-1 shows in diagrammatic form the key symptoms that laypeople associate with colds and flu. The thickness of the lines between the concept nodes express the value of a coefficient of co-occurrence between a reference to any given symptom (in fifty-four research interviews) and any other symptom mentioned. The diagram also displays links between the symptoms and the two key entities of

---

*During the H1N1 pandemic of 2009, virological testing was available as a public health monitoring tool, but it is currently rarely used in screening for routine seasonal influenza.

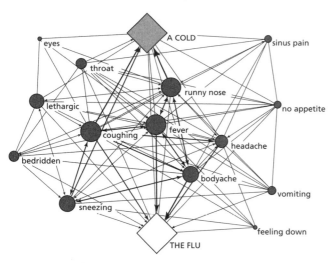

Figure 12-1. The size of nodes is proportional to the total number of references to a symptom in fifty-four interviews. Line thickness expresses a coefficient of association between symptoms (and symptoms with cold and flu) as linked by respondents at interview. *Adapted from Prior et al. (2011)*

"cold" and "flu." The size of each node is proportional to the total number of references to each concept in the fifty-four interview transcripts that were gathered during the research process. Looking at figure 12-1, we see that there is a range of entities deployed for the purpose of diagnosis. These include affected parts of the body (nose, throat, eyes); physiological processes (coughing, sneezing, vomiting, fever); behavioral processes (being bedridden); and to a lesser extent psychological processes (feeling down, lethargy). Note that most, but not all, of the symptoms are common to both conditions.

Laypeople naturally weave these entities into their accounts in idiosyncratic ways, but this diagram contains all of the components that respondents required to distinguish between a cold and the flu. Essentially, the diagnosis of a cold focuses on symptoms in the head because colds are associated almost entirely with the head. (Headache, however, is viewed primarily as a symptom of flu, as is evident from the detail in fig. 12-1). So when respondents were asked to distinguish between colds and flu, they would say, "I think colds [are] just in the head and runny nose and stuffy nose," or refer simply to "a head cold." Unsurprisingly, also seen in figure 12-1, the nose (and sneezing) is particularly prominent in the symptom pattern for cold, though associated sites such as the sinus, throat, and eyes also figure in the diagnostic frame. This is in marked contrast to flu, which is invariably viewed as a whole-body illness characterized by "body ache" (fig. 12-1). Interestingly, a number of respondents also referred (usually in a dismissive manner) to a third category of illness, "the sniffles," which seemed to relate to mild forms of rhinorrhea and associated nasal symptoms. The following extracts from various interviews illustrate some of the ways in which laypeople differentiate colds from flu.

Well, flu, you get all your aches and pains. You feel lethargic, that type of thing, but with a cold, it's usually a head cold and plenty of coughs, sneezes and such like that you don't always get with the flu. I feel the flu is more in the whole of the body.

Always the question is, I mean my daughter's about 44 but I said, um, is your body aching all over? Yes or no? "Yes." You've got flu then. If it's not, you've got a heavy cold and that's it.

I think with flu you're aching all over, aren't you? You go, you get hot and then you get cold and you're aching all over whereas if it's a cold you're sneezing. You have a sort of a heady cold. I think it's a big difference, isn't there?

Well the influenza usually affects your stomach. It usually affects aching all over the body. And you usually have a higher temperature. You feel a lot worse with flu, obviously.

As suggested by the third of the above respondents, flu is strongly associated with fever. In addition, it is predominantly associated with myalgia, and exclusively related to being bedridden or to an inability to undertake routine, normal duties. It is sometimes associated with vomiting and correlated stomach pain. Above all, to have flu is to be "really ill"; flu is "more of an illness than a cough or a cold." And "when you've got the flu, you're really ill. When you've got a cold you can manage you know." It is possible to "shake off a cold," but not the flu; flu "knocks you off your feet." It is often the severity of the discomfort that enables a person to diagnose one from the other. So, "flu is woof, bang wallop, out, you're gone." In short, the flu necessitates withdrawal from normal and routine social intercourse, and as such, flu is more "serious" than a cold. But respondents also made clear that, on occasion, colds can develop into flu, which is why the behavioral features can be so crucial in diagnosing one from the other. And perhaps it is this unique capacity of

flu to remove an individual from everyday affairs that warrants the invariable use of the definite article in discussions of the one (the flu) as compared to the more probable use of the indefinite article (a cold) in discussions concerning the other. In any event, the possibility of a cold metamorphosing into flu serves to highlight the dynamic, "wait-and-see," and emergent aspects of lay diagnosis with respect to both upper and lower respiratory tract infections such

> The process [of diagnosis] is dialectical—from the confusion arising out of the jumble of information that naturally exists in and around the sick person, a disease category (the diagnosis) is chosen. Then the abstract knowledge about the diagnosis is brought back and integrated with what has, at the same time, become known of this sick person to produce a more rounded, individualized, and whole interpretation of the disease . . . Too often what is lacking [in clinical practice] is this last step of integration. (Cassell 2004, 169)

as pneumonia. Wait-and-see is of course a strategy that can be (and often is) adopted by doctors as well as by patients (e.g., when considering whether to prescribe specific treatments such as antibiotics), and in a world of predictive diagnostic testing and the emergence of what Blaxter (2004, 123) has called "diseases-in-waiting," wait-and-see is steadily emerging as a new mode of being ill.

There is a school of thought suggesting that laypeople (especially older people) who focus predominantly on individual symptoms of illness are not too concerned with diagnosis and are more concerned with treatment (see, e.g., Arcury et al. 2012). Yet an assessment of symptoms alone is usually insufficient for laypeople to develop appropriate treatment strategies. It is only diagnosis that can connect things in a narrative form and explain why things developed in the way that they did, how things are now, and (most important of all) how things are likely to unfold in the near future. In that sense, diagnosis is key not merely to understanding illness, but also a trigger for action—whether to rely solely on lay knowledge and experience in the management of a disorder or to seek professional knowledge and care. Before going any further, let us consider what happens when the symptoms of an illness are not clearly connected.

USING THE LANGUAGE: DIAGNOSING STRESS

Diagnosing and understanding depression in primary care settings is not an easy business for doctors (Chew-Graham et al. 2002), and there are various disputes as to whether primary care physicians underdiagnose or overdiagnose depression. Our concern is with lay diagnosis of disorders, including common psychiatric ones. A persistent claim of researchers and campaigners concerned with depression in community settings is that laypeople often feel stigmatized by labels of depression and therefore fail either to declare their symptoms or to seek medical help (see, e.g., Givens et al. 2007). It could be, however, that laypeople simply do not recognize the symptoms of depression and consider such symptoms as a normal part of the life process. Or it could be that they do recognize such symptoms but fail to regard emotional disorders as "real" illnesses.

Naturally, the best way to discover an answer to the problem of recognition is to ask laypeople for their views. In research on a range of different Welsh communities (urban, rural, affluent, and deprived) during the early 2000s, Prior et al. (2003) asked 127 patients randomly selected from primary care practice lists for such views in a series of interviews and focus groups.

One of the techniques used to elicit responses from the sample involved the use of vignettes like the following:

> Miss Jones is a 29-year-old single parent with two small children. They live on a fairly run down [housing] estate and rely on [welfare] benefits. She feels low in energy, has lost weight, is not sleeping properly and feels terrible in the mornings. She also feels that she has no self-confidence and that the future holds nothing for her. At times, if it were not for the children she wonders if it would be worth going on. Her relatives visit her from time to time but they are not prepared to contribute to childcare.

> Mr. Edwards, a 38-year-old factory worker married with two children, has been feeling tired irritable and lacking in energy for about three months. There has been a lot of uncertainty about the future of the company he works for. He has trouble getting to sleep and has chronic backache, stomach pains and aching legs. This has affected his ability to care for his children and enjoy their company. He prefers to sit around the house watching television.

These vignettes are closely based on ones used as components of a psychiatric interview by Lloyd et al. (1998), and they are in many ways similar to Rorschach inkblots in the sense that one can read (or project) almost anything in to them.

In the research referred to here, the vignettes were used to ask research participants to comment on "what, if anything was wrong" with the person depicted in the vignette, and whether that person should seek professional medical help for their problems. Note that no diagnostic terms are contained in the vignettes, nor were any such terms introduced to participants by the researchers; participants consequently focused on symptoms and how such symptoms might be connected. They discussed whether symptom A (say, backache) might cause symptom B (sleeplessness), or whether living on a run-down housing estate might affect sleep patterns and so forth. For the most part they felt that the array of symptoms set before them needed "further investigation," and the symptoms they focused on primarily were the somatic rather than the emotional ones. Even the presence of suicidal ideation was considered by almost all participants as less important than chest pain, breathlessness, and backache. When we asked respondents both as members of a group and as individuals to place some thirteen different symptoms in rank order of "things to take to the doctor," suicidal ideation was ranked only fourth overall.

Figure 12-2 displays the results of the ranking exercise. Node size is proportional to the position of the symptoms in the rank order (1 to 13). Chest pain, breathlessness, and backache all trump suicidal thoughts in importance, while weight loss closely follows suicidal ideation. In order to trace how these evaluations relate to the variables of sex and age, nodes for men and women, as well as for three age groups, are also included in the diagram. The ranking of symptoms in illness significance is more or less common to all groups, but there are some notable differences. Men, for example, tended to downplay suicidal ideation as something to be taken seriously, and only one third of older men regarded it as a symptom to be concerned about in any way at all. Men were also slightly more concerned about chest pain and breathlessness, and older people were more concerned with weight loss than younger people. Note again that there are no references to diagnosis in figure 12-2, though of the 127 lay participants in the various focus groups, some ventured diagnoses, including "depression." But depression was not the most frequently offered diagnosis; rather, it was "stress" that was referred to most often. Stress often surpassed depression as a diagnostic category in two different respects; it was mentioned more frequently and it was also believed to be a common cause of depression. Yet, as Pollock (1988) has indicated, stress is not a recognized disease category in any sense; rather, it is a useful—and relatively recent—

metaphor that people draw upon to account for suffering. Its function is to make sense of the various personal troubles that afflict people in their everyday lives, to connect dis-ease to an understandable cause.

So what can we learn from this example? The low estimation of the seriousness of emotional symptoms and the heightened concern about somatic symptoms (in a predominantly white European population) clearly stand out. So, too, does the general inability to "see" the potential for depression in the vignettes or even to understand that somatic symptoms might be a product of emotional disturbance. But it was also clear from the focus group discussions

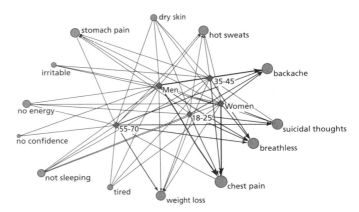

Figure 12-2. The size of the vertices (nodes) is proportional to the rank order of the symptoms calculated on the basis of 117 questionnaire responses from primary care patients. Arc (line) thickness is proportional to the percentage of men, women, and members of three age groups who considered the symptom "worth taking to the doctor." *Adapted from Prior et al. (2011)*

that there was a need for an overarching explanation for the symptoms—things were connected, but how they were connected was puzzling. The vignettes needed a key, an organizing frame, a diagnosis. For most (probably all) people in the focus groups, providing a diagnosis was regarded as a task for the doctor, though in the absence of any medical diagnosis, stress was the preferred candidate explanation. Stress tied together the symptoms and linked the diverse elements into a meaningful narrative; stress linked illness to biography and to action. The significance of biography and narrative for an understanding of illness is discussed below.

THE PLACE OF DIAGNOSIS IN A FORM OF LIFE

As contributors to this volume have indicated, one of the functions of diagnosis, according to Balint (1957), is that it transforms a set of unorganized symptoms into an organized illness—diagnosis should not only connect symptoms and signs, but should also explain why things are connected in the way that they are. And that position resonates clearly with the first example above.

However, we know that there are occasions when no rational cause for a patient's symptoms can be identified, as was the case in the second example above. It is also possible that even after extensive clinical investigation symptoms can remain unexplained. Medically unexplained symptoms, or MUS, are seen across general medicine and even represent the most common diagnosis in some specialties (Nimnuan et al. 2001). Kroenke and Rosmalen (2006) suggest that around one third to one half of the physical complaints brought to outpatient encounters are medically unexplained. In such instances the symptoms remain disorganized and the patient is left in a state of **liminality** (see chap. 3) and uncertainty, and under those conditions patients often self-diagnose (Copelton and Valle 2009). When they do, they sometimes connect symptoms of illness that would (and perhaps should) otherwise remain unconnected.

A research project during 2003–5 looked at people who attended a university medical clinic with MUS and who had self-diagnosed a condition known as myalgic encephalomyelitis (ME). The objective of the study was to improve systems of support and care for these patients. ME is often referred to in the medical literature as chronic fatigue syndrome (CFS) or sometimes as chronic fatigue immune dysfunction syndrome (CFIDS). In the 2002 Report to the Chief Medical Officer for England on CFS/ME—a report by a working group of lay sufferers and medical professionals—the condition was described as follows:

> CFS/ME is a quite common, very heterogeneous condition of adults and children that lacks specific disease markers but is clinically recognizable . . . The characterising features are overwhelming fatigue, related effects on both physical and cognitive functioning, and malaise, accompanied by a wide range of other symptoms. The fatigue is evidently very different in character from everyday tiredness and is accompanied by a profound lack of energy; it is commonly described as like no other in type and severity. (CFS/ME Working Group 2002, Annex 6, 1)

The fact that patients often prefer to use the term ME, while physicians refer to CFS, is indicative of controversy about the nature of the illness, its causes, and its treatment. This chapter does not delve into such controversy or what might be called the politics of the disease (Banks and Prior 2001); suffice it to say that ME/CFS offers an excellent site for investigating the kinds of conflicts that arise when laypeople and medical professionals disagree over the nature of an illness (see chap. 12 for further discussion of contested diagnoses).

A. B. was a forty-one-year-old married mother of two children. She was interviewed as part of a research project that was focused on understanding CFS from the patient's point of view. In the course of a research interview, A. B. explained that during her adult life she had been afflicted with various maladies and had consulted with numerous medical specialists. She mentioned her contacts with dentists, specialist dental surgeons, primary care physicians, locum physicians, gynecologists, psychiatric nurses, physiotherapists, and also the physician headed the university clinic that she was attending at the time of the research. Among the interventions that she had been offered (and sometimes accepted during previous decades) were removal of some of her teeth, surgery on her abdomen, hysterectomy, an introduction to a graded exercise program, prescriptions for antidepressants and muscle relaxants, and medication for abnormal blood pressure.

She reported that most of the medical professionals were often baffled by her symptoms and sometimes suggested that there was no medical problem to investigate. Of her toothache some twenty-three years previously, for example, she stated, "they said there was nothing wrong with the tooth or the jaw and when they took the tooth out . . . I still had the pain afterwards and it never went away and it's always been there." Of the hysterectomy, she stated, "as if all the problems will go away once you get a hysterectomy . . . but I've still got the pain in my side and it comes and goes, you know, as it always has."

The patient was also critical of some of the diagnoses that had been suggested to her, especially diagnoses of psychiatric conditions. In that context she cited the words of a psychiatric nurse who had spoken to her some years previously. " 'Oh you're not very depressed,' she [the nurse] said, 'in fact you're a lot less depressed than I think you should be with what you've got, and had to put up with,' she said." Indeed, A. B. wished to account for her chronic pain and suffering entirely in physical terms, and she sought a diagnosis that would connect the various (chronic) symptoms—acquired throughout the adult life course—in a coherent manner.

> From antiquity until the nineteenth-century, the word "symptom" (from the Greek for coincidence) meant any manifestation of disease . . . Only in this era have symptoms come to be seen as purely subjective and signs as objective. Further, the word "objective" has come to have the connotation of real, in contrast to subjective things which are "only mental" and therefore unreal. This shift in meaning of the word "symptom" and the derogation of symptoms because of their subjective nature are results of the influence of scientific ideals on medicine. (Cassell 2004, 90)

Figure 12-3 displays the range of symptoms to which A. B. referred during her interview, together with some of the associations that she made between them.

The size of the nodes is proportional to the number of references that she made to a given entity. It shows that "pain" loomed large in her discussion and therefore exists as the largest node. She also referred to her nose and throat as sites of diverse problems. On occasion she referred to a localized pain (rather than just pain), in which case a line connects pain to a specific part of her body. The thickness of the lines linking two entities is a reflection of the association between any two entities; the thicker the line, the more likely the two things in question are to be associated. So "the right-hand side" of her body is mentioned a lot in relation to "pain," as well as her jaw, joints, and muscles. Other anatomical sites mentioned included her legs, hips, hands, arms. Her face was mentioned in relation to a "sun rash" and "itching." In most cases these symptoms (such as the sun rash and the pains in the right-hand side and jaw) had lasted since she was eighteen years old. She also referred to tiredness (and fatigue) and "weakness" as relatively common features of her life.

As has already been suggested, A. B.'s medical advisers had often failed to identify any structural pathology to explain her symptoms, and one of the reasons she was attending her university clinic was that her primary care physician had referred her for further investigation of the pain that she was experiencing in the right-hand side of her body. Kroenke and Rosmalen (2006) suggest that in cases of this kind it is important to treat both psychological and somatic symptoms systematically.

In addition to the symptoms that A. B. described in her interview, figure 12-3 also contains reference to two candidate diagnoses. The diagnoses connect to each other and to some of the aforementioned symptoms, including pain. One diagnosis was what A. B. called "shogun syndrome" (previously unheard of by the author, and possibly a mispronunciation of Sjögren syndrome or a reference to scleroderma), and the other was ME. According to her own account, she had to "discover" these conditions for herself. As she stated, "Well, I just think, it comes to something when you've got to diagnose yourself." She felt in particular that the dental surgeon ought to have diagnosed "shogun syndrome" before she did. She was also somewhat put out by the fact that her primary care physician thought little of ME as a diagnosis. In reference to the aforementioned report of the CFS/ME Working Group (2002) to the Chief Medical Officer for England—which had stressed that CFS/ME is a "genuine" and "real" illness—she added that "the government announced that doctors should be taking ME seriously and dealing with it." Note that although she also mentioned "depression" and "anxiety" during her interview, she made no connection between these conditions and her other symptoms—depression was something

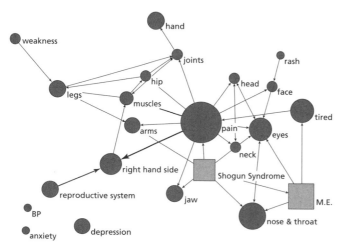

Figure 12-3. The size of the vertices (nodes) is proportional to the frequency of mention in interviews. Arc (line) thickness is proportional to the association of entities as made by the respondent. *Adapted from Prior et al. (2011)*

that other people (such as nurses and primary care physicians) had suggested to her.

Cassell (2004) has argued that modern medicine has little to offer patients like A. B. precisely because it focuses on diseases rather than on suffering. A focus on suffering, he suggests, implies understanding the person rather than the disease. Instead of viewing symptoms as a direct manifestation of underlying bodily pathology, symptoms are to be considered in the context of the patient's biography. In short, he suggests, we need to study illness as a form of life rather than as disease and to engage in what Balint (1957, 53) called "deep diagnosis." There are a number of ways in which that argument resonates in the data of our case. It seems as if A. B. sought an explanation for her pain and suffering not in terms of discrete episodes of illness but in terms of the entirety of her adult life. She has suffered her pains "since she was 18"; they have never gone away and therefore any reasonable diagnosis would have to account for those decades of discomfort. In addition, a suitable diagnosis would have to connect and provide cohesion to what are seemingly unconnected and diverse symptoms, to give cohesion to her narrative and her biography (her history). For underlying the individual symptoms is a condition, and it is the correct diagnosis of that condition that will (at least) explain her suffering in a satisfactory manner. To find this condition she has had to self-diagnose, and it was self-diagnosis that helped her to organize her illness and to make sense of disparate symptoms. In that respect the diagnosis serves as a *weltanschauung*, or comprehensive worldview and a vantage point from which the chronology of illness could be understood. A. B. was "amazed" when she first read of "shogun syndrome," which seemingly explained her pain (especially in her eyes and jaw) in a meaningful way. In comparison, the alternative diagnoses that had been offered to her over the years simply lacked the power required to account for decades of pain. In such a context, figure 12-3 well represents the nature of A. B.'s illness. It is an illness in which almost everything is connected; the presence of "shogun syndrome" and ME illustrates how even vague, imprecise, and chimerical diagnostic terms function to organize the experience of illness.

THE NATURE OF NARRATIVE

The case of A. B. above provides an important clue to understanding the role of diagnosis in everyday life in general, for diagnosis explains disorder. A given person is well at time t^1 and is unwell at time t^2 (and possibly for many days, weeks, months, or years later); something caused that change, and something is needed to explain that change. For both laypeople and medical professionals the diagnostic categories provide a plausible account as to how otherwise disparate symptoms might be connected and why the person moved from a state of wellness and health into a state of illness. In that role, diagnosis provides an excellent example of what the philosopher Arthur C. Danto (2007) referred to as narrative explanation. Illness symptoms point to an observable or noticeable change in biophysical functioning (the *explanandum*), and the diagnosis points to a cause for that change (the *explanans*). In the words of Danto (2007, 249), narrative renders the *explanandum* "intelligible or justifiable."

The body is not mute, but it is inarticulate; it does not use speech, yet begets it. The speech that the body begets includes illness stories; the problem of hearing these stories is to hear the body speaking in them. (Frank 1995, 27)

Narratives are central to the ways in which both laypeople and professionals understand disease and illness. Medical students are, after all, still trained to take the histories of their patients as a precursor to diagnosing malady.

Taking one's history (i.e., the narrative) is a central component of doctor-patient interaction (Good and Good Delvecchio 2000). Narrative techniques have also been adapted for use in clinical contexts and allied to concepts of healing (Charon 2006), and various social scientific studies have helped underline the significance of narratives for understanding disease and illness in the everyday world (Frank 1995; Hydén 1997).

According to Ricoeur (1984), our basic ideas about narrative are best derived from the work and thought of Aristotle, who in his *Poetics* sought to establish "first principles" of composition. Of particular interest to Ricoeur is the emphasis that Aristotle (Halliwell 1995, 56) placed on the notion of "plot" (*muthos*), and on the way to construct such plots. Ricoeur subsequently lays emphasis on "emplotment" as one of the most important features of narrative form. For Ricoeur (1984), as for Aristotle, plot ties things together; it "brings together factors as heterogeneous as agents, goals, means, interactions, circumstances, unexpected results" (65) into the narrative frame. For Aristotle, it is the ultimate untying or unraveling of the plot that releases the dramatic energy of the narrative.

In short, diagnosis functions in lay illness narratives as a kind of plot. It is diagnosis that ties together (connects) the diverse symptoms, signs, events, and experiences that people come to know as illness. And although symptoms are mainly addressed by the sufferer and his advisers in their considerations as how they will treat and manage any episode of illness, it is the act of diagnosis that ultimately helps them make sense of what has occurred in the past, what is occurring now, and what will unfold in the days (and sometimes months and years) ahead. It is, one assumes, why A. B. was "amazed" when she discovered "shogun syndrome."

RETICULATING SYMPTOMS, ILLNESS, AND BIOGRAPHY

Diseases as well as people have biographies—histories—and so, too, have episodes of illness. Illnesses unfold through time, symptoms appear sequentially, and it is to symptoms that sufferers initially attend. Yet at some stage laypeople also require explanations as to what their symptoms "mean," as well as answers to those invariant and universal questions: Why me? Why now?

In the unfolding story of illness—the illness narrative—diagnosis has the role of gluing the disparate elements together. It functions as something akin to Aristotle's plot, of which he suggests there are three parts: reversal (a change in the state of things), recognition (a change from ignorance to knowledge), and suffering (an action that involves destruction and pain). In any illness narrative there will be many characters: symptoms, people, places, causative agents, and therapies. But the characters on their own are insufficient to explain the illness; only diagnosis fulfills that role, and it is why diagnosis is so often central to the lay experience of illness; that is, precisely, its use in the language. Ultimately, diagnosis is an indispensable net that holds together the connections between people's bodily symptoms, illnesses, and biographies.

TAKEAWAY POINTS

- Patients require diagnoses to make sense of the symptoms that they experience and to shape their strategies for managing an illness.
- A lay diagnosis—whether in accord with a professional diagnosis or not—is central to a patient's understanding of illness and helps to explain the origins of dis-ease as well as the nature and trajectory of disease.
- Engaging with lay diagnosis involves listening to the patient's narrative of illness as well as a report on symptoms.
- Such narratives invariably inform doctors as to how any given pathology connects to this particular person and to this particular body.

DISCUSSION QUESTIONS

1. Consider the last time you were ill. Did you think you knew what your diagnosis was? Did your doctor agree? Now, reverse the situation, and put yourself in the place of a diagnostician; how would or could you respond to your patient's proposed diagnosis?
2. What are some conditions where self-diagnosis would be desirable? Why?
3. What are some conditions where self-diagnosis would not be desirable? Why?

REFERENCES

American Psychiatric Association. 1995. *Diagnostic and Statistical Manual of Mental Disorders: DSM-IV.* Washington, DC: American Psychiatric Association.

Arcury, Thomas A., Joseph G. Grzywacz, Rebecca H. Neiberg, Wei Lang, Ha Nguyen, Kathryn Altizer, Eleanor P. Stoller, A. Bell Ronny, and Sarah A. Quandt. 2012. "Older Adults' Self-Management of Daily Symptoms: Complementary Therapies, Self-Care, and Medical Care." *Journal of Aging and Health* 24: 569–97.

Balint, Michael. 1957. *The Doctor, His Patient and the Illness.* London: Pitman Medical.

Banks, Jonathan, and Lindsay Prior. 2001. "Doing Things with Illness: The Micro-Politics of the CFS Clinic." *Social Science and Medicine* 52: 11–23.

Blaxter, M. 2004. *Health.* Cambridge: Polity.

Cassell, Eric J. 2004. *The Nature of Suffering and the Goals of Medicine.* 2nd ed. New York: Oxford University Press.

CFS/ME Working Group. 2002. *A Report to the Chief Medical Officer of an Independent Working Group.* London: Stationery Office.

Charon, Rita. 2006. *Narrative Medicine: Honoring the Stories of Illness.* New York: Oxford University Press.

Chew-Graham, Carolyn, Sean Mullin, Carl R. May, Scott Hedley, and Hannah Cole. 2002. "Managing Depression in Primary Care: Another Example of the Inverse Care Law?" *Family Practice* 19: 632–37.

Copelton, Denise A., and Guiseppina Valle. 2009. "'You Don't Need a Prescription to Go Gluten-Free': The Scientific Self-Diagnosis of Celiac Disease." *Social Science and Medicine* 69: 623–31.

Danto, Arthur C. 2007. *Narration and Knowledge.* New York: Columbia University Press.

Donaldson, Liam. 2003. "Expert Patients Usher in a New Era of Opportunity for the NHS." *BMJ* 326: 1279–80.

Evans, Meirion R., Hayley Prout, Lindsay Prior, Lorna M. Tapper-Jones, and Chris C. Butler. 2007. "A Qualitative Study of Lay Beliefs about Influenza Immunization in Older People." *British Journal of General Practice* 57: 352–58.

Frank, Arthur. 1995. *The Wounded Storyteller: Body, Illness, and Ethics.* Chicago: University of Chicago Press.

Frankel, Richard M. 2001. "Clinical Care and Conversational Contingencies: The Role of Patients' Self-Diagnosis in Medical Encounters." *Text* 21: 83–111.

Gill, Virginia T., Anita Pomerantz, and Paul Denvir. 2010. "Pre-Emptive Resistance: Patients' Participation in Diagnostic Sense Making Activities." *Sociology of Health and Illness* 32: 11–20.

Givens, Jane L., Ira R. Katz, Scarlett Bellamy, and William C. Holmes. 2007. "Stigma and the Acceptability of Depression Treatments among African Americans and Whites." *Journal of General Internal Medicine* 22: 1292–97.

Good, Byron J., and Mary-Jo Good Delvecchio. 2000. "'Fiction' and 'Historicity' in Doctors' Stories: Social and Narrative Dimensions of Learning Medicine." In *Narrative and the Cultural Construction of Illness and Healing*, edited by C. Mattingly and L. Garro, 50–69. Berkeley: University of California Press.

Halliwell, S., trans. 1995. *Aristotle's Poetics.* Cambridge, MA: Harvard University Press.

Heikkinen, Terho, and Asko Järvinen. 2003. "The Common Cold." *Lancet* 361: 51–59.

Hydén, L. C. 1997. "Illness and Narrative." *Sociology of Health and Illness* 19: 48–69.

Jutel, Annemarie. 2011. *Putting a Name to It: Diagnosis in Contemporary Society.* Baltimore: Johns Hopkins University Press.

Jutel, Annemarie, Michael G. Baker, James Stanley, Q. Sue Huang, and Don Bandaranayake. 2011. "Self-Diagnosis of Influenza during a Pandemic: A Cross-Sectional Survey." *BMJ Open* 1(2): e000234, doi:10.1136/bmjopen-2011-000234.

Kroenke, K., and J. G. M. Rosmalen. 2006. "Symptoms, Syndromes, and the Value of Psychiatric Diagnostics in Patients Who Have Functional Somatic Disorders." *Medical Clinics of North America* 90: 603–26.

Lloyd, K. R., K. S. Jacob, V. Patel, L. St. Louis, D. Bhugra, and H. A. Mann. 1998. "Explanatory Model Interview (SEMI) and Its Use among Primary-Care Attenders with Common Mental Disorders." *Psychological Medicine* 28: 1231–37.

McChlery, Susan, Gordon Ramage, and Jeremy Bagg. 2009. "Respiratory Tract Infections and Pneumonia." *Periodontology 2000* 49: 151–65.

Nimnuan, Chachana, Matthew Hotopf, and Simon Wessely. 2001. "Medically Unexplained Symptoms: An Epidemiological Study in Seven Specialties." *Journal of Psychosomatic Research* 51: 361–67.

Pollock, Kristian. 1988. "On the Nature of Social Stress: Production of a Modern Mythology." *Social Science and Medicine* 26(3): 381–92.

Prior, Lindsay, Meirion Evans, and Hayley Prout. 2011. "Talking about Colds and Flu: The Lay Diagnosis of Two Common Illnesses among Older British People." *Social Science and Medicine* 73: 922–28.

Prior, Lindsay, Fiona Wood, Glyn Lewis, and Roisin Pill. 2003. "Stigma Revisited, Disclosure of Emotional Problems in Primary Care Consultations in Wales." *Social Science and Medicine* 56: 2191–200.

Ricoeur, Paul. 1984. *Time and Narrative.* Vol. 1, translated by K. McLaughlin and D. Pellauer. Chicago: University of Chicago Press.

Scheff, Thomas J. 1984. *Being Mentally Ill: A Sociological Theory.* 2nd ed. New York: Aldine.

Wittgenstein, Ludwig. 1958. *Blue and Brown Books.* Oxford: Blackwell.

World Health Organization. 2008. *International Statistical Classification of Diseases and Related Health Problems.* 10th ed. Geneva: World Health Organization.

Researching the Social Aspects of Diagnosis
Answers for Clinical Practice

Sandra H. Sulzer

STARTING POINTS

- Randomized control trials and other comparative, experimental, and epidemiological research help doctors to know what treatments are the most effective.
- Research is the cornerstone of evidence-based practice.
- Medicine may rely on science, but it does so with subjective actors in social contexts.

Concepts like **medicalization**, authority, diversity, and the many other topics covered in this book do not necessarily lend themselves to the most prominent research methods in medical education. The previous chapters of this book have introduced new concepts and ways of understanding the diagnostic experience. The next step is to learn more about how these findings are constructed. This chapter explores the research methods that help elucidate and solve the kinds of problems surrounding the implementation and practice of medicine. Sociological research may seem a few steps removed from the critical goals of understanding and responding to disease processes. But the dilemmas and contradictions clinicians face in their efforts to save lives go far beyond the effectiveness of any particular pharmaceutical or treatment regimen. What do you do with a **patient** who doesn't speak English and won't follow your instructions? How exactly do you tell a patient that she has months left to live in a way that is as clear and beneficial to them as possible? How do you decide whether to tell a patient that she has an incredibly stigmatizing diagnosis? There is a wealth of social science literature to respond to these and other concerns. This chapter explores these questions and more to demonstrate how sociological research is tremendously useful to physicians.

I refer to what Mary Ebeling called "the crowded examination room" in chapter 9 to explain that the problems outlined above are not just about the individual patient and the individual doctor. Even in the exam room, the patient and clinician are both shaped by a wide array of social factors. Expanding your research literacy to include social science approaches will provide you with additional resources in your pursuit of effective, patient-centered care.

Doctors are inevitably situated in specific hospitals and clinics wherein they must provide care. The social context in which medicine takes place becomes incredibly important. As the Association of American Medical Colleges (2011) states, "improving the health of the public involves addressing health disparities and ensuring patient safety, as well as engaging the social and political aspects of health care governance, financing, and delivery" (5). Medicine doesn't occur in a void—it happens among real people, dealing with real budgets and real constraints set by the politics of health care. Medicine is carried out by practitioners who remain subjective beings, even in the most critical of contexts. These are social, not simply medical, considerations.

This chapter will help you to be a discerning clinician whether you engage in research practices or not. I review the distinctions between methodologies and methods, and then present a series of vignettes illustrating particular challenges a clinician might face in everyday work practices. Through these cases you will learn how different social science research approaches can be used to undertake a systematic and rigorous analysis of these problems. These examples offer robust research findings upon which you can buttress your own practice, in the same way that the odds ratios of a well-designed randomized control trial (RCT) might provide you with direction in your therapeutic challenges. You will be presented with a range of different methodologies and methods that are generally not emphasized in medical education but nonetheless have the potential to help answer different questions pertinent to your everyday work. This chapter is a short introduction to some of the many methods available to researchers and physicians.

Social research questions demand specific methods. When studying how individual and social mechanisms interface with effective public health campaigns to prevent coronary disease, Charlie Davison and his colleagues used semi-structured qualitative interviews and observations to develop a general explanatory framework to describe how lay communities account for common chronic illness. They argue effectively that problems of prevention are not simply individual phenomena, but are anchored in the collective realities and beliefs of communities (Davison et al. 1991).

METHODOLOGIES: CHOOSING THE MEDIUM

Every research project has a methodological orientation, which can be broken down into three parts: methodology, research design, and method. The methodology paints the broad strokes of how to proceed and is based on your perspective on how best to understand the social world. The research design is like a map of how to answer your research question. The methods are the particular data collection instruments that you might use. So the chosen methodology might be primarily quantitative, qualitative, or even philosophical. Quantitatively, the world can be understood as something that you can apprehend in a detached and neutral way, that you can measure and count. Qualitatively, you might view the world as one constructed out of the interactions between people, and in which the research process itself is an act of interpretation. And finally, philosophically, you might be more interested in the relationship between ideas and their argumentation than in observations of phenomena. Your research design might be an RCT or a case control study where analysis starts after all the information has been collected. Or it could be one that evolves as you collect and interpret the data, and test your ideas through the next bout of data collection. And your methods may involve the use of online questionnaires, face-to-face interviews, or observation.

The kinds of questions we ask drive the kind of methodology we use. Asking how many or how often, for example, sets up the researcher to explore the world in a quantitative way. Asking how, more simply, often demands a qualitative inquiry. This simple distinction is how most scholars think about methodology: by dividing the world into qualitative and quantitative. While that formulation is too simple to capture the full range of differences in approaches, it makes intuitive sense in many cases.

For example, asking "how does an engine run?" demands examination of an engine or a technical manual, both of which are qualitative approaches. One would probably not need to observe a hundred identical engines to determine how one operates, and this is where the number of cases in qualitative research is often different from quantitative. It is not because qualitative research is less rigorous, but because the kinds of evidence that are sufficient to answer a question thoroughly are often different. Asking, on the other hand, "how many fan belts break each year?" demands a quantitative analysis. Another way of thinking about this distinction is whether an inquiry is intensive, requiring a deep understanding of a narrow area, or extensive, requiring a more superficial understanding of a broad range of information and where the representation of occurrences alone is adequate (Sayer 2010).

Methodologies can become more specific, laying out a general trajectory of how research will proceed. Some examples of methodologies include ethnography, ethnomethodology, participatory action or community-based research, discourse analysis, and grounded theory (see Dew 2007), many of which will be discussed at greater length in the examples below. You may see article authors mentioning their methodology in passing, likely because there often isn't a great deal of space in journals for discussion of research practices. To complicate matters further, in scientific writing, "method" and "methodology" are sometimes conflated or used interchangeably. Accordingly, it is not terribly important to worry about which is which when you're reading research. There is some definitional creep between the terms. For the sake of conceptual clarity, however, method and methodology are presented here as distinct concepts.

METHODS AND PROCESSES: THE DEVILISH DETAILS OF DOING RESEARCH

Methods and research design constitute the actual business of doing research. They take scholars from a general starting point, such as survey methodology, to the real practicalities. Researchers must be prepared to answer many questions, including: Whom will they talk to? What will they say? How will they say it? How will they make sure participants are informed about their rights as research participants? Even the plan for analysis affects what data need to be collected. In addition to being able to answer these questions, a researcher must be able to defend her choices as the best that could have been made, given the constraints of attempting to answer complex questions within the resources available.

While in basic science it may be possible to control for outside events, or to create an entire universe within a petri dish, this is simply not the case when studying all of society or even just one clinic. For obvious ethical reasons, we cannot restrict humans to large petri dishes, nor can we examine a clinic as an entire contained universe without creating some kind of prison in the process. As a result, the research design involved in social sciences is necessarily complex. There are three important areas of design that must be planned for: sampling, instrument design, and implementation. A strong research design addresses all three.

Unexplained illness challenges both the patient and the clinician. The tension between the certain symptoms and the uncertain diagnosis can be stigmatizing, demoralizing, and frustrating. For the clinician, understanding what the patient experiences, how she responds, and what matters to her may provide tremendous insights for better care. Annika Lillrank collected written narratives from sufferers of chronic back pain, a condition for which measurable findings are often elusive despite serious pain. The narrative analysis consisted of what Elliot G. Mischler calls "reconstructing the told from telling" and provides a richness of insight that other forms of analysis could not provide (Lillrank 2003).

1. *Sampling.* Before selecting a sample, a researcher must know his population or group of interest. Perhaps it is an entire nation of people. Or perhaps it is women over the age of forty who have congestive heart failure. Maybe it is every ambulatory clinic in the tristate area. Once the population is determined, a sample from within that population must be selected for study. In most cases it simply isn't feasible to study absolutely every single person from a population (as with a census), so researchers use a sample to try to understand trends that happen within the entire population or a piece of the population. Accordingly, the sample selection involves choices about how many or which people or clinics or other unit of analysis from which to choose. Researchers may choose to randomly sample because they'd like something representative of the whole that is generalizable. Or they might use a variety of other strategies, including choosing the most contrasting cases in order to illuminate the range of possibilities (Stinchcombe 2005). Perhaps they are working with a difficult-to-reach population and will take anyone they get their hands on, which is also known as "convenience sampling." In that case, researchers often continue to recruit until they reach "saturation" (Charmaz 2008), a point at which they learn no new information from continuing to talk with respondents.

2. *Instrument design.* The type of instrument employed may include a survey, or interview guide. Sometimes projects involve secondary data analysis only, and then rely on the survey or interview data of another researcher. Some

scholars, such as ethnographers, may go into the field with nothing but themselves as the instrument. The instrument must be well matched to the type of sample selected. It would be difficult, for example, to conduct two-hour interviews with five thousand participants. And it would be relatively meaningless to give a survey to three people.

3. *Implementation*. Research is carried out through implementation. It includes everything from making sure participants have given or waived their informed consent to participate, to purchasing and administering incentives, to data management strategies. This step is often relatively invisible to the reader of a journal article, but it encompasses many key decisions about how a project can be done, and done well. Failing to have some participants consent to participate (if consent is required), for example, is an ethics violation. And the storage of names or addresses to deliver incentives for participation can lead to concerns about confidentiality. Data management becomes ever more important, particularly when using any data that have identifiers. Having the appropriate staff and resources to carry out the research is essential to ensure that each step of the research process is conducted with a high level of efficacy. Unfortunately, as a reader, it may be unclear to how well any given research team handles these issues, except to the extent that they discuss them as weaknesses of their project in the limitations section of an article.

Health-care providers likewise face a series of challenges. Below are some examples of dilemmas that illustrate how social science research can provide the clinician with robust research to provide insight on the social factors affecting the problem. Through the following examples you will become familiar with a variety of research strategies that are not typically considered medical in nature but are valuable in negotiating the social issues surrounding diagnosis.

SOCIAL RESEARCH EXAMPLES
Lack of Diagnostic Compliance

What do you do when you face language or cultural barriers that prevent you from communicating effectively with your patients? Anne Fadiman (1997) explores exactly this issue in her book *The Spirit Catches You and You Fall Down*, where she catalogues the experience of a Hmong family and their daughter with epilepsy. Through in-depth interviews, a translator, and spending many hours taking notes as she followed this family and their doctors, Fadiman captures a profound linguistic and cultural clash between patient and provider. Such research is called ethnography, and it can involve months or years at a research site trying to understand complex questions. Rather than relying exclusively on self-reports such as in survey research, the researcher is able to observe events from an outside perspective. Ethnography often allows multiple, and sometimes discordant, perspectives to emerge.

Fadiman (1997) captures the difficulty of patients who have different cultural backgrounds than their doctors. "According to Dr. Small," she writes, "the Hmong are highly uncooperative obstetrical patients. 'They don't do a damn thing you tell them,' he said" (73). Fadiman explains, "because they were approximately as fond of most doctors as Robert Small was of them, Hmong women . . . tended to avoid prenatal care" (73). She records the words of another doctor who describes the tension: "'I have the same standard of care for the Hmong as I have for everyone else,' she said. 'My hands are just tied to provide it. So I give them suboptimal care. Sometimes you can find a middle ground and try to understand where they are coming from, which is hard, but not impossible'" (75).

While Fadiman may not be able to respond conclusively to what should be done about cultural differences, she is able to explain in an in-depth way how both parties come to the encounter with their underlying assumptions. By illuminating the different expectations of each group, she can point to where disconnects are happening. The patient in this research, Lia, who is epileptic, loses all ability to walk and talk by the end of the narrative. Fadiman (1997) goes on to say, "I have come to believe that her life was ruined not by septic shock or noncompliant parents but by cross-cultural misunderstanding" (263). She explains that the doctors who cared for Lia were equipped to treat "white middle-class patients who always took their medicine and whose insurance companies always paid on time" (265). What doctors were not trained for were house calls, communicating within a belief system where all discussions with the family went through the father, or learning to wish a family to have many blessings before asking questions.

This research method allowed the scholar to much more intensively understand the many factors—in particular cultural barriers—that went into noncompliance. While there are no simple answers, Fadiman includes a discussion of the need for cross-cultural education among doctors. She provides examples of research that have been done where Hmong shamans were allowed to conduct healing ceremonies preceding any medical intervention, and notes the health outcomes. Ultimately she concludes that the biomedical model of allopathic medicine is concerned most with the body of the patient, while some patients ultimately care more about their souls.

Another example of ethnographic research helping to give insight into issues of diagnosis is Rayna Rapp's study of the problems faced by patients and clinicians with prenatal diagnostic technologies, discussed in her book *Testing Women, Testing the Fetus: The Social Impact of Amniocentesis in America*. Paul Atkinson (1997), in his book *Clinical Experience: The Construction and Reconstruction of Medical Reality*, uses an ethnographic approach to understand the distinctive nature of medical training, including how the training transforms people.

Doctor-Patient Communication

How do you communicate painful or negative news to patients? How do you talk to patients about the most difficult news of all: the possibility of their death? Physicians must communicate with their patients about diagnosis and prognosis in the course of the consultation. Sometimes the news they must convey is particularly bad or difficult to share. There is a great deal of research that speaks to exactly these issues. Doug Maynard (2003) explored how physicians communicate difficult news to patients in his book *Bad News, Good News: Conversational Order in Everyday Talk and Clinical Settings.* Maynard examined the communication of good news and bad news to patients by carefully analyzing transcripts of clinical encounters. This kind of work is considered a form of microsociology, in which the data are examined at great depth. Using this method, Maynard was able to examine how physicians cope with the difficult process of communicating bad news to patients and how patients prefer to be spoken to.

One important contribution of Maynard's (2003) work is its finding that patients prefer to be informed about a diagnosis (even if it is bad news) than not to be told. The act of being told a diagnosis unites a patient and provider into a shared reality. It becomes a "bad but somewhat intact world capable of being known-in-common" (16). In this way microsociology can connect small conversational exchanges into larger **social structures**, and it can be a powerful tool to analyze social interactions.

This method, conversation analysis, draws from an understanding that the social world is constructed and co-created through interactions between people. A diagnostic encounter unfolds through the conversations a clinician and patient have. Words are not just language, but ways people do social life. When a patient denies that she smokes, for example, she is doing the work of upholding herself as a morally sound individual, since smoking is often perceived as bad. When a doctor asks a series of questions that might be considered invasive had they been asked in an informal setting, she is enacting her role of being a doctor, because doctors have privileged access to all kinds of personal information about patients. These interactions are shaped around roles in a specific social context and can be understood through a method that captures in vivo conversation.

Another researcher went beyond the question of communicating bad news and examined the specific task of communicating prognosis, particularly death. In *Death Foretold: Prophecy and Prognosis in Medical Care*, Nicholas Christakis (1999) explores the difficulties doctors face in answering some of the hardest questions from patients. He describes patients asking if they will make it until next Christmas or major life event and says: "these questions pained me, and not just because they touched on the ineffable sadness of deadly disease or the efforts the dying often make to stay connected to the living. They pained me as well because it was so difficult, yet at the same time so essential, to answer them" (xi). Much of how Christakis approached studying how doctors provide answers to patients came from survey data, textual analysis, prospective studies, as well as interviews and recordings of clinical events similar to what Maynard and Fadiman used in their studies. This survey data included a random sample of 1,500 internists in the United States who self-reported their prognostication practices and responded to how they would approach different patient vignettes. Christakis's textual analysis included a study of how medical education textbooks addressed a condition that was historically untreatable with a poor prognosis. His prospective study required over five hundred doctors to make specific mortality predictions about patients in hospice in Chicago. The patients were then followed for two years to determine the accuracy of clinician prognosis.

Christakis found that doctors had a set of **norms** that drove their prognostic practices. These norms included that doctors (1) favor nondisclosure of pessimistic prognoses over disclosure; (2) should keep any predictions to themselves; (3) should not tell predictions to patients unless directly asked; (4) should not be specific; (5) should not be extreme; and (6) should be optimistic. You can see how these clinical practices are not aligned with what Maynard (2003) found patients wanted, which was to be told the truth, however horrible. But Christakis also found that physicians were overly optimistic about patients' prognoses, greatly overestimating their likelihood of survival. On top of not being direct with patients about "bad news," the bad news providers would have planned to convey was also overly rosy.

These two in-depth studies combine a great variety of methodological choices to weave a complex web of description, theory, and explanation around how providers choose to communicate difficult news to patients. Not only do Maynard and Christakis depict a disconnect between clinical practice and patient preference, they also link these practices to the structure of medical education, **socialization**, and the role of being a doctor. They point to a need for doctors to have a better understanding of statistical probabilities, and more open communication strategies with patients.

There is a strong tradition of using conversation analysis, often combined with other methods, to explore diagnostic issues. For example, Schwabe et al. (2007) looked at the diagnosis of nonepileptic seizures, which can be difficult to distinguish from epileptic seizures, but the distinction is important in terms of treatment plans. Conversation analysis was undertaken of interviews between physicians and patients in cases where the physician was unable to make a clear diagnosis. The conversation analysts predicted the correct diagnosis in all cases, suggesting that attending to the fine-grained features of communication can be clinically important. Conversation analysts have examined many health-related issues, including how patient "candidate" diagnoses are responded to (Stivers et al. 2003) and the role of the clinicians' commentaries during patient examination in preparing for diagnostic news (Heritage and Stivers 1999).

Mystery Illnesses

What do you do when a patient is sick, perhaps seriously, and you can't figure out what is wrong? Social sciences scholars have had surprising success tackling what might otherwise be understood as strictly "hard science" questions when it comes to identifying tricky conditions. Consider the story of the hantavirus laid out by the first female Navajo surgeon Lori Alviso Alvord. In 1993, national news sources reported on the "Navajo mystery virus" that began to infect many people with a flu-like illness. Healthy young Navajo began to die, and alarmed citizens filled hospitals. The U.S. Centers for Disease Control and Prevention (CDC) and a dozen other laboratories began an urgent investigation into this mystery illness, which caused acute respiratory distress and in many cases death. The national media drew on *stereotypes* of "dirty Indians," yet the best epidemiologists, doctors, and scientists in the country could not find the cause of the sudden wave of lethal sickness.

A Navajo medicine man had informed the CDC that the excess rainfall that year had caused a bumper crop of piñon nuts, which in turn led to a robust mouse population. Unsurprisingly, Western scientists did not take the warnings of this medicine man seriously, even though a Navajo medical doctor reported his findings to them. How could excess rain lead to the deaths of otherwise healthy young men and women? The CDC ultimately determined that the sickness was caused by the hantavirus, which was carried by rodents. The excess numbers of mice could be attributed to the excess rainfall and unusually large crop of food. The susceptibility of the Navajo primarily had to do with their geographic location and poverty (Alvord and Van Pelt 1999). It turns out the medicine man was right: the excess rainfall had caused the deaths of so many.

This process of identifying the cause of an immediate community issue is actually part of a research method called participatory action research (PAR) or community-based research. This method generally begins with participant co-construction of the research question, and participants weigh in on the best methods, as well. They also review the data, so if an individual is interviewed, the researcher sends him a transcript to see if he would like to modify any of what was said. Each stage of the process emphasizes collaboration between the community and the researcher, and as a result community members gain empowerment and knowledge about each stage in the process. This method can produce powerful information that is undetectable through other methods, and it can bring attention to inherent social inequalities often embedded in research practices such as racial and ethnic biases (Stoecker 2005).

The hantavirus case has shown how the power of listening to nonscientists and valuing their lived knowledge, even in research studies, can uncover and co-create powerful information. This is a strength of this kind of research, but a drawback is that it is hard to integrate into the scientific conversation. Questions often arise from issues in the community rather than a gap in the literature. Not only is there limited funding for this kind of research, and few places that provide training, but this method requires flexibility on the part of the researcher to work with the time line of the community. In the hantavirus case, there was no time available to apply for grant funding in twelve months of the urgent effort to understand the cause of so many unexpected deaths.

PAR is often used in situations where there are concerns about equity and social justice, so those who are marginalized in society are empowered through the research. But PAR has been widely used in health-care settings. A PAR process led to the development of a screening tool for at-risk psychiatric patients in an emergency department (Heslop et al. 2000). PAR-influenced research has also facilitated improvement in diagnostic accuracy of malaria in sub-Saharan Africa (Allen at al. 2010).

Managing Stigma

Some diagnoses carry tremendous **stigma**. How do you decide whether to tell a patient that he has a label that might be damaging? There are many different methods that can be used to explore exactly this question, but one particularly fruitful method is institutional ethnography (IE). I used this methodological orientation to examine how mental health clinicians did their everyday work of telling (or not telling) patients with borderline personality disorder their diagnoses. Founder Dorothy Smith (2005) explains that IE "deploys many of the traditional skills of sociological ethnographers but supplements them with an incorporation of texts grasped 'in action' in the local settings of people's work" (181). Institutional ethnography often draws from texts such as insurance forms and policy documents to illustrate the institutionalization of power. Some documents "travel" across **institutions** of power, defining the realm of possible choices in any given situation. If a diagnosis does not exist in writing, for example, it generally cannot be used in a clinical setting, so tools like the *Diagnostic and Statistical Manual of Mental Disorders* (DSM) shape the realm of the possible across many individual encounters. The declaration of illness actually happens through documents that travel across both institutional contexts and time to certify the reality of the illness (Hak 1998). Institutional ethnography has meaningful differences from ethnography. The first is that the focus is on texts and documents rather than a specific locality, geography, or group. The second important difference is that IE works to connect the day-to-day practices of something like making a diagnosis to institutional structures, which is not an explicit goal of ethnography, though some ethnographers do make social critiques on the foundation of their local research site.

Researchers have used this strategy in the past to understand how providers bestow diagnoses. Godderis (2011) interviewed three mental health practitioners and tracked the many forms and kinds of paperwork they used with clients. What she found is that communicating a diagnosis with a patient may only take a moment, but that moment is only one of a series of communications, many of which happen with third parties. "'Diagnosis' does not happen at a particular instant in time, such as when a psychiatrist makes a pronouncement, but rather is an institutional process that occurs over a period of time and in a variety of locations" (139).

I extended this research, examining the particular case of borderline personality disorder (BPD; Sulzer 2012), which some providers and scholars have described as the most stigmatizing condition in the mental health field (Nehls 2000). My findings included evidence that much of the time most providers do not disclose the BPD diagnosis to patients. Their reticence to tell their patients their diagnosis was a direct result of fears of the damage the label could inflict. Providers worried that patients would receive inferior care from other providers, be denied treatment, or would look up their diagnosis and feel stigmatized.

By interviewing patients as well as reading their memoirs and online message board postings, I was able to gather information about how patients responded to these institutionalized communication practices. My findings suggested that the primary thing patients wanted from providers was honesty. In fact, some patients who had been given a diagnosis of BPD without their knowledge subsequently learned that they had been so diagnosed from their charts or billing documents. Upon making this discovery, these patients categorically left treatment. While not everyone who received the label agreed with it, even those who disagreed tended not to debate their fit with criteria, but with the terms of the DSM and psychiatry itself. They posed many of the same questions that prominent researchers have about whether this disorder is a jumble of several diagnoses, and whether there is really evidence to suggest it is an affliction of the personality. In other words, even if patients pushed back against providers, they didn't push back against the diagnosis itself so much as they began to question why there was so much stigma within the mental health field toward people with the label. They provided a clear and resounding answer to the question of whether to communicate a profoundly stigmatizing diagnosis with patients: yes.

In this way, IE offers an opportunity to understand how the everyday work practices of providers can affect even treatment adherence. Ultimately, patients wanted honesty. Without a larger sample size and an outside researcher, it would have been difficult, if not impossible, for any one mental health provider to have discovered that patient preferences did not mirror professional practices.

Institutional ethnography has been used in many other health-related studies. Townsend et al. (2003) used IE to understand the barriers occupational therapists faced in providing patient centered care. And McGibbon et al. (2010) examined texts in action to understand the different kinds of stresses nurses faced in providing effective care.

Patient Self-Advocacy

You're confronted with a patient brandishing a stack of Internet research, some of it at odds with your medical beliefs. How do you manage to practice as you feel you should? This particular issue comes up frequently with contested illnesses. A patient may find an online group that claims a disease or syndrome exists, but the majority medical community has not yet verified it, or perhaps it has even been debunked. The patient may then self-diagnose as possessing this illness, which you as a provider do not believe is real. Such conflict can present problems as you try to communicate with them about their underlying symptoms, while simultaneously wanting to discourage their reliance on information that has yet to be vetted by scientists.

With the growth of online information available to patients, the need for Internet research is growing. If patients are frequently relying on Internet sources, researchers must understand what exactly is contained in online information and how it is influencing care. Internet research can include anything from reading online news sources to studying websites (Fair 2010). Internet research may encompass many methods, but it is a unique category in that the rules of doing research online and off can be dramatically different. Sampling may be determined by a search engine or by which groups have informative webpages. Online research can be a way to recruit subjects to interview offline, or the entire inquiry may center on online persons or texts. Researchers can focus on what is being stated in Internet discussions and also on what people might take from the Internet in their diagnostic sense making. In the case of contested illnesses, Internet research can be particularly useful.

Fair (2010) used online webpages as well as news sources to document how Morgellons disease has been diagnosed differently across time. Initially, the term "Morgellons" was adopted by a layperson who sought an explanation for the appearance of small fibers in her son's skin. Doctors did not initially use this term with patients, but by following the historical usage of the term, Fair discovered that at one point in time doctors began using the term "Morgellons" with patients. They did this in spite of the fact that the doctors in question did not generally believe that Morgellons was a real disease.

What Fair discovered is that using the term with a patient was designed to build rapport, even while doctors spoke openly about their conviction that the diagnosis was more accurately delusional parasitosis. Fair's research then demonstrated the important disconnect between a diagnosis as a "real" category and a diagnosis as a social tool to ease compliance with a treatment regimen of psychiatric medications. Physicians began to use Morgellons as a lay term, not because they agreed with it much of the time, but because it was a way to connect with patients over the information they were finding online. By doing so, clinicians were able to increase treatment compliance among their patients. In this way, in the case of a particular contested illness, an inquiry based on Internet data led to real answers about how doctors cope with the information patients find online. While ethical questions may still remain about when or how a physician should use a diagnostic label they do not believe is real, Internet research offered helpful insights into how providers have coped with this decision in the past.

Internet research has been used for a variety of other reasons. Harshbarger et al. (2009) examined pro-anorexia (or "pro-ana") websites, some of which contest the view of anorexia nervosa as a disease, instead seeing it as a lifestyle choice. By studying the pro-ana websites the researchers were able to identify important issues related to diagnosis, such as tips provided on some websites on how to conceal symptoms. Internet research of online discussion groups has also been used to understand the progression from diagnosis to death in breast cancer patients (Wen et al. 2011).

KNOW YOUR RESEARCH

Social science research methods have a great deal to contribute to the discussion of how clinicians can resolve everyday dilemmas. There is a vast array of research methods for answering difficult social questions. While this chapter provides only a simple introduction into a handful of approaches, it is a taste of what methods can provide better answers than a randomized control trial for certain kinds of questions. This chapter highlights just how many questions a clinician faces in the everyday course of practicing medicine that require innovative and varied approaches.

Doctors are often not explicitly trained in research methods in the course of their already intensive medical education programs. Becoming literate in the basics of various methods will allow you to find your own answers to the questions that arise in your everyday work practices. The next time you read a qualitative research study with a small *n*, you will understand that the size of a study is important in having the power to find statistical significance, but not in describing intensively the inner workings of a specific setting. You will also already be familiar with many of the most common social science approaches to research, which will allow you to digest findings more quickly and efficiently. When looking at research articles it is important to consider what kind of research question is being asked and if the best approach has been taken to answer it, rather than only asking whether the sample is representative and the statistical analyses are appropriate. When attempting to understand the social nature of diagnosis, many different research approaches are relevant, important, and revealing. And, given the social nature of ascertaining a diagnosis, the information that emerges from social science research studies may be just as important in the provision of medical care as dosage information and randomized control trials.

TAKEAWAY POINTS

- Researching social processes requires different approaches but still must be systematic and rigorous.
- Research methods that do not figure in the evidence-based practice "hierarchy of evidence" may nonetheless make an important contribution to the goals and practice of medicine.
- When wanting to understand an issue involving the social context, experiences, meanings, or activities, the research approach needs to be carefully matched to the research question.

DISCUSSION QUESTIONS

1. Following a clinical audit you have found that a particular group of patients is less likely to comply with medical advice than others. What research approaches might you consider to find out why this is the case?
2. Have you ever participated in a social research study? How did you react to that participation?
3. Why might a conversation analyst or linguist be better at diagnosing certain conditions on the basis of a consultation interview than a clinician? What type of conditions do you think this difference in capability might apply to?
4. How might you use the Internet or social media as data sources?

REFERENCES

Allen, Lisa, Erin Hetherington, Mange Manyama, Jennifer Hatfield, and Guido van Marle. 2010. "Using the Social Entrepreneurship Approach to Generate Innovative and Sustainable Malaria Diagnosis Interventions in Tanzania: A Case Study." *Malaria Journal* 9(42): doi:10.1186/1475-2875-9-42.

Alvord, L. A., and E. C. Van Pelt. 1999. *The Scalpel and the Silver Bear: The First Navajo Woman Surgeon Combines Western Medicine and Traditional Healing*. New York: Bantam.

Association of American Medical Colleges. 2011. *Behavioral and Social Science Foundations for Future Physicians*. Washington, DC: Association of American Medical Colleges.

Atkinson, Paul. 1997. *Clinical Experience: The Construction and Reconstruction of Medical Reality*. Aldershot: Ashgate.

Charmaz, Kathy. 2008. "Reconstructing Grounded Theory." In *The Sage Handbook of Social Research Methods*, edited by Pertti Alasuutari, Leonard Bickman, and Julia Brannen, 461–79. London: Sage.

Christakis, Nicholas. 1999. *Death Foretold: Prophecy and Prognosis in Medical Care*. Chicago: University of Chicago Press.

Davison, Charlie, George Davey Smith, and Stephen Frankel. 1991. "Lay Epidemiology and the Prevention Paradox: The Implications of Coronary Candidacy for Health Education." *Sociology of Health and Illness* 13(1): 1–19.

Dew, Kevin. 2007. "A Health Researcher's Guide to Qualitative Methodologies." *Australian and New Zealand Journal of Public Health* 31(5): 433–37.

Fadiman, Anne. 1997. *The Spirit Catches You and You Fall Down: A Hmong Child, Her American Doctors and the Collision of Two Cultures*. New York: Farrar, Straus, and Giroux.

Fair, Brian. 2010. "Morgellons: Contested Illness, Diagnostic Compromise and Medicalization." *Sociology of Health and Illness* 32(4): 597–612.

Godderis, Rebecca. 2011. "From Talk to Action: Mapping the Diagnostic Process in Psychiatry." In *Sociology of Diagnosis*. Vol. 12, *Advances in Medical Sociology*, edited by P. J. McGann and D. J. Hutson, 133–52. Bingley: Emerald.

Hak, Tony. 1998. "There Are Clear Delusions: The Production of a Factual Account." *Human Studies* 21: 419–36.

Harshbarger, Jenni, Carolyn Ahlers-Schmidt, Laura Mayans, David Mayans, and Joseph Hawkins. 2009. "Pro-Ana Websites: What a Clinician Should Know." *International Journal of Eating Disorders* 42: 367–70.

Heritage, John, and Tanya Stivers. 1999. "Online Commentary in Acute Medical Visits: A Method of Shaping Patient Expectations." *Social Science and Medicine* 49: 1501–17.

Heslop, Liza, Stephen Elsom, and Nyree Parker. 2000. "Improving Continuity of Care across Psychiatric and Emergency Services: Combining Patient Data within a Participatory Action Research Framework." *Journal of Advanced Nursing* 31(1): 135–43.

Lillrank, Annika. 2003. "Back Pain and the Resolution of Diagnostic Uncertainty in Illness Narratives." *Social Science and Medicine* 57(6): 1045–54.

Maynard, Douglas. 2003. *Bad News, Good News: Conversational Order in Everyday Talk and Clinical Settings*. Chicago: University of Chicago Press.

McGibbon, E., E. Peter, and R. Gallop. 2010. "An Institutional Ethnography of Nurses' Stress." *Qualitative Health Research* 20(10): 1353–78.

Nehls, Nadine. 2000. "Recovering: A Process of Empowerment." *Advances in Nursing Science* 22(4): 62–70.

Rapp, Rayna. 2000. *Testing Women, Testing the Fetus: The Social Impact of Amniocentesis in America*. New York: Routledge.

Sayer, Andrew. 2010. *Method in Social Science: A Realist Approach*. 2nd ed. New York: Routledge.

Schwabe, Meike, Stephen Howell, and Markus Reuber. 2007. "Differential Diagnosis of Seizure Disorders: A Conversation Analytic Approach." *Social Science and Medicine* 65: 712–24.

Smith, Dorothy E. 2005. *Institutional Ethnography: A Sociology for People*. Lanham, MD: Altamira.

Stinchcombe, Arthur L. 2005. *The Logic of Social Research*. Chicago: University of Chicago Press.

Stivers, Tanya, Rita Mangione-Smith, Marc Elliott, Laurie McDonald, and John Heritage. 2003. "Why Do Physicians Think Parents Expect Antibiotics? What Parents Report vs What Physicians Believe." *Journal of Family Practice* 52(2): 140–48.

Stoeker, R. 2005. *Research Methods for Community Change: A Project-Based Approach*. London: Sage.

Sulzer, Sandra H. 2012. "Borderline Personality Disorder: Clinical Navigation of Stigma, Communication and the Reimbursable Patient." PhD diss., University of Wisconsin, Madison.

Townsend, E., L. Langille, and D. Ripley. 2003. "Professional Tensions in Client-Centered Practice: Using Institutional Ethnography to Generate Understanding and Transformation." *American Journal of Occupational Therapy* 57(1): 17–28.

Wen, Kuang-Yi, Fiona McTavish, Gary Kreps, Meg Wise, and David Gustafson. 2011. "From Diagnosis to Death: A Case Study of Coping with Breast Cancer as Seen through Online Discussion Messages." *Journal of Computer-Mediated Communication* 16: 331–61.

Diagnosis as Problem and Solution

Lisa Sanders

Shirley's familiar rasp sounded discouraged and a little breathless in my cell-phone. "Doctor, I'm not any better." The tough eighty-three-year-old retired factory worker had severe emphysema and was dependent on three liters of oxygen running through nasal prongs. Without it, she'd be too breathless to get out of her chair or even talk. She had called me the week before, complaining of a bad cough and wheezing that her medicines couldn't calm. She felt tired and short of breath. I'd tried to get her to come see me at my office, but she didn't want to go out into the wintery streets. I prescribed an antibiotic and a five-day course of prednisone, assuming that her latest symptoms were just one more typical exacerbation of her terrible lung disease.

Now on the last day of her steroids, she called to tell me that she was no better. She was still short of breath, still coughing, and I could hear that she was still wheezing. This time I suggested she go to the hospital. "No," she told me without hesitation, "I'm never going to the hospital again." And when I suggested that she come see me in my office, she again refused, saying she felt too short of breath to go anywhere. I called in a higher dose of steroids and arranged to make a house call the next morning.

Even before I had a chance to ring the bell on the double-wide trailer home, I heard Shirley croak, "Come on in." She was in the living room propped up on a full sized sofa and covered by a colored afghan and a long, skinny tabby cat. A canary twittered a nervous greeting. Clear oxygen tubing snaked around the room, linking her to one of several large cylinders. A large-screen television and an oxygen condenser commandeered the rest of the tiny room.

I could see that Shirley was breathing much more rapidly than normal and I didn't need my stethoscope to hear the wheeze. I clipped the oxygen saturation monitor to her index finger, and almost immediately the alarm began to sound. As I suspected, her oxygen level was low despite the three liters of oxygen piped into her nose. What I hadn't expected was that her heart rate was also low. Crazy low. Her heart was beating at a rate of thirty beats per minute, less than half the normal rate.

It was immediately clear to me that I had made the wrong diagnosis. It wasn't her lungs making her miserable—not this time. It was her heart. And that changed everything.

Over the years, Shirley and I had many conversations about the inevitable progression of her lung disease. She had made it clear to me and to the grandchild she'd made her health proxy that she would never want to be kept alive on a breathing machine. She also said that she would rather die at home with her family than at a hospital. That's why I had been willing to treat her at home. She thought it might be the end. And so had I.

Seeing her now, it was clear to me that she really was dying, but she was dying of another disease. I knew her lungs would do her in some day, but today it was bradycardia that was causing the problem, and I wasn't willing to give her heart the same leeway. No matter what was causing her heart to slow down, I knew we could fix it. She had to go to the hospital. She simply had to.

"I was wrong," I told her. "You need to go to the hospital. Right now." I explained that what was making her so sick was, unlike her lungs, fixable. I didn't know how long she would live with a heart that beat at the right speed, but I was certain that if she didn't go to the hospital now she would die very soon.

The story above illustrates the essential task of diagnosis. Correctly identifying a disease in progress can save a life just as overlooking disease, or seeing the wrong one, can lose one. My initial diagnosis had been wrong, but standing in her living room, I knew that Shirley could (and should!) live. I didn't have a full diagnosis (I didn't know why her heart was slow), but I knew it could be fixed and that we could save her life. Once Shirley understood, she agreed to go to the hospital. She was discharged to short-term rehab a couple of days later with a brand new pacemaker and now she's back at home. All in all, a satisfying day's work!

DIAGNOSIS IS JOB NUMBER ONE

In twenty-first-century medicine, making the right diagnosis allows a doctor to choose the right treatment in order to intervene in a disease process and to go as far as saving a life, or at least improving the **patient**'s lot. And although medicine is centuries old, the diagnosis-treatment link is relatively new.

The process of cataloging and identifying disease dates back at least to 400 BCE and the work of a man (actually probably a whole school of men) known as Hippocrates. This father of medicine believed that diseases had an earthly cause and were not the consequence of some deity intervening in human life. The doctor's job was to correctly identify that earthly disease process. But Hippocrates wasn't a big fan of treatment because in his era there were no effective treatments. Hippocrates understood and preached that all medicine could really do with that data was to predict the future. In particular, he understood that recognizing who would live and die from their disease was essential.

Hippocrates started his work titled *Prognosis* with a description of how to judge the extent of illness by looking at the patient's face. "If the patient's normal appearance is preserved, this is best; just as the more abnormal it is, the worse it is." He goes on to describe the face of someone who is going to die: the nose is sharp, he tells us, the eyes sunken, the temples fallen in, the skin stretched and dry with a dusky color. "By realizing and announcing beforehand which patients were going to die," he writes at the end of that first chapter, the physician "would absolve himself from any blame."

Recognizing the natural history of a disease gave doctors the almost magical power to predict the future, but the diagnostic and therapeutic technology of his day allowed for few ways to distinguish between diseases with a similar presentation, and virtually no way of changing the outcome beyond what nature provides. That wouldn't be possible for another couple of millennia.

The stethoscope, our first piece of diagnostic equipment beyond our five senses, was invented in 1816, the blood pressure cuff in 1855, the X-ray in 1896. The Gram stain, the earliest effort to identify infectious bacteria, was developed in 1884. The CT scanner didn't appear until 1963. The wealth of tests that characterize twenty-first-century medicine grew from humble beginnings. Our tools for treatment are even newer. Joseph Lister first noticed that some molds prevented bacteria from forming in urine in the 1870s. The first antibiotic drug was developed in 1881. Penicillin wasn't identified until 1928 and didn't become widely used until the Second World War.

Now a decade into the twenty-first century, diagnosis and treatment are the twin pillars that make up contemporary medicine. It is the basis of our training, the essence of what we do that makes us doctors. It is so much of who we are and what we do that, like the air we breathe, we no longer really think about diagnoses and treatments. We march through our days taking histories, performing exams, ordering tests, making a diagnosis, and prescribing the therapy, like an ox so used to his yoke that we no longer attend to the larger world beyond this farm, this field, this row.

And yet we must. Medicine, we are told, is both a science and an art: a science because of the extensive research that supports so many of our decisions, and an art because it's clear that there is more to the practice of medicine than just measurements, lab tests, and technology. And if you asked most clinicians where that art resides, they would probably tell you that it is situated in the individuals we see in daily practice their physical, social, and emotional differences. We know, and for the most part accept, that our patients have to be seen on a larger stage than the one that reveals the symptoms they describe and the pathology we find.

But this new approach to the study of diagnosis makes the argument that our medical science also has to be seen in the context of the society that has produced it. Understanding the diagnoses we make, along with their origin and function in society around us, is also part of the art of medicine, a part that is too often overlooked.

THE "DISEASIFICATION" OF OBESITY

When I first went into practice, I started a once-a-week clinic where I saw obese and overweight patients who wanted to lose weight. I felt comfortable assuring them that their weight really was a medical problem. And they were glad to hear it.

But it turns out that, for the most part, I was wrong. We were all wrong.

In Western culture, obesity has long been seen as a moral failure. Gluttony was one of the original deadly sins first described in the fourth century by the Christian ascetic Evagrius Ponticus. In the twentieth century that moral opprobrium ex-pressed itself as a medical concern. In the 1990s Americans were suddenly flooded with messages about the obesity epidemic. During just that decade, the rate of obesity in the United States increased from less than 15% of the population to nearly 25%. Small wonder we thought of obesity as some kind of deadly epidemic. Yet when we tried to study how weight loss improved health and fitness, the results were puzzling. When studied, overweight folks were shown to have the lowest mortality, and those who went on diets seemed to gain the most in longevity when they did not lose weight. Strangest of all, those who were most successful at losing weight had the highest mortality. We figured there had to be something wrong with the way these studies were being conducted. Again, we were wrong.

In 2005 Kathleen Flegal, a researcher at the U.S. Centers for Disease Control and Prevention, published a study showing that being overweight did not in-crease mortality or even morbidity. It seemed to show that individuals who were overweight—those with a body mass index (BMI) between 25 and $30 \, \text{kg/m}^2$—actually lived longer than people with a "healthy" weight. Flegal published a second study in early 2013 showing that even those who are obese are no more likely to die than those with normal weight. It is only those who are morbidly obese—with a BMI greater than $35 \, \text{kg/m}^2$—who face an increased risk of death.

The newest research also suggests that it's not even the additional weight that causes the increased risk to these morbidly obese individuals but reduced physical activity. Several recent studies suggest that aerobically fit obese adults have a lower risk of death than those who are not fit at any weight. Interestingly, Kathleen Flegal, who first made these counterintuitive observations about relationship between obesity and mortality, is not a physician. She's a statistician.

Yet we still talk of an obesity epidemic. According to a search of PubMed, from 1990 to 2000 there were only a handful of articles published in the medical litera-ture with the phrase "obesity epidemic" in the title. Starting in 2003, the number of articles published each year more than tripled from twenty-two to about eighty. The research has shown that the obesity epidemic is for the most part not a medi-cal problem, but we don't seem to be listening.

Doctors want to practice medicine based on science. But our understanding of what we do is inevitably shaped by the society we live in. These assumptions are so deeply ingrained that, unless we deliberately look for society's fingerprints on what we think, we will never see them.

A wonderful researcher at Yale and my advisor in medical school, Alvan Fein-stein, was an important force in the development of clinical epidemiology—that is, using data gathered at the bedside to formulate and sometimes test medical hy-potheses. Feinstein prided himself on his ability to separate fact from assump-tions. When the Women's Health Initiative, the study that first investigated the utility of postmenopausal estrogen replacement, was launched in 1991, Feinstein loudly and publicly ridiculed the study. "Why study what we already know to be true?," he asked repeatedly. I'm sorry that he didn't live to see the surprising results of that study. The study was designed to evaluate some of the common recommen-dations for women's postmenopausal health, particularly the effectiveness of hormone replacement therapy (HRT). To universal surprise, the study showed that the use of HRT caused more harm than good. Feinstein would have been shocked and fascinated by these results.

I wish I could tell you that I gave up my obesity practice once I saw that being overweight and obese were not health issues. Actually, I gave up that practice long before the 2005 study because, even though most of my patients began to pay more attention to what they ate and exercised more regularly, they didn't lose weight. I gave it up because I was a failure as a weight-loss doctor. It turns out that it is much easier to get fit than to get thin. Lucky for my patients, and most of the rest of us, it's really the former that matters after all.

MORE THAN JUST A WORD

"Doctor, it's just not right. You gotta help me," the familiar baritone pleaded on my voicemail. "What is wrong with me? Do I have AIDS?" My heart sinks a little; I don't have to write down the phone number he leaves when I call him back. It's David, a patient of mine for over a decade, and we have this chat every day. It wasn't always this way. But for the last two years, rarely a day goes by without some version of this conversation.

David is fifty-six. He's obese, he smokes, and usually has a gentle, thoughtful manner. Medically he has diet-controlled diabetes (probably brought on by the psychiatric medications he had to take for years), chronic low back pain, and a severe anxiety disorder. Three years ago he decided to stop taking his psychiatric medications. He felt that they just made him tired and stupid. He has continued to see his psychiatrist every week or so.

Not long after stopping his psychiatric medications, David began to lose weight. At first I was delighted, because his central obesity was clearly contributing to his low back pain. He continued to lose weight slowly but steadily. Over the past two years he has lost over seventy-five pounds. He's moved out of the obese category into the merely overweight. And he's terrified.

For the first year or so I tried to reassure David that it was all due to the discontinuation of the antipsychotics he had taken for years. When he started those medications, he, like most patients, put on twenty to thirty pounds. As he continues to lose weight, I continue to think that it is most likely the reestablishment of his "natural" weight now that he's off these obesogenic drugs. I suspect his untreated anxiety disorder is also a part of his weight loss, but I make sure he is up to date on all the screening tests he should have given his risk factors. I've also tried to think broadly about what else could be driving this persistent weight loss. I got a CT scan, controversial in the United States, to look for lung cancer because he smokes. Nothing.

David is convinced that he has HIV. He has a history of intravenous drug use and homemade tattoos from a risk-filled youth. I have tested him for HIV—twice—as well as hepatitis C and several other diseases. All of his test results have been normal. Except for his continued smoking, David is in pretty good shape.

Nothing hurts, and everything seems to work right. But he is worried. And he continues to slowly lose weight.

At this point David is consumed with anxiety about his weight loss. So he calls my office every day. And every day we have the same conversation where he expresses his concern and I try to reassure him by pointing out what we have done so far to look for serious causes. But he believes, and it's certainly true, that it's not normal to lose weight without trying in this country. "Doc, I just need a diagnosis," he tells me day after day.

It's an all too familiar complaint to me.

I write a monthly column for the *New York Times Magazine* called "Diagnosis." Every month I tell the story of a patient who seeks medical attention because of some (often exotic) symptom. I show my readers what happens to the patient and the doctors as they pursue of the usually elusive cause of these symptoms. A diagnosis is always found. The patient is treated and often cured. It's been a popular feature in the magazine for over a decade and was the inspiration for the popular television drama *House, M.D.*

After each column is published, I get a flurry of emails. Many are from people sharing their experiences of having the same odd symptoms or diseases I wrote about. But maybe half are from readers who tell me they—like David—are in desperate need of a diagnosis. They share with me their terrible stories of pain and suffering. They send me scanned records and test results, time lines of onset and development of their odd symptoms. Often these patients have foregone therapy intended to treat the symptoms. Therapy seems to some of them merely a way to mask the underlying problem rather than finding the particular disease and treating it—the way it works with the patients I write about.

I usually write back to say that I can't diagnose them over the Internet, and for the most part they understand that. I tell them that they need to work with their doctor to figure out the cause of their symptoms and that, at the same time, it is imperative to work out a therapy so that they can get on with their lives. Because, while it is terrible when illness takes over one's health, it is tragic when it takes over one's life as well.

Until recently I used to tell these people who were suffering in need of a diagnosis that a diagnosis was just a word, and that the purpose of that word was simply to lead doctors to a treatment in order to relieve suffering. The focus on finding a name for this thing that caused them so much suffering seemed strange to me. If you could fix the symptom, why worry about the cause (once you were certain, of course, that it wasn't going to kill you)? Most of the people who wrote me could have that certainty. They had been suffering for years, far too long to be in danger of dying of their disease.

It was David who finally taught me that there is more to a diagnosis than just getting relief from a symptom. I see now that a diagnosis is a way of giving meaning to their suffering. Not just from the illness they feel but have not been able to name, but also from the sea of uncertainty they are now forced to swim. A diagnosis was, to them, so much more than just a word. Like David, these writers felt that their nameless illness has taken them from their work, from their intimate relationships, from their children, and from their lives. For them, a diagnosis is more than a direction for treatment—it is a reason in what has become for them an unreasonable world. It has medical, emotional, and practical utility. To ignore these dimensions is to miss the true meaning of making a diagnosis.

I still respond to people who write me with this desperate plea. I still suggest that they work with their internist, because for chronic and longstanding symptoms, partnering with your doctor is probably the best way to unravel this kind of mystery. But I no longer tell them to get over their need for a label. I understand that they would if they could. Because for these patients, as for David, a diagnosis is so much more than just a word.

I'm deep into that process with David. I still think that his anxiety is likely behind this weight loss, but I certainly recognize that patients don't always have the most likely illness. And David won't accept that diagnosis at all. Although he is on disability due to his psychiatric illness, he denies it. He's not anxious, he tells me—sometimes angrily—he's just worried about his health. And though his behavior, with his constant calls to my office and need for daily reassurance, suggests an anxiety that cannot be contained, there is a possibility that he has an additional condition that I simply haven't considered.

Recently I suggested that David seek a second opinion. I am sending him to a physician I admire. I've sent only the results of the studies we have done and a letter explaining the course of his illness. I have tried to keep my own tentative diagnosis out of it. I need this doctor to approach David with a fresh set of eyes. If he thinks of something I didn't think of, great. I'm happy to pursue a fresh lead. If not, at least I can be more comfortable in the watchful waiting mode that this possibly unexplained weight loss requires.

Every patient is a teacher. And as doctors, if we're paying attention, we're constantly being forced to learn and relearn stuff we thought we mastered long ago—about medicine, about our patients, and sometimes about ourselves. On my first day of medical school at Yale, when we were presented with our crisp, new white coats, Dean Gerard Burrows stood before my class of one hundred to tell us, "Half of what we teach you these next four years will be wrong. Unfortunately, we don't know which half." What he didn't tell us then was that this tendency to be wrong continues long after medical school and after specialty and subspecialty training. Maybe the ratio eases up a bit, but our patients, colleagues, and world require us to be constantly relearning what we thought we knew.

David is my CME in diagnostic uncertainty, my ongoing refresher course in the multiple meanings of diagnosis. Time will tell if there is any additional medical intervention required. Until then, my job is to be the doctor I describe to my readers, and to partner with David in managing the multiple uncertainties of his illness—whatever the diagnosis—until it's manageable. Our job is to reduce suffering, even when we don't understand the cause. It's really why our patients came to us in the first place.

When Diagnosis Goes Wrong
Connecting and Dissecting Diagnostic Errors

Gordon Schiff

As covered in multiple places and ways throughout this book, diagnosis—rather than being absolute or objective, with only one "right" or "wrong" diagnostic explanation—is instead often contingent, contextual, confusing, and complicated. But that does not mean that diagnosis does not matter. Making a correct diagnosis can be critical. As Lisa Sanders illustrated (chap. 14), having the right diagnosis can mean the difference between death and life. Had Dr. Sanders not made the house call (common in an earlier era but an extraordinary act in 2013) or listened to her *patient*'s heartbeat, she would not have detected serious arrhythmia and the patient would have succumbed to the wrong diagnosis.

In recent years there has been a growing awareness of the fact that diagnoses are often wrong or delayed, often with no (but at other times serious) consequences. Building on lessons from a broader patient safety movement centered around the historic *To Err Is Human Report* (which estimated an annual incidence 44,000 to 98,000 deaths occurring in the United States due to medical error), diagnostic error in medicine is now recognized as a neglected patient safety problem (Kohn et al. 1999; McDonald et al. 2013; Schiff et al. 2005, 2009; Tehrani et al. 2013; Wachter 2010). Depending on the diagnosis, error definitions, and intensity of surveillance, it has been conservatively estimated that 5–15% of diagnoses are either delayed or mistaken (Berner 2009; Schiff et al. 2005). Over the past decade, there have been a series of studies, initiatives, and conferences attempting to learn from and reduce diagnostic errors. These initiatives have brought together a number of streams of work in both patient safety and systems quality improvement, along with efforts to better understand cognition and to minimize frequently demonstrated biases in the diagnostic reasoning process (Croskerry 2003; Graber et al. 2005; Schiff and Leape 2012; Singh et al. 2012; Wachter 2010).

Lacking in this important and growing movement has been an explicit discussion of how understanding the social context of diagnosis and diagnostic error reduction efforts can help us better understand and prevent diagnostic errors. In the pages that follow, I deploy the language and lens of sociology—its perspectives and tools—to help better describe, explain, and understand diagnosis errors with the aims of both helping readers become better diagnosticians as well as collectively improving diagnosis safety and outcomes.

This chapter defines and discusses a series of concepts and insights to help readers understand diagnostic errors: what are they, how they can be detected, why they occur, ways they can be prevented, and how their harmful effects can be mitigated. Finally, this chapter covers broader questions regarding where the diagnostic error in medicine movement has come from and where it should be going.

DIAGNOSIS ERRORS AND DELAYS ARE CONTEXTUAL AND TEMPORAL CONSTRUCTS

Diagnostic errors have been variously defined, but one useful operational definition includes the following language:

> A diagnostic error is any mistake or failure in the diagnostic process leading to a misdiagnosis, a missed diagnosis, or a delayed diagnosis. This includes any failures in the process of care, including timely access in eliciting or interpreting symptoms, signs, or laboratory results; formulating and weighing of differential diagnosis; or lack of timely follow-up and specialty referral and evaluation. A diagnostic error is a construct that is usually based on reference to a subsequent test, clinical outcome, consultant's diagnosis, or autopsy—gold standards that are themselves often imperfect or unavailable. (Schiff and Graber, "Hospital Medicine," chap. 8 in McKean 2012)

This definition is useful, yet it is curious. Unlike other constructs in medicine that one can define and measure in the here and now, this definition is one that mostly revolves around hindsight: looking backward to label earlier acts as missed, delayed, or misdiagnosis. This means that "diagnosing a misdiagnosis" represents a rather subjective judgment, subject to well-known hindsight biases ("should have known it all along," "obvious in retrospect," "should never have missed") as well as difficulties knowing and re-creating the exact conditions and findings present at some earlier point in time (are we sure the "missed" spleen enlargement or breast mass was really present at the time the first doctor examined the patient and missed this finding?).

The term "delayed diagnosis," by definition, introduces a dimension that medical textbooks and teachings often lack when listing the features of a disease or constructing a differential diagnosis: time. When is a diagnosis timely, and when is it delayed? There is no question that we're talking about delay if diagnosis is not made and therapy not immediately initiated when a child presents with a fever and rash typical of meningococcal meningitis in the emergency room. But when the rash is atypical or not yet present and the patient is sent home without the diagnosis, the consequences of delay in diagnosis and treatment may be just as lethal, although more easily forgiven by all but the grieving parents.

The question of delay is just as potentially harmful for patients, but far less clear-cut in the cancer diagnosis. The leading cause of malpractice suits against physicians, particularly in the outpatient setting and in primary care, is missed and delayed diagnosis of cancer (Gandhi et al. 2006; Tehrani et al. 2013). Yet in practice, if we consider when the first abnormal or cancerous cells divide to be the moment a diagnosis is first present, every cancer diagnosis is delayed for months, years, or even decades, depending on the so called "doubling time" of that particular tumor.

DIAGNOSTIC ERROR: A TWO-TAILED BEAST

When surveyed, one out of three people have either personally experienced a missed or delayed diagnosis or know someone who has. And when we surveyed physicians, nearly every one could readily recall multiple cases of diagnostic errors that either they or a colleague had committed (Schiff et al. 2009). The situation represented by these examples almost invariably depicts cases where a diagnosis— either a common or rare diagnosis—was missed and subsequently discovered.

Often unstated or unclear from such reports is the kind of misdiagnoses in question. In some cases, a misdiagnosis occurs when the doctor did not think the patient was ill at all (also known as a "nondiagnosis"). Sometimes misdiagnoses occur when doctors have dismissed a symptom or misattributed it to a common, more benign cause ("it's just . . . the flu, heartburn, anxiety, stress, etc."). But misdiagnosis can also be a serious, mistaken "false positive" or overdiagnosis, illustrated by the dramatic case of Linda McDougal. A surgeon performed a bilateral mastectomy on McDougal before realizing the biopsy specimen showing breast cancer actually came from a different person.

Another type of overdiagnosis has become the subject of major interest in recent times. Such overdiagnosis is evident when a disease unlikely to cause symptoms or death during a patient's lifetime is diagnosed and treated. As repeatedly illustrated in this book, such diagnostic labels can turn healthy people into patients and lead to unnecessary or even harmful treatments in addition to needless psychological distress. The disease is diagnosed correctly, but the diagnosis is irrelevant. It most frequently occurs with the diagnosis of cancers that are increasingly being detected by evermore sensitive diagnostic laboratory and imaging tests (e.g., prostate-specific antigen, or PSA; computed tomography, or CT; magnetic resonance imaging, or MRI; and mammograms). While always a theoretical concern, such overdiagnosis had been largely trumped by patients' and physicians' desires to not miss a treatable disease. This issue has now been thrust into national policy debates, however, as data show the enormous costs and long-term psychosocial harm related to screening testing and incidentally discovered lesions. In the case of breast cancer, for example, a Cochrane review concluded that it is "not clear whether screening does more good than harm," and for every 2,000 women screened one will have her life prolonged by ten years of screening, while another ten healthy women will undergo unnecessary breast cancer treatment (Gøtzsche and Nielsen 2009). Is this misdiagnosis?

IS MISDIAGNOSIS AN ERROR?

Missed, delayed, and misdiagnosis are not necessarily the result of errors, whereas many diagnostic errors often occur with no resulting misdiagnosis. There is much confusion and controversy regarding whether a misdiagnosis is an error. As represented by the Venn diagram below (fig. 15-1), many errors occur regularly in the diagnostic process but do not result in a wrong diagnosis or patient harm (Schiff and Leape 2012). Should the public be frightened or reassured by this fact? Many thousands of laboratory and pathology specimens are mixed up every day, but few result in a tragic outcomes such as unnecessary bilateral mastectomy.

The field of patient safety, borrowing from nonmedical accident theory, engineering practices, and high-reliability organizational safety culture, has introduced several concepts that can help us approach these questions of sorting out the "process error-misdiagnosis-harm" triad of overlapping circles. Several of these interacting concepts are worth noting to better understand diagnosis error, including near misses or intercepted errors, mitigation and recovery, and a blame-free organizational culture.

Near Miss or Intercepted Error

A near miss or intercepted error refers to a situation where something goes wrong in the diagnostic process but gets detected and intercepted, or for various other reasons does not result in a misdiagnosis or harm. Such detection or buffering mechanisms are often deeply woven in organizational culture, behaviors, and processes and highlight the

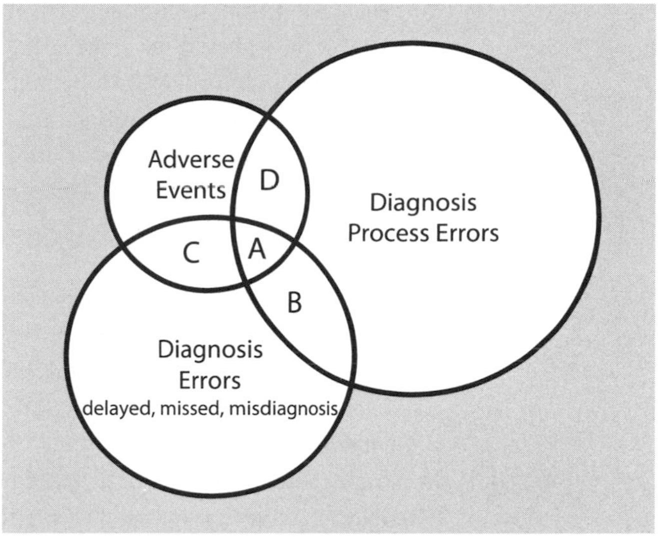

Figure 15-1. Venn diagram illustrating relationships between diagnostic process errors, delayed diagnoses and misdiagnoses, and adverse outcomes. Group A had adverse outcome resulting from error-related misdiagnosis. For example, the pathology specimens are erroneously mixed up (diagnostic process error), resulting in the wrong patient being given a diagnosis of cancer (misdiagnosis), who then undergoes surgery with an adverse outcome (adverse event). Group B experienced delayed diagnosis or misdiagnosis due to process error. Perhaps a positive urine culture was overlooked, meaning a urinary tract infection was not diagnosed, but the patient has no symptoms or adverse consequences. Group C had an adverse event due to misdiagnosis, but no identifiable process error. For example, the patient dies from acute myocardial infarction, but had no chest pain or other symptoms that were missed. Group D experienced harm from an error in the diagnostic process (such as a colon perforation from a colonoscopy done on the wrong patient), but no misdiagnosis.

multiple structures, people, and practices involved in preventing propagation of an error and its likelihood of causing harm. We see related constructs from organization safety in high-reliability organizations. These are organizations that have high levels of "situational awareness," where individuals and teams are trained and poised to anticipate and expect errors, and hence are on the lookout for early warnings of errors (Kohn et al. 1999; Shojania 2008).

Mitigation and Recovery

Building on the above organizational culture and mechanisms preventing error, mitigation and recovery efforts represent the next line of defense for minimizing harm to patients from diagnostic error. There are multiple interacting components to such protection, including a well-informed patient who is educated to look for clues that the illness is not responding to therapy as expected. Another mitigation safety net domain might include practices related to the timely informing of patients about errors, the administration of antidotes, or the withdrawal of therapy that may have been started for an incorrect diagnosis.

Blame-Free Organizational Culture

Errors will not be readily detected nor can their harm be prevented when those involved are fearful of being punished if their errors are discovered. With fear, organizations loose the opportunity to learn from their mistakes. It is impossible to overestimate the power and importance of removing blame and fear and replacing it with a search for learning and organizational improvement. Efforts to isolate a single cause or person are replaced by a paradigm that sees errors as multifactorial and systematic, requiring both a commitment from leadership to help remedy error-producing conditions and support for and from frontline staff to delve into the causes of problems (Leape et al. 2012).

PATIENTS AS CO-PRODUCERS RATHER THAN MERELY CONSUMERS OF DIAGNOSIS

Patient engagement and empowerment is a largely unexplored aspect of diagnosis error and its improvement. Patients play a key, often poorly acknowledged and appreciated role in preventing or mitigating diagnostic errors. We need to turn our attention to patients and doctors not simply to understand and improve their respective roles, but also to better understand the interactions between the two (Hart 1997, 2006).

Patients need to be engaged and have strong, continuous relationships with their clinicians to improve diagnosis. Patients must seek timely access for worrisome symptoms, provide accurate and thorough histories, have their hunches about possible exposures or etiologies heard, be vigilant about making sure their test results are reported back to them, and give feedback when diagnosis and response to treatment does not go as expected.

Here "blame-free" trusting relationships again become a key for unlocking mitigation, healing, learning, and improvement when inevitable mishaps occur. A culture of "defensive medicine," where many physicians state they order excessive and unnecessary diagnostic tests (leading to potential overdiagnosis, excessive radiation, and costs), prevails in U.S. medicine. It is antithetical to a system where patients and physicians work together in trusting relationships to practice conservative, cost-conscious, safer diagnosis. Such collaborative coproduction of safer, more reliable diagnosis requires trust and continuity. Unfortunately this kind of collaboration is being potentially undermined by various forces that are shaping health care in the United States, such as questionably ethical financial incentives to withhold tests and treatments from patients who in turn may understandably distrust advice to watch and wait or to avoid questionable screening tests when doctors may be biased by financial incentives (Reason 2000).

MISDIAGNOSIS: A SYMPTOM OF INFORMATION DEARTH AND OVERLOAD

When I was a medical intern three decades ago, retrieval of needed past and current information about my patients required enormous effort. I'd spend many hours each week on hold calling the laboratory for blood test results, waiting in long lines while X-ray clerks searched for films (often having difficulty finding even that day's X-rays and almost never being able to retrieve old ones), and undertaking time-consuming, often unsuccessful, efforts to retrieve past medical records (and if lucky enough to secure the old chart, I would often search in vain through reams of handwritten notes and lab results for sought-after pieces of data such as old pathology or operative reports). Today I can retrieve all of these things in my hospital in seconds with only a few mouse clicks. Many errors have doubtless been prevented by instantaneous access to information that at times can be decisive for accurate diagnosis. Consider the value and errors prevented by instant access to a patient's old pathology report to correctly recall the cell type of a cancer, or an old X-ray showing that the 7-mm lung nodule was the same size ten years ago, or getting a complete past medical history for a patient in a coma, including a complete listing of which drugs they were taking (Schiff and Bates 2010).

Why or how could I or anyone complain after reaching this medical information retrieval nirvana? It turns out that much electronic medical information is stored in silos, locked away in different hospital and laboratory databases that are not interoperable, meaning that our hospitals' computers do not connect with those of the hospital across the street. This lack of interoperability is in part technical, but mostly driven by political, financial, and social issues that underlie our fragmented health-care system. While there have been U.S. federal governmental efforts in recent years to overcome these barriers (though the Office of the National Coordinator for Health Information Technology), progress in connecting disparate systems has been slow, in large part because private vendor systems each use their own proprietary software and have little incentive to facilitate easily switching (data or systems) to their competitors' products (Buntin et al. 2010).

Ironically, as challenging as is this problem of barriers to information access, it is dwarfed by an even bigger problem impacting diagnosis: information overload. Busy clinicians are now bombarded with thousands of test results, past notes, X-ray reports, streams of data from patient monitoring systems, consultation notes, and increasingly emails or portal messages from their staff and patients. Without highly reliable, well-designed systems, it is easy for a problem or test result or trend in a patient's condition to get overlooked. Even if this happens for only 1% or 0.1% of critical test results, it means, given the high volume of tests and information, that many balls will be dropped each month. One group of Harvard physicians estimated that on average they each missed critical test results fourteen times a year (Poon et al. 2004, 2012).

"Cognitive overload" is a frequent complaint among physicians practicing in busy emergency rooms or primary care clinics. They simply do not have enough time to review and process and weigh all the information coming their way (some have likened the challenge to drinking from a fire hose). Although smart health information technology design can go a long way to helping busy clinicians by organizing, filtering, and customizing displays as well as providing timely decision support alerts, most current systems fall short (Schiff and Bates 2010). In fact, many of the alerts are so problematic that 90% or more are typically ignored or overridden. Similarly, the hope that computers using artificial intelligence algorithms (the so-called "Greek oracle" model of computer diagnosis, whereby one types in the symptoms and the computer magically spits out the diagnosis) could help physicians make the correct diagnosis and avoid diagnostic errors, or even remind them of ones to consider, has thus far not realized this alluring potential (Garg et al. 2005; Miller 1994).

DIAGNOSIS, MISDIAGNOSIS, AND THE PROBLEM OF TIME

Recent surveys have shown that physicians perceive lack of time as the most important constraint in preventing better diagnosis. Time is needed to take careful histories; to weigh different diagnostic possibilities (especially for more complex patients); to consult with colleagues, textbooks, or other reference materials; and to carefully document and follow up with patients and unanswered questions (Schiff 2008). Cognitive researchers point to two systems of mental functioning to make diagnoses efficiently and accurately. The first system involves rapid decision making, quick pattern recognition, and mental heuristics (shortcuts) to efficiently make quick best guesses. The second system requires clinicians to slow down and carefully think through patients' problems, which obviously takes additional time (Croskerry 2003; Elstein 2009; Graber et al. 2012; Poon et al. 2012).

Getting to know patients personally, to better sort out their mix of psychosocial and medical symptoms, also takes time and may become harder if panel sizes increase as physicians assume more of a team manager role (e.g., overseeing nurse practitioners) rather than a direct caregiver role for each of their patients. And getting to know patients over time takes time. Patients' and clinicians' busy schedules also introduce other disruptions in care continuity relationships. There can be continuity breaks due to patient or doctor mobility and employment or employer switches in health insurance plans (a frequent occurrence in the United States).

Areas for Improving Diagnosis and Minimizing Errors

- Improved, coordinated, systematic follow-up and feedback of patients and problems.
- Enhanced role for patients in coproducing diagnosis by better tapping into their observations of their symptoms and responses to therapies and by playing an active role as collaborators in the diagnostic process.
- Closer longitudinal relationships with patients and caregiver teams, with better continuity supporting better personal knowledge of patients, so that problems don't get lost and assuring timely access, trust, and ability to choose tests wisely, conservatively, and appropriately for each patient.
- Reengineered health information technology, particularly to support clinical documentation of assessments, uncertainties, and streamline access to key clinical and reference information resources.
- Streamlined consultations for real-time answering of questions and consultations to colleagues, specialists, and other caregivers.
- Better appreciation, understanding, and data on the role and limitations (e.g., false positive and false negative rates) of diagnostic testing (along with better tests). More reliable systems for tracking test results and ensuring appropriate follow-up.
- Improved learning from and sharing of diagnostic errors. Need for a blame-free culture and forums, such as enhanced morbidity and mortality conferences that emphasize uncovering system factors, follow-up investigation and correction, and standardized approaches to facilitate learning across cases.

WEAVING IT ALL TOGETHER

Exactly how these contextual, organizational, health information technology, and work organization trends will affect diagnosis quality can only be speculated. But their complex interactions mean that the conditions, constraints, and enablers of diagnosis accuracy as well as contributors to diagnosis errors will continue to evolve. They point to various areas where improvements can be made to thoughtfully weave together the social context of diagnosis and the opportunities to improve how we approach diagnosis and avoid errors and harm.

REFERENCES

Berner, Eta S. 2009. "Diagnostic Error in Medicine: Introduction." *Advances in Health Sciences Education* 14: 1–5.

Buntin, Melinda Beeuwkes, Sachin H. Jain, and David Blumenthal. 2010. "Health Information Technology: Laying the Infrastructure for National Health Reform." *Health Affairs* 29(6): 1214–19.

Croskerry, Pat. 2003. "The Importance of Cognitive Errors in Diagnosis and Strategies to Minimize Them." *Academic Medicine* 78(8): 775.

Elstein, Arthur S. 2009. "Thinking about Diagnostic Thinking: A 30-Year Perspective." *Advances in Health Sciences Education* 14(1): 7–18.

Gandhi, Tejal K., Allen Kachalia, Eric J. Thomas, Ann Louise Puopolo, Catherine Yoon, Troyen A. Brennan, and David M. Studdert. 2006. "Missed and Delayed Diagnoses in the Ambulatory Setting: A Study of Closed Malpractice Claims." *Annals of Internal Medicine* 145(7): 488–96.

Garg, Amit X., Neill K. J. Adhikari, Heather McDonald, M. Patricia Rosas-Arellano, P. J. Devereaux, Joseph Beyene, Justina Sam, and R. Brian Haynes. 2005. "Effects of Computerized Clinical Decision Support Systems on Practitioner Performance and Patient Outcomes." *JAMA* 293(10): 1223–38.

Gøtzsche, Peter C., and Margrethe Nielsen. 2009. "Screening for Breast Cancer with Mammography." *Cochrane Database of Systematic Reviews* 4(1): CD001877, doi:10.1002/14651858.CD001877.pub4.

Graber, Mark L., Nancy Franklin, and Ruthanna Gordon. 2005. "Diagnostic Error in Internal Medicine." *Archives of Internal Medicine* 165(13): 1493.

Graber, Mark L., Stephanie Kissam, Velma L. Payne, Ashley N. D. Meyer, Asta Sorensen, Nancy Lenfestey, Elizabeth Tant, Kerm Henriksen, Kenneth LaBresh, and Hardeep Singh. 2012. "Cognitive Interventions to Reduce Diagnostic Error: A Narrative Review." *BMJ Quality and Safety* 21(7): 535–57.

Hart, Julian Tudor. 1997. "Cochrane Lecture 1997: What Evidence Do We Need for Evidence Based Medicine?" *Journal of Epidemiology and Community Health* 51(6): 623–29.

———. 2006. *The Political Economy of Health Care: A Clinical Perspective.* Bristol, UK: Policy Press.

Kohn, Linda T., Janet M. Corrigan, and Molla S. Donaldson. 1999. "To Err Is Human." In *Building a Safer Health System.* Washington, DC: National Academy Press.

Leape, Lucian L., Miles F. Shore, Jules L. Dienstag, Robert J. Mayer, Susan Edgman-Levitan, Gregg S. Meyer, and Gerald B. Healy. 2012. "Perspective: A Culture of Respect, Part 2: Creating a Culture of Respect." *Academic Medicine* 87(7): 853–58.

McDonald, Kathryn M., Brian Matesic, Despina G. Contopoulos-Ioannidis, Julia Lonhart, Eric Schmidt, Noelle Pineda, and John P. A. Ioannidis. 2013. "Patient Safety Strategies Targeted at Diagnostic Errorsa Systematic Review." *Annals of Internal Medicine* 158(5.2): 381–89.

McKean, Sylvia C. 2012. *Principles and Practice of Hospital Medicine.* New York: McGraw-Hill.

Miller, Randolph A. 1994. "Medical Diagnostic Decision Support Systems—Past, Present, and Future a Threaded Bibliography and Brief Commentary." *Journal of the American Medical Informatics Association* 1(1): 8–27.

Poon, Eric G., Tejal K. Gandhi, Thomas D. Sequist, Harvey J. Murff, Andrew S. Karson, and David W. Bates. 2004. "'I Wish I Had Seen This Test Result Earlier!': Dissatisfaction with Test Result Management Systems in Primary Care." *Archives of Internal Medicine* 164(20): 2223.

Poon, Eric G., Allen Kachalia, Ann Louise Puopolo, Tejal K. Gandhi, and D. M. Studdert. 2012. "Cognitive Errors and Logistical Breakdowns Contributing to Missed and Delayed Diagnoses of Breast and Colorectal Cancers: A Process Analysis of Closed Malpractice Claims." *Journal of General Internal Medicine* 27(11): 1416–23.

Reason, James. 2000. "Human Error: Models and Management." *BMJ* 320(7237): 768.

Schiff, Gordon D. 2008. "Minimizing Diagnostic Error: The Importance of Follow-Up and Feedback." *American Journal of Medicine* 121(5): S38–S42.

Schiff, Gordon D., and David W. Bates. 2010. "Can Electronic Clinical Documentation Help Prevent Diagnostic Errors?" *New England Journal of Medicine* 362(12): 1066–69.

Schiff, Gordon D., Omar Hasan, Seijeoung Kim, Richard Abrams, Karen Cosby, Bruce L. Lambert, Arthur S. Elstein, Scott Hasler, Martin L. Kabongo, and Nela Krosnjar. 2009. "Diagnostic Error in Medicine: Analysis of 583 Physician-Reported Errors." *Archives of Internal Medicine* 169(20): 1881.

Schiff, Gordon D., Seijeoung Kim, Richard Abrams, Karen Cosby, Bruce Lambert, Arthur S. Elstein, Scott Hasler, Nela Krosnjar, Richard Odwazny, and Mary F. Wisniewski. 2005. "Diagnosing Diagnosis Errors: Lessons from a Multi-Institutional Collaborative Project." In *Advances in Patient Safety: From Research to Implementation*, 2:255–64. Rockville, MD: Agency for Healthcare Research and Quality.

Schiff, Gordon D., and Lucian L. Leape. 2012. "Commentary: How Can We Make Diagnosis Safer?" *Academic Medicine* 87(2): 135–38.

Shojania, Kaveh G. 2008. "The Frustrating Case of Incident-Reporting Systems." *Quality and Safety in Health Care* 17(6): 400–402.

Singh, Hardeep, Mark L. Graber, Stephanie M. Kissam, Asta V. Sorensen, Nancy F. Lenfestey, Elizabeth M. Tant, Kerm Henriksen, and Kenneth A. LaBresh. 2012. "System-Related Interventions to Reduce Diagnostic Errors: A Narrative Review." *BMJ Quality and Safety* 21(2): 160–70.

Tehrani, Ali S. Saber, HeeWon Lee, Simon C. Mathews, Andrew Shore, Martin A. Makary, Peter J. Pronovost, and David E. Newman-Toker. 2013. "25-Year Summary of U.S. Malpractice Claims for Diagnostic Errors 1986–2010: An Analysis from the National Practitioner Data Bank." *BMJ Quality and Safety* April: doi:10.1136/bmjqs-2012-001550.

Wachter, Robert M. 2010. "Why Diagnostic Errors Don't Get Any Respect—and What Can Be Done about Them." *Health Affairs* 29(9): 1605–10.

Table C-1 The CLASSIFY Mnemonic

C **ertainty:** How important is it to be certain? Is your patient at risk in the absence of certainty? Can he or she be satisfied without it? What additional information might bring certainty, and should it be pursued?

L **abel:** Does the label improve the patient's perception of their condition? Do they need it to have access to the sick role, or to gain access to services or treatments? Are there alternatives means of access? What is the impact of the label?

A **lternate:** are there alternate belief systems that either complement or compete with the diagnosis and treatment offered by Western biomedicine? What accommodation can help integrate biomedicine with alternate belief systems?

S **ocial context:** What is your patient's social context? Social identity? How does the diagnosis affect their status or ability to interact within this group? How does the group understand the disease (causation, interpretation, status, interactions, impact on daily life, timing)?

S **tigma:** Is the diagnosis likely to cause stigma or to be perceived as casting an unfavorable light on your patient's moral status? Is your patient likely to tell you so? How can the stigmatizing effects be reduced?

I **nformation:** Where has your patient sought information about this illness? Has he or she shared this information with you? What are the limitations of these sources? What does this information tell you about the patient and their beliefs?

F **inancial:** Who's paying? Does anyone stand to benefit or to suffer financially from this diagnosis? What are the potential health-care costs?

Y **ou:** How do certainty, labels, alternative belief systems, social group, stigma, information, and finances influence your thinking about your patient, your practice, and yourself? CLASSIFY yourself! Go through this mnemonic again, but this time ask the same questions about your perspective instead of your patient's.

Conclusion

Annemarie Goldstein Jutel and Kevin Dew

The doctors' views on the preceding pages underline the importance that social factors play in the actual job of diagnosing. They highlight the pressures, the challenges, the potential false clues. But they also punctuate the opportunities that are present in every challenging diagnosis and the important role that diagnosis can play in the preservation of health and the management of disease. Every diagnostic process offers an opportunity for you to learn more about the **patient**, yourself, and your values and skills.

Atul Gawande (2010) wrote about this opportunity in his *New Yorker* essay "Letting Go." He described the discussion of the diagnosis of a terminal disease with a patient as being predominantly about figuring out the patient, rather than sorting out the illness. Who would have thought that the diagnosis was not actually about disease?

We hope that what the chapters in this book have led you to think about will confirm the extent to which diagnosis is about so much more than pathophysiology. This social overlay should resonate with you, whether it be now or later. The noncompliant patient may remind you about how diagnosis can be a contest with resources and legitimization at stake. The diagnosis you miss may punctuate twenty-first-century reliance on technology and its limitations (which you may now be able to enumerate). And the way that the diagnosis refuses to comply with its textbook picture, raising questions in your mind, and in your patient's as well, may even lead you to question whether diagnosis is actually the goal you should be pursuing. How about just looking after your patient? Annemarie has written about this in the *Journal of the American Medical Association* (Jutel and McBain 2012). Even something as technically easy to diagnose as a broken bone need not always be identified. If the treatment doesn't depend on an accurate diagnosis, and if you've ruled out the stuff that matters, do you really need to know?

The chapters in this book shed light on diagnosis in order to reveal just how much the seemingly discrete and insular process of diagnosis hinges upon myriad social conventions and relations. Your diagnostic role, be it diagnoser or diagnosed (and don't overlook the fact that diagnosticians regularly find themselves on the other side of the table), is often about far more than just the two parties. Mary Ebeling in chapter 9 refers to the "crowded room" in which diagnosis takes place—it is a metaphor we find quite apt and hope you will keep in mind.

But you may already find diagnosis to be a messy business. It's not just that Dr. Google keeps raising his head, or that you can't find an explanation for persistent nonspecific symptoms in a difficult patient. You may have a clear-cut case with the clinical picture, history, and labs all in agreement. There may be a straightforward treatment and an agreeable patient. Yet diagnosis doesn't always work seamlessly. The theoretically graceful relationship between diagnosis and treatment fails to manifest. Your patient seems to understand the therapeutic regimen, the treatment is tried and true, but the outcomes are unexpected and disappointing. Why?

The solution may well be in the social, rather than psychological or biophysical, realm. Is your patient's agreement with the plan simply a consulting room sign of respect for the authority of your position as opposed to an acceptance of its constraints? Is your view of the plan clouded by your own belief systems or understandings of culture, gender, or ethnicity? Where does your patient turn for information or interpretation? What does the diagnosis mean for this particular patient? Does it change her perspective of herself, or her social group's perspective of her in a way that is not palatable?

You have been or will be taught that diagnosis is a cognitive act, and you will likely think about cognition in terms of your own synapses and mental pictures. But diagnosis is always more than just a thought process. It is a social process, and failing to recognize its sociality will hinder the potential favorable outcomes enabled by the important task of diagnosis. Lest the clinician forget the social content and implications of diagnosis, we provide the CLASSIFY mnemonic table on page 230. It attempts to capture the range of factors a diagnoser should consider in order to ensure optimal results for the individuals under their care.

Social awareness is often a difficult goal to attain because we are all so embedded in the society and the social groups of which we are members. To be a thinking and effective clinician, however, it is an undeniable attribute to understand how your patients live in and see the world around them, and how their diagnoses shape and are shaped by their experiences.

REFERENCES

Gawande, Atul. 2010. "Letting Go: What Should Medicine Do When It Can't Save Your Life." *New Yorker*, August 2.

Jutel, Annemarie, and Lynn McBain. 2012. "Do We Really Need to Know?" *JAMA* 308(15): 1533–34.

Glossary

Agency   The capacity of an individual to act independently. Agency is often referred to in contradistinction to *social structures* that are organizational facets of society, shaping and influencing individual actions, often in subconscious ways.

Aversive racism   The social awkwardness or discomfort that an individual might experience when interacting with someone from a different cultural or ethnic group.

Biographical disruption   A concept developed by Michael Bury to describe how chronic illness creates an abrupt disjuncture in the way an individual experiences his life story, changing its structures and the experiential knowledge upon which it is based.

Biopower   A term developed by French social theorist Michel Foucault to describe how modern nations manage the behavior, practices, and bodies of their citizens through a range of institutional techniques, knowledge practices, and forms of control. Important in biopower specifically (and Foucauldian theory generally) is the notion of self-control, which emerges from these techniques as citizens emulate the desired social outcomes as opposed to being forced to assume them.

Biosociality   A term coined by the anthropologist Paul Rabinow to describe the potential for shifts in social relations emerging from increasing knowledge of, and awareness about, genetic makeup and other aspects of biomedicine.

Branding   A marketing practice that uses language, names, labels, design, symbols, and imagery to identify and distinguish one product from another. Branding aims to establish a significant and loyal relationship with consumers by attributing emotional and affective attributes to products.

Cultural capital   A term developed by the French sociologist Pierre Bourdieu to describe the social assets that provide status and advancement within a particular social group. Closely linked to the concepts of *habitus* and *field*, cultural capital is not fixed, as it varies according to each field and what they respectively consider valuable and legitimate.

Definition of the situation   In symbolic interactionism theory, a definition of the situation refers to the way in which people frame particular situations so that the various participants understand the expectations, roles, and behaviors within the interaction.

Demedicalization   The process by which a physical or mental state deemed a medical problem is reclassified as either a healthy state or a nonmedical problem. One example of demedicalization is homosexuality. Once identified in the *Diagnostic and Statistical Manual of Mental Disorders* as a diagnosis, homosexuality was eventually removed in response to political and intellectual debate.

Diagnostic limbo   A term used by Juliet Corbin and Anselm Strauss to describe the experience of having poor or declining health without a diagnosis. The term can also be applied to named conditions, such as irritable bowel syndrome, where there is a known pattern of symptoms but no definitive medical explanation for its cause.

Diagnostic moment   The point in time at which a specific disease label emerges from the process of narrative, physical, and technological exploration of illness.

Direct-to-consumer   An approach to advertising and marketing that is aimed at consumers to promote new drugs or devices. Direct-to-consumer advertising is not authorized in many countries and has not always been legal in countries where it is currently authorized (in the United States and New Zealand, for example).

Disease awareness marketing   The commercial promotion of symptoms, disease definitions, and disease categories. This type of marketing seeks to raise public consciousness about a disease in order to promote the sale of its associated remedy (drug or medical device).

Disease monger   One who attempts to promote a disease label, to raise social concerns about the disease, and to increase the desire for treatment for a particular condition, sometimes before a diagnosis has been medically validated.

Empiricism   The view that knowledge comes from observations of the world. Empiricism is at the base of experimental science and is in contrast with the view that knowledge can come from theorisation, speculation, or intuition.

Environmental health movements   Social movements—often driven by laypeople, *patients*, and supportive medical specialists—that lobby to reduce toxic chemical levels in the environment, to raise awareness of the dangers of toxins, to initiate medical studies, and to hold government and industry accountable for environmental illnesses.

Epistemology   The branch of philosophy that studies knowledge. It emphasizes the field specificity of knowledge and examines the perspective through which a given discipline or profession understands the world. Different disciplines apply different tests to determine what counts as knowledge. An empiricist would count as true knowledge things that can be experienced and measured, while a theorist would count as true those arguments that are logically and conceptually cohesive.

Evidence-based medicine   A practice developed in the early 1990s encouraging medicine to use empirical research to underpin clinical decision making. One feature of evidence-based practice is a hierarchy of research designs, which privileges experimental methodology over other forms of research.

Field   Linked with the concepts of *habitus* and *cultural capital*, the concept of field was developed by Bourdieu and describes an organized body or institution, such as medicine, law, and the academy, with rules and practices that are replicated by its members and maintained by tensions within (and relative to) cultural capital.

Gold standard   A metaphoric term, borrowed from the standard weight at which gold is fixed, referring to generally accepted best practices to which clinicians are expected to conform by their licensing bodies.

Habitus   Linked with the concepts of *field* and *cultural capital*, the concept of habitus was developed by Bourdieu and describes the set of skills, approaches, dispositions, and activities acquired and experienced by individuals within their own specific social and cultural settings. It describes the ways individuals navigate the structural constraints of the fields of which they are members.

Health social movements   Groups of people engaged in organized collective action related to health concerns.

Identity   A sense of self that is anchored in continuity. Identity links the past, present, and future by a meaningful self-narrative. It emerges from the personal and the social, and involves being part of a social network with a particular set of normative expectations, including support and reciprocity.

Illness-disease dichotomy   The difference that can exist between lay and professional perceptions of dysfunction (illness is the subjective perception of an ailment perceived to be medical in nature, while disease is a formal classification for a medically recognized disorder). This sometimes-irreconcilable difference is couched in the fact that not all illnesses can be attributed to a disease state, and that not all disease states may manifest as illness.

Institutions   A cohesive and enduring pattern of social activity that includes multiple roles for those participating in that activity, such as schools (with teachers and pupils), hospitals (with patients, orderlies, and doctors), and workplaces (with employers and employees).

Liminality   A term used to refer to a state of transition between one state and another. In anthropology, liminality refers to a rite of passage. In sociology, it may be used to refer to situations where one's role or status is not clearly identified; for example, between being healthy or sick.

Medicalization   The process by which a particular condition, which was previously not considered to be medical in nature, is placed under medicine's authority. The mechanisms by which this occurs are varied and may not issue from medicine itself, but from lay advocacy, commercial interests, or the biomedical industry.

Moral philosophers of the private   A term developed by Rayna Rapp in 1999 to describe women who, after receiving diagnostic results about the condition of their unborn, are required to make a difficult ethical decision about what course of action to undertake. As a result of new diagnostic technologies (particularly those used in antenatal screening), more expectant parents must make challenging moral decisions.

Norms   Behaviors and activities that are seen as acceptable and expected within a particular social or cultural group. Behavior that does not conform to these norms is referred to as "deviant" and is likely to be sanctioned or justified.

Ontology   The study of things that exist. In diagnosis, ontology is an important question when it comes to defending the idea that diseases are discrete, nameable entities separate from the individual who experiences them.

Paternalism   A fatherly approach to people. Often used in reference to a particular medical tradition of caring, in which the doctor takes responsibility for the well-being of the *patient*, often at the expense of patient autonomy.

Patient   An individual who perceives herself to be ill (or who is perceived by others to be ill) and who receives care from a clinician or care that is imposed. The use of the term suggests a submissive relationship to the caregiver, in which the individual is a passive recipient of care, rather than an active partner.

Positivism   A term originally coined by Auguste Comte in the nineteenth century premised on the idea that science is the source of true knowledge. It purports that the social world may be studied in the same way as the natural world; that is, in a neutral, detached way where concepts are operationalized, theories tested, and analysis undertaken without bias.

Professional socialization   A concept used to describe the way individuals learn and assume the roles of the professional groups to which they belong (see *socialization*).

Professions   Vocational groups with specific educational standards and high social status. Historically, the professions included only medicine, law, and divinity. Today, however, professions include many groups with high educational requirements, autonomy over their practice, and supportive state regulation. The legal ability to diagnosis is a powerful professional tool that, while initially the preserve of medicine, is now extended to other health professionals.

Reductionism   Understanding complex systems as a result of the sum of parts. Medicine is often critiqued as reductionist in understanding ill health as the outcome of a single knowable causation (e.g., a genetic defect), rather than taking a more holistic approach.

Reification   To treat an abstract concept as if it had a natural, material existence. For example, the market is an abstract concept that we may treat as a natural, external force that has a power all of its own, but the market in reality is people making decisions about buying and selling.

Sick role   A concept developed by Talcott Parsons that identifies the social benefits and responsibilities of being ill. On the one hand, the sick role permits the individual to overlook certain social obligations such as going to work, dressing, and getting out of bed. On the other, it requires the individual to dedicate effort to becoming well again and to being compliant to medical instruction.

Social construction   A theory arguing that there is no uniform social reality, stressing that even material objects and facts are socially framed and negotiated. This means that the ways we understand the world are historically and culturally specific. Knowledge of reality is the product of interactions between people. Even scientific "facts" (diagnosis included) are the product of social processes involving negotiation between people.

Socialization   The way individuals learn to fit in and take on particular roles in within society.

Socially embedded   A term describing the relationship between technology and humans. Technology exists within social and institutional networks, which shape the development of the technology and influence how the technology will be used. In turn, technologies can shape the networks within which they exist. Technology is an integral part of the social world of humans.

Social structure   A stable organizational facet of a society that enables interactions between members, as well as the maintenance and reproduction, of the society. Social structures include language, kinship, class, and gender.

Sociotechnical network   In relation to diagnosis, an assemblage of health-care workers, medical technologies, and *patients* that form during the process of a diagnosis. A diagnosis is the product of the complex interactions within a sociotechnical network.

Statistical discrimination   The way in which decisions are made about individuals on the basis of information known about the group that the individual is thought to belong to.

Stereotype   To make generalizations that are applied to particular groups.

Stigma   The experience of shame and disgrace that result from an individual's behavior or state of being deviating from social *norms* and expectations. Stigma may be health related, and particular diseases or disabilities may be particularly stigmatizing. Psychiatric diagnoses and even gout, for example, may be considered unacceptable to those so diagnosed because of their stigmatizing nature.

Subjectivity   The perspectives and feelings of a specific individual. In scientific research, subjectivity is often referred to as a bias that interferes with interpretation of findings. In philosophy, however, subjectivity refers to the autonomy of the individual to feel and to think. In the case of the care of the ill person, the subjective experience represents a needed perspective for capturing the individual's perspective and achieving optimal health outcomes.

Thought collectives   Groups who are, according to Ludwik Fleck, locked into ways of thinking called *thought styles*. Thought collectives and their ways of thinking build upon extant ideas of truth.

Thought styles   The way of thinking of a particular *thought collective*, as argued by Ludwik Fleck. Truth in science is a function of the particular style of thinking that has been accepted by the thought collective. To be correct is to be accepted collectively.

Index